Minimally Invasive Endonasal Sinus Surgery

Minimally Invasive Endonasal Sinus Surgery

Principles, Techniques, Results, Complications, Revision Surgery

Werner G. Hosemann, M.D.
Department of Otorhinolaryngology
Regensburg University Hospital
Germany

Rainer K. Weber, M.D.
Department of Otorhinolaryngology
Head, Neck, and Facial Plastic Surgery
Communication Disorders
Hospital Fulda
Department of Otorhinolaryngology
Magdeburg University Hospital
Germany

Rainer E. Keerl, M.D.
Department of Otorhinolaryngology
Head, Neck, and Facial Plastic Surgery
Communication Disorders
Hospital Fulda
Germany

Valerie J. Lund, MS, FRCS, FRCS Ed
Professor in Rhinology
Honorary Consultant Otorhinolaryngologist
University College London Medical School
Institute of Laryngology and Otology
Great Britain

Foreword by Wolfgang Draf

83 illustrations

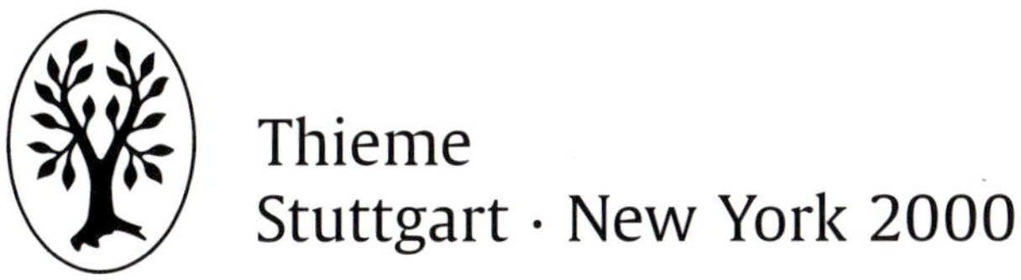

Library of Congress Cataloging-in-Publication Data is available from the publisher

Important Note: Medicine is an ever-changing science undergoing continual development. Research and clinical experience are continually expanding our knowledge, in particular our knowledge of proper treatment and drug therapy. Insofar as this book mentions any dosage or application, readers may rest assured that the authors, editors, and publishers have made every effort to ensure that such references are in accordance with the state of knowledge at the time of production of the book.

Nevertheless, this does not involve, imply, or express any guarantee or responsibility on the part of the publishers in respect of any dosage instructions and forms of application stated in the book. Every user is requested to examine carefully the manufacturer's leaflets accompanying each drug and to check, if necessary in consultation with a physician or specialist, whether the dosage schedules mentioned therein or the contraindications stated by the manufacturers differ from the statements made in the present book. Such examination is particularly important with drugs that are either rarely used or have been newly released on the market. Every dosage schedule or every form of application used is entirely at the user's own risk and responsibility. The authors and publishers request every user to report to the publishers any discrepancies or inaccuracies noticed.

All endoscopic photographs included in this book were produced using Karl Storz products.

Any reference to or mention of manufacturers or specific brand names should not be interpreted as an endorsement or advertisement for any company or product.

Some of the product names, patents, and registered designs referred to in this book are in fact registered trademarks or proprietary names, even though specific reference to this fact is not always made in the text. Therefore, the appearance of a name without designation as proprietary is not to be construed as a representation by the publisher that it is in the public domain.

Cover drawing by Martina Berge, Erbach-Ernsbach

Typesetting and printing by Gulde, Tübingen

Printed in Germany

ISBN 3-13-124611-1 (GTV)
ISBN 0-86577-907-4 (TNY)

1 2 3 4 5 6

Preface

The application of the microscope to endonasal surgery and the introduction of a new generation of endoscopes as diagnostic and therapeutic tools in the treatment of chronic rhinosinusitis led to a renaissance in endonasal sinus surgery, building on the expertise of some gifted surgeons working at the turn of the last century using just a headlight and the naked eye. The routine use of the rigid endoscope for more detailed examination of the anatomic structures of the nasal cavity has increased our knowledge about both the physiology and pathophysiology of the nose and sinuses while modern anesthesia provides a surgical field with minimal bleeding, facilitating the most sophisticated and least traumatic surgery. This has been combined with a significant drop in the risk of more severe complications. As a logical consequence, patients no longer accept the classic so-called "radical" sinus operations with their associated morbidity.

Endonasal micro-endoscopic sinus surgery, also known as functional endoscopic sinus surgery, has spread throughout the world as the gold standard of surgical treatment for inflammatory sinonasal disease. Meanwhile, the spectrum of endonasal endoscopic surgery has been widened significantly. This book is a result of a European cooperation of centers representing a vast experience in rhinology. Based on personal experience and a review of more than 1000 references, the principles, techniques, results and complications are described in considerable detail. This publication is not only a fascinating mirror, reflecting how an old technique comes once again into focus as a result of new technical developments and their application to surgery, it is also a most practical guide to this challenging minimally invasive surgery.

I would like to thank the authors for their devotion and enthusiasm combining their personal experience with a comprehensive updated review of the literature.

I hope this book is welcomed by the many readers it deserves.

Wolfgang Draf, MD, FRCS, Ed
Department of Otorhinolaryngology
Head, Neck, and Facial Plastic Surgery
Communication Disorders
Fulda Hospital
Germany

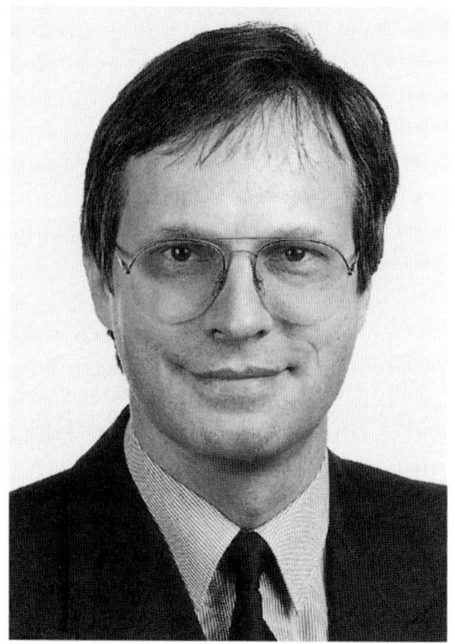

Werner G. Hosemann
werner.hosemann@klinik.uni-regensburg.de

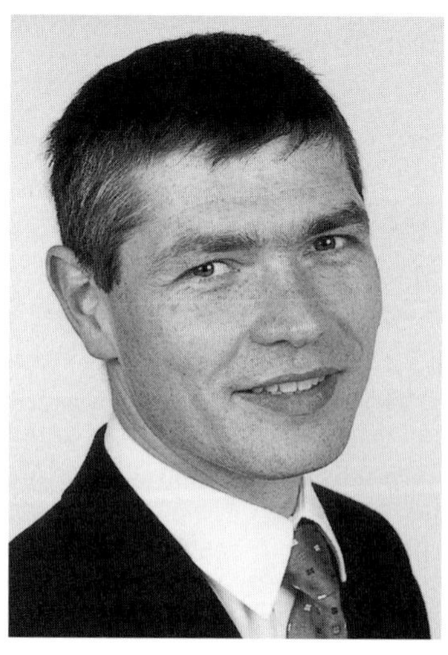

Rainer K. Weber
rainer.weber@medizin.uni-magdeburg.de

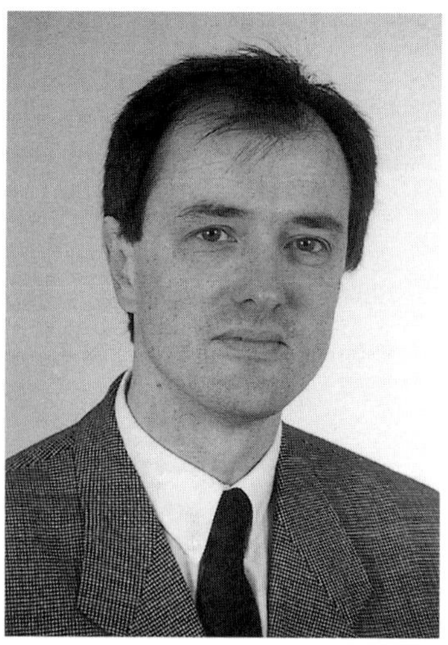

Rainer E. Keerl
rainer.keerl@t-online.de

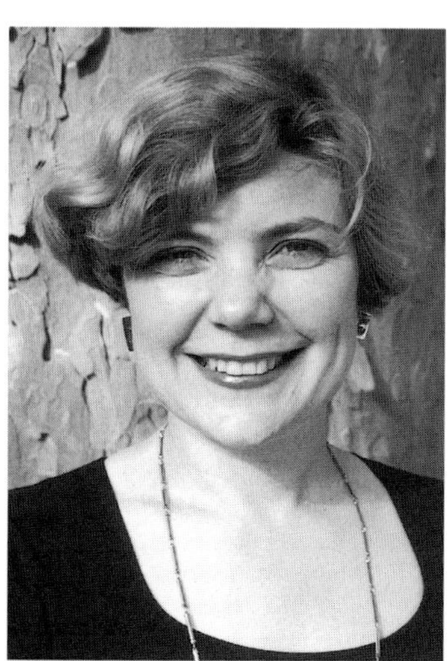

Valerie J. Lund
v.lund@ucl.ac.uk

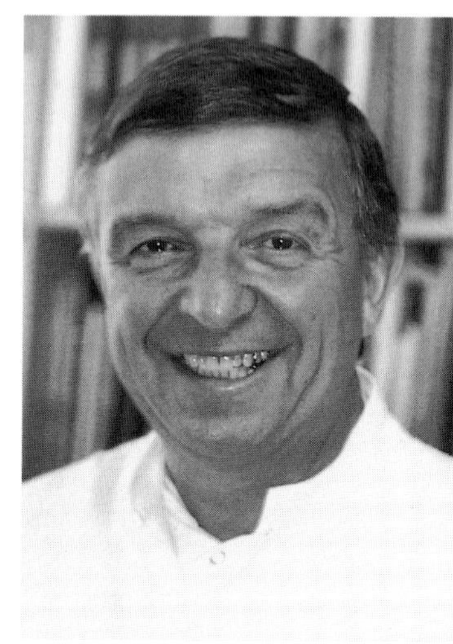

Wolfgang Draf
Wdraf@aol.com

Contents

1 Introduction

It is not clear why human beings have paranasal sinuses. There has been speculation about their physiological significance since antiquity. Some have proposed that their purpose is to reduce the weight of the skull, others that they have an effect on voice quality or help to increase the moisture content and the temperature of inhaled air, while still others have suggested that they represent a potential enlargement of the olfactory region or provide shock absorption or thermal insulation to protect the central nervous system. The paranasal sinuses have been credited with having a special architectural role in the construction of the facial skeleton and have been seen as evolutionary relics or air-filled cavities serving no useful purpose. In summary, if there was any potential evolutionary advantage in the development of the sinuses, it remains as yet completely obscure [277].

In contrast to these speculations, diseases of the paranasal sinuses, especially the chronic inflammatory conditions, have always represented a very definitive therapeutic problem [419, 708, 938]. Five to twelve percent of the population suffer from the complaints of chronic rhinosinusitis [500, 937]. These patients' lives are often highly restricted [276]. Our profession has therefore frequently addressed issues of sinus surgery either as a topic in its own right or in connection with other subjects. Papers on suppurative inflammation of the paranasal sinuses have been published throughout this century. Draf presented a survey on the surgical treatment of inflammatory diseases of the paranasal sinuses in 1982 and this book based on that paper. It aims to complement, expand upon and update the 1982 paper, focusing exclusively on endonasal sinus surgery conducted with the assistance of optical aids, primarily the endoscope.

A number of monographs have been published on this topic: Draf 1978 [171], 1983 [172a]; Messerklinger 1978 [599]; Rice and Schaefer 1988, 1993 [750]; Wigand 1989 [996]; Stammberger 1991 [860]; Terrier 1991 [908]; Denecke et al. 1992 [153]; Klossek and Fontanel 1992 [460]; Lusk 1992 [534]; Anand 1993 [12]; Levine and May 1993 [506]; Mehta 1993 [594]; Stammberger and Hawke 1993 [866]; Paulsen 1995 [701]; Messerklinger and Naumann 1995 [602]; Donald et al. 1995 [168]). The broad range of different surgical approaches and the specific steps of the operations are impressively and comprehensively described in these papers. The present volume aims to provide an up-to-date overview of the approaches and techniques, including a review of the most recent literature, but it is not intended as a substitute for reading the original publications. The luminaries of modern endonasal surgery include Messerklinger, Wigand, Draf, Stammberger, Terrier and Kennedy, while the works by Buiter, Friedrich, Grünberg, Hellmich, Heermann, Herberhold, Illum, von Riccabona, Rosemann, Timm and others promoted these developments. Clearly it is not possible to pay full tribute to all these individuals in the context of the present volume. Modern endonasal endoscopic surgery is based on systematic research in microanatomy and physiology. During the last hundred years, anatomists, physiologists and clinicians such as van Alyea, Dixon, Grünwald, Hajek, Halle, Hartmann, Heymann, Hilding, Ingal, Kasper, Keros, Killian, Lothrop, Messerklinger, Mosher, Mouret, Neivert, Ohnishi, Onodi, Proetz, Schaefer, Siebenmann, Uffenorde, Whitnall, Yankauer and Zuckerkandl have presented a series of standard works and individual papers of exceptional importance reviewed by Lang in 1988 [478]. Again a detailed discussion of the general anatomy of the region is not included in the present text. None the less, sinonasal surgery has undergone a substantial renaissance during the last 30 years and was given further impetus by the spread of the Messerklinger school in the United States with the introduction of the term "functional endoscopic sinus surgery" by Kennedy et al. in 1985 [435] in recognition of physiological concepts. Although endonasal sinus surgery developed out of maxillary sinus endoscopy [172], we have chosen to give the latter limited attention in the present text while including some of the extended applications of endoscopic surgery in the adjacent areas of the orbit and skull base. Furthermore, we have chosen to concentrate on the surgical management of chronic rhinosinusitis that has failed to respond to medical therapy.

2 Endonasal Sinus Surgery: Basic Principles and Approaches

Surgical Aspects of the Pathophysiology of Chronic Sinusitis

It is very likely that the term chronic sinusitis in fact covers a number of different disease processes due to a range of pathogeneses (Fig. 2.**1**). These chronic diseases include, for example, the circumscribed, chronic recurrent paranasal sinusitis that develops as a consequence of a definable anatomic obstruction. An extreme form is the diffuse nasal polyposis occurring in patients with the ASA triad (polyps, asthma, aspirin sensitivity). As yet, the causal and formal pathogenesis of nasal polyposis is still poorly understood.

Circumscribed forms of chronic recurrent sinusitis develop generally as a result of microanatomic anomalies, especially narrow passages or clefts and areas of pathological mucosal contact. These occur mainly in the middle nasal meatus in the region of the central "ostiomeatal unit" and result in a disturbance of mucociliary clearance and ventilation of the functionally dependent paranasal sinuses (see Fig. 2.**3**). The functional term "ostiomeatal unit" was introduced by Naumann [653] and refers to the anatomic region lateral to the anterior two-thirds of the middle turbinate. It includes the uncinate process, the hiatus semilunaris, the bulla ethmoidalis, the remaining anterior ethmoidal cells and the frontal recess, and the ostium of the maxillary sinus. The maxillary and frontal sinuses are functionally subordinate to the anterior ethmoid complex. The effects of the narrow clefts are potentiated by disturbances of mucociliary clearance associated with areas of tissue contact or inflammatory cell reactions associated with the release of mediators. In addition to the above factors, microbial colonization, dysregulation of transepithelial fluid transport and the immigration of inflammatory cells result in a vicious circle consisting of obstruction of the ostium, followed by changes in the milieu of the dependent sinuses and further mucosal congestion.

The diagnosis of chronic, treatment-resistant sinusitis is made on the basis of a review of the patient's specific history and complaints in conjunction with the findings on endoscopic examination of the nasal cavity and the condition of the functionally dependent sinus mucosa. The functional condition of the mucosa is conventionally equated with the degree of congestion and determined by imaging techniques (CT or MRI).

In circumscribed forms of the disease, surgical treatment is in principle based on the identification and targeted elimination of anatomic bottlenecks. Areas of mucosa that appear to be irreversibly damaged are simultaneously removed. When optimal ventilation and drainage have been restored, the remaining sinus mucosa is allowed to heal spontaneously.

What microanatomic bottlenecks or pathological anatomic variants can be defined? The list below gives a summary of the most common anatomic variants that are considered responsible in the literature for triggering or maintaining chronic paranasal sinusitis. The anatomy of the paranasal sinuses is diverse and unique to each individual. Accordingly, the list of possible bottlenecks is infinite effectively [448, 449]. A pathogenically significant obstruction can only be diagnosed in an individual case on the basis of extensive experience of the microanatomy and with a knowledge of a number of clinical principles. Thus, the presence of a concha bullosa alone, as is found in 14–50% of the population, is not necessarily synonymous with obstruction [112, 190, 512, 1026]. Only the individual shape and a critical overall size, in combination with the adjacent anatomic structures, determine whether there is a surgically relevant obstruction [64, 1019, 1026]. In practice, only pneumatization that extends to the inferior portion of the middle turbinate appears to be of pathogenic significance [64, 930]. The situation is similar with Haller's cells (infraorbital cells) which occur in 10% (8–20%) of the population [190, 403]. The microanatomic changes are sometimes complex and interconnected. Thus, Earwaker [190] distinguished six different types of alteration of the ostiomeatal complex. To date, CT screening has generally been unsuccessful in providing unequivocal evidence of the pathogenetic significance of any anatomic variants of the ethmoid bone or establishing threshold values for their significance [64, 94, 512, 513, 1019]. Many variants are also found in healthy individuals [527]. Table 2.**1** gives a breakdown of the incidence of anatomic variants in patients with paranasal sinusitis complaints. Table 2.**2** summarizes the results of several studies in healthy individuals, patients with chronic sinusitis and children.

Nasal septal deviations over and above a certain critical size and position also result in an increased incidence of inflammation of the paranasal sinuses [94, 513, 716]. Deviations at the level of the ostiomeatal unit appear to be especially relevant [1019]. Septal deviations are frequently associated with further anatomic variants of the ethmoid bone [527]. Areas of opacification in the anterior and posterior ethmoid complex have been observed in association with sep-

Table **2.1** Incidence of anatomic variants in patients with paranasal sinusitis complaints [437]

Anatomic variant	Incidence in patients with complaints
Concha bullosa	36% (bilateral in 44% of cases)
Septal deviation	21%
Paradoxically bent middle nasal turbinate	15%
Haller's cells	10%
Large bulla ethmoidalis	8%
Lateral rotation of the uncinate process	3%
Pneumatized uncinate process	0.4%

Table **2.2** Incidence of anatomic variants of the paranasal sinuses in healthy individuals (H) and patients with chronic sinusitis (P) and children (C)

	Lloyd [512]	Stoney et al. [890]	Lloyd et al. [513]	April et al. [15]
Concha bullosa	14% (H)	30% (P)	24% (P)	19% (C, P)
Paradoxical. middle nasal turbinate	17% (H)	24% (P)	15% (P)	7% (C, P)
Haller's cells	2% (H)	7% (P)	15% (P)	18% (C, P)
Agger nasi cells	3% (H)	15% (P)	14% (P)	–

tal deviations [94], as have opacifications in the contralateral sinus system [1019]. Moreover, inflammatory changes in the mucosa of the paranasal sinuses are frequently associated with hyperplasia of the nasal turbinates [716].

Anatomic variants that foster the development of paranasal sinusitis

- Septal deviation: convexity, septal spur [858]
- Variants of the middle nasal turbinate: concha bullosa; paradoxically convex or bent turbinate; juxtaposition against the lateral wall and the middle meatus [190, 403, 405, 527, 858, 865]
- Variants of the uncinate process: rotation particularly medial or anterolateral; displacement following fracture, contact with the middle nasal turbinate; pneumatization [190, 403, 405, 527, 858, 865, 1019]
- Variants of the bulla ethmoidalis: variations in shape or size [403, 405, 527, 858]
- Variants of the agger nasi: pneumatization with crowding of the frontal recess [403, 527]
- Haller's cells [403, 405, 527]

Radiological studies on the incidence of the anatomic obstructions reveal that these are only one of many

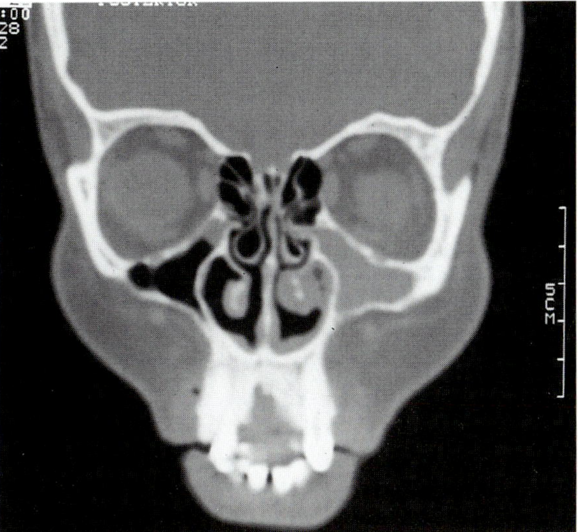

a

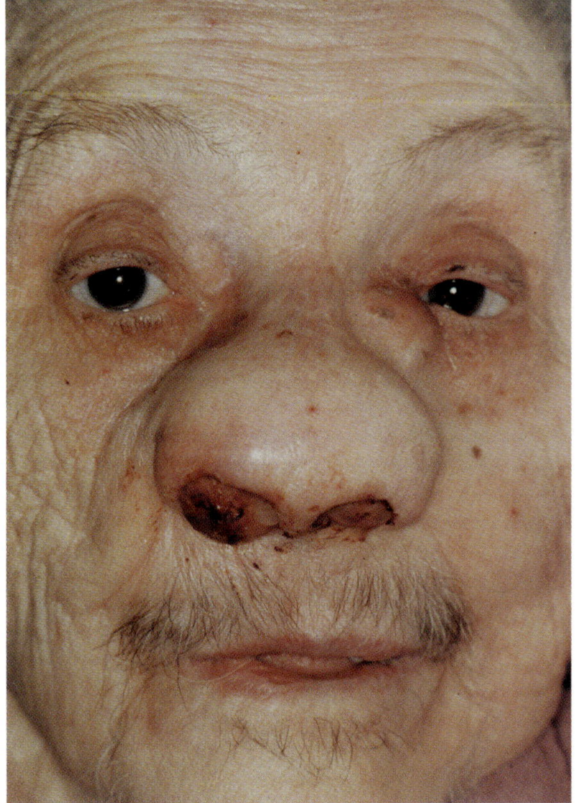

b

Fig. 2.**1a,b** **Types of chronic rhinosinusitis**
(**a**) Coronal CT of chronic rhinosinusitis associated with anatomic narrowing (medially deviated uncinate process and concha bullosa on both sides) in the middle nasal meatus. (**b**) A 91-year-old woman with extreme nasal polyposis. Secondary mucocele of the lacrimal sac on the left side

factors involved in the development of chronic sinusitis [433, 512]. Neither the concept of the ostiomeatal unit nor functional endoscopic sinus surgery can be applied indiscriminately in all forms of chronic sinusitis. [212]. On the other hand, not every area of obstruction is necessarily detectable on the CT. Certain individual factors and variations can be established only by a thorough endoscopic examination [860].

Hyperplastic pansinusitis, in particular, cannot be explained by radiologically or endoscopically detected areas of obstruction alone. Other conditions are necessary for nasal polyps to develop. The origins of many polyps are located beyond these obstructions, in the superficial portions of the middle meatus, but similarly, different forms of polyp growth have been observed, including diffuse involvement of the entire sinus system [483].

The paranasal sinuses are dependent upon undisturbed drainage of secretions and unobstructed ventilation. Mucociliary flow follows fixed transport pathways out of the frontal and maxillary sinuses and the anterior ethmoidal cells through the narrow clefts of the ostiomeatal unit into the middle meatus. Compromising factors (inflammation, anatomic variants with narrow passages and secondary mucositis) are most frequently encountered in the region of the anterior ethmoid. They result in a secondary obstruction of drainage of the dependent sinuses and thus in a rhinogenic or centrifugal spread of disease. If the underlying pathogenetic factors are eliminated, ventilation and mucociliary drainage are restored and the mucosa of the dependent sinuses can recover without any further intervention [866].

The functional concept of the ostiomeatal unit has been confirmed by radiological studies. The functional dependence of the peripheral areas of the sinuses on the middle meatus has been demonstrated in screening studies [659]. Marked opacification of the frontal or maxillary sinuses was always associated with swelling of the mucosa in the adjoining sinus system (anterior ethmoid, frontal recess, ethmoidal infundibulum) [188]. Obstructions in the middle nasal meatus led to an increased incidence of opacification of the dependent frontal and maxillary sinuses [309, 513]. This relationship has been demonstrated particularly clearly for the ethmoidal infundibulum and adjacent maxillary sinus [64]. Circumscribed areas of opacification in the ethmoidal cell system without reactions in the adjacent sinuses are not uncommon in healthy individuals and are then often of no pathological significance [512].

Reventilation of inflamed sinuses has also been revealed as the most reliable guarantee of spontaneous mucosal healing in *animal studies* [620]. If irreversibly altered areas of the mucosa have to be removed, the rest of the sinus system recovers when normal mucociliary transport pathways are restored [48, 345]. However, in animal studies this functional restitution often proves to be of inferior quality. The number of ciliated cells is smaller and the rate of mucociliary flow is reduced compared to normal [45, 621]. In addition, extirpation of ethmoidal cells in young animals leads to reduction in the growth of the ipsilateral visceral cranium [544]. This has not been shown in clinical studies. For these reasons, in functional endoscopic sinus surgery, areas of the peripheral sinus mucosa that are only mildly affected are left to heal spontaneously once optimal ventilation and drainage have been restored. Unfortunately, it is not possible intraoperatively to distinguish reliably between reversible and irreversible changes of the mucosa on the basis of the endoscopic appearance [551].

Respiratory Allergy and Chronic Sinusitis

Generally, in patients with a type I allergic affection, opacification of the sinuses is rare or not very pronounced [376, 513]. However, especially in children, a nasal allergy can be associated with radiological changes of the mucosa in the paranasal sinuses and may then trigger episodes of *acute recurrent sinusitis* [44, 255]. Accordingly, specific allergic therapy improves the chances of success of surgical treatment, thereby reducing the need for primary and revision surgery [796].

In contrast, the role of allergy in *chronic hyperplastic sinusitis* remains controversial. The incidence of seasonal rhinitis is not greater in patients with nasal polyposis [181, 455]. In most of these patients, skin tests and serological tests are negative or comparable with those of control groups [659, 817]. Patients with allergy account for only 6% of all cases undergoing paranasal sinus surgery for nasal polyposis [142]. The prevalence of nasal polyps is the same in patients with and without allergic rhinitis [382]. The conclusion drawn from these data is that immunoglobulin E (IgE)-mediated reactions do not play an important role in the pathogenesis of chronic hyperplastic sinusitis [181, 455]. Specific hyposensitization before or after ethmoidectomy has not been shown to influence the rate of adhesions, polyp recurrences or ostium stenoses [214, 382, 837].

This last opinion has not remained unchallenged, however. Other authors have observed roughly 40% positive skin tests in patients with polyposis [232, 382]. It is possible that the observed damage to the epithelium of the hyperplastic mucosa promotes the absorption of allergens [378]. An increased rate of allergies to the house dust mite, in particular, is found in sinusitis patients [382, 795]. Other IgE antibodies not detected in serological or skin tests are also found in polyp tissue [232]. Various authors have reported good results with antiallergic treatment of patients following sinus surgery [128, 162, 996].

In summary, the role of type I allergy in the pathogenesis of nasal polyposis in the literature remains uncertain. At all events, it is unlikely that seasonal allergy plays an appreciable pathogenetic role. For the specific diagnosis of sinusitis it is important that the presence of tissue eosinophilia in the nose cannot be taken as an indication of respiratory allergy [142].

Aspirin Intolerance and Chronic Sinusitis

About 10% (6–35%) of patients with nasal polyposis suffer from aspirin intolerance [78, 218, 627, 698]. This intolerance usually applies to all nonsteroidal anti-inflammatory drugs (NSAIDs). While the prevalence of simple, chronic hyperplastic sinusitis is higher in men, the ASA triad (a combination of bronchial asthma, aspirin intolerance, and chronic sinusitis) in particular affects a higher proportion of women [208]. Different reaction types of aspirin intolerance have been observed, bronchospasm being by far the most frequent form.

Intolerance usually develops after a preliminary phase of eosinophilic rhinitis and becomes manifest after the age of 40 years [519]. Over 90% of these patients show opacification on sinus radiographs [885]. In skin tests these patients do not as a rule react to the conventional seasonal and perennial allergens [207].

The currently assumed mechanism of action of aspirin intolerance is inhibition of the cyclooxygenase pathway in the breakdown of membrane phospholipids (Fig. 2.**2**). This leads to preferential breakdown of arachidonic acid by the unaffected lipoxygenase and, consequently, to a shift in the overall profile of metabolites towards leukotrienes [88, 885].

The association between bronchial asthma, nasal polyposis and aspirin intolerance is 25 times stronger than would be expected statistically [791]. Patients with intolerance and polyposis usually suffer from a severe form of sinusitis (see Chapter 4). Accidental administration of nonsteroidal anti-inflammatory drugs to patients with aspirin intolerance can lead to substantial side effects with medicolegal consequences. For these reasons, aspirin intolerance has special significance for rhinologists. The elucidation of its pathobiochemistry could become the key to understanding nasal polyposis. If the biochemical feedback systems could be influenced by medication, this would pave the way for concomitant drug therapy of chronic sinusitis. The therapeutic use of adaptive desensitization is already a first step in this direction (see Chapter 8, p. 105).

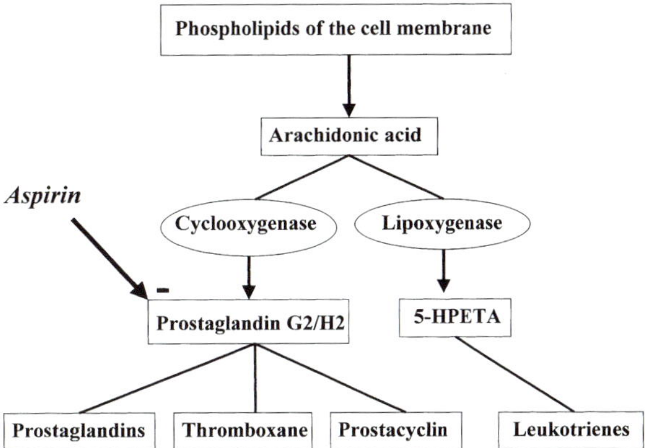

Fig. 2.**2** **Metabolism of the eicosanoids** (prostaglandins, prostacyclin, thromboxane, leukotrienes); simplified diagram modified after Stevenson [885]. Cyclooxygenase is an essential component of prostaglandin synthesis. It is inhibited by aspirin and other nonsteroidal anti-inflammatory drugs (NSAIDs). This leads to preferential use of the alternative metabolic pathway via lipoxygenase, which remains uninfluenced, and hence to increased production of leukotrienes with histamine-like and leukotactic action. This mechanism is considered to be responsible for the pulmonary reactions of patients with aspirin-induced asthma. It is also assumed to play a role in the pathogenesis of chronic rhinosinusitis. 5-HPETA = 5-hydroperoxyeicosatretraenoic acid

To date there exists no in vitro test for aspirin intolerance. If the patient has a negative history, diagnosis is only currently possible by means of oral, nasal or bronchial provocation. These tests are complicated and may be associated with serious side effects. No standardized test procedure is yet available [760, 885, 886].

In the treatment of patients with chronic sinusitis and a history of aspirin intolerance, the use nonsteroidal anti-inflammatory drugs should be strictly avoided. This applies to all substances, including the usually better tolerated paracetamol. In patients with asthma who have a negative history and whose sinus CT shows no signs of pathology, aspirin intolerance is unlikely. The same applies to a lesser extent to patients with an unequivocal diagnosis of allergic rhinitis. If a patient has taken a tablet of a nonsteroidal anti-inflammatory drug without negative consequences during the previous two months, tolerance of this group of drugs may be assumed [88, 885].

Principles of Endonasal Surgery

Indications for Endonasal Surgery of the Paranasal Sinuses

The main indication for endonasal sinus surgery is *chronic sinusitis* that has failed conservative treatment. This is characterized by findings and symptoms that persist over a period of two to three months despite appropriate medication. A special form of chronic sinusitis in which the indication for surgery is usually unequivocal is diffuse nasal polyposis. *Recurrent acute sinusitis* presents as periodic episodes of acute sinusitis with complete remission in the intervening periods [530]. Depending on the symptoms and frequency of the episodes, surgical management is indicated if conservative treatment fails to have any lasting effect. Treatment-resistant opacification of the sinuses in the CT scan without concomitant symptomatology should be investigated by means of a diagnostic and therapeutic operation, depending on the patient's history and the endoscopic findings. In isolated cases, surgical intervention may be indicated even if endoscopy reveals no pathological findings or where radiology shows aerated sinuses as, for example, in suspected recurrent barosinusitis. The spectrum of possible presenting signs and symptoms in sinusitis is broad, ranging from headache and facial pain, obstructed nasal breathing, nasal and postnasal secretion to ocular, pharyngeal, bronchial and middle ear symptoms.

In all endonasal surgery the operative procedure is planned on the basis of appropriate imaging after taking a thorough history and performing careful intranasal endoscopy. The necessary postoperative care is included in the treatment plan. In the surgical management of uncomplicated sinusitis the endonasal technique has completely supplanted external routes of access. The same applies to the saccular and postsaccular stenoses of the lacrimal ducts. In the last few years the range of indications has also constantly been extended (see below) and it is often no longer possible in these "borderline cases" to give a generally valid indication for endonasal surgery. In such cases, the choice of the procedure is determined by the respective anatomy and pathology, the personal experience of the surgeon, the equipment available, and the informed patient.

In the case of nasal polyposis, some authors prefer standard intranasal polypectomy as the initial operation [482]. It has been reported that more extensive sinus surgery can be avoided or postponed in 50% of cases simply by giving systemic and topical corticosteroids, in some cases in high doses [921]. Treatment with cortisone in combination with polypectomy has been reported to lead to a lasting improvement in symptoms in 65% of patients for up to four years [482]. In individual cases where there is circumscribed formation of polyps within the middle meatus, it is understandable that polypectomy alone is successful. However, in over 70% of cases, recurrent polyps are observed within two years [699, 700]. With repeated polypectomy, permanent scarring is more likely. This results in the obscuration of important landmarks, an increase in intraoperative blood loss and an unfavorable prognosis in patients with hyposmia [353]. In principle the chances of cure after appropriate ethmoid surgery are good, even after previous polypectomy [195].

Approaches to Endonasal Surgery in Chronic Inflammation of the Paranasal Sinuses

In the more recent literature, preservation of the respiratory mucosa is generally recommended and the high incidence of spontaneous healing of secondarily altered areas of mucosa is emphasized. Thus, all the surgical procedures presented below center on conservative removal of mucosa aimed at reventilation the sinuses and allowing regeneration of mucociliary clearance [866, 990]. Notwithstanding this, a range of different approaches to endonasal sinus surgery have developed.

Functional Endonasal Sinus Surgery (FESS)

Defined microanatomic obstructions within the ethmoid system, especially in the anterior middle meatus, can lead to a persistent disturbance of mucociliary drainage and ventilation of the dependent paranasal sinuses. As a result of a pathophysiological vicious circle of local congestion and irritation, this inflammation may become chronic and spread in a centrifugal pattern. Most cases of chronic sinusitis can be attributed to a pathological mechanism of this kind. Where appropriate, it is often sufficient to eliminate the obstructed areas by cautiously excising grossly hyperplastic areas of mucosa. Messerklinger's investigations on the self-cleansing mechanism of the sinuses [599] played a formative role in the development of this approach, now generally referred to as "functional endonasal sinus surgery," in which these bottlenecks are visualized under endoscopic guidance and eliminated. The aim is to optimize ventilation and drainage. Any mucosal reactions in the adjoining sinuses are left to heal spontaneously. The extent of the operative procedure is dictated by the intraoperative findings. The endoscope thus has simultaneous diagnostic and therapeutic functions [857, 859, 860].

The direction of dissection is mainly anterior-to-posterior. Depending on the respective requirements, retrograde dissection along the base of the skull is also possible [437].

The extent of surgery is established by the preoperative CT scan and the intraoperative endoscopic findings, but is also guided by probable or known areas of obstruction based on a thorough knowledge of the microanatomy. The surgical procedure is complete when all mucosal changes visible in the CT scan have been exteriorized, which is ensured by opening into the next ethmoid cells with normal mucosa [433]. There is no attempt to create a standardized cavity and thus each is individual. This is deliberate and has the advantage of causing minimal trauma. On the other hand, it can be a disadvantage when it comes to evaluating outcome and comparing different procedures.

The mucosal reactions in the sphenoid, maxillary and frontal sinuses usually play a less important role in the specific planning of functional endonasal sinus surgery. The sphenoid sinus is opened only if its mucosa is clearly significantly involved in the disease process. Similarly, complete endoscopic evaluation of the maxillary sinus is not mandatory even if there is radiological evidence of mucosal thickening. At all events, manipulations of the maxillary sinus are kept to a minimum [433]. Some authors create a second, transoral opening, in order to be able to keep the surgical opening through the middle nasal meatus small [433, 866]. Other authors create an endonasal window in the maxillary sinus measuring 1.5 × 2 cm while otherwise using the same technique [503]. Manipulations in the region of the frontal sinus recess are also avoided where at all possible. If the patient has massive, diffuse polyposis, individual polyps in the ostium of the frontal sinus can be left so to avoid causing damage to the mucosa and provoking secondary circumferential scarring. These polyps may be removed later as an outpatient procedure [433]. Similar caution is exercised with regard to septal deviations, which are only included in the surgical treatment plan if they obstruct endoscopic manipulation with a 4-mm endoscope. In such cases the operation on the septum is sometimes performed in advance. If the patient still has symptoms following this operation, ethmoidectomy is carried out a few weeks later. Only in cases of massive polyposis are correction of the septum and sinus surgery performed in a single session [865].

In advanced disease the boundaries between circumscribed functional endoscopic surgery and complete ethmoidectomy are fluid. However, the fundamental principle of functional endoscopic surgery remains limited surgery based on the microanatomy of the lateral nasal wall and sinus system. A 0° straight endoscope is the preferred optical instrument for this procedure.

Pansinus Rehabilitation by Functional Compartment Surgery

Wigand [996] presented a global treatment approach for the paranasal sinuses consisting of a specific series of surgical steps performed on the basis of the pathophysiological obstructions and an intimate knowledge of the local microanatomy.

In principle, no fixed direction of operation is stipulated. However, in more extensive ethmoid surgery an early sphenoidotomy is frequently performed [993]. The roof and lateral wall of the sphenoid sinus can then be used as landmarks for posterior-to-anterior dissection. The removal of septa, division of scar tissue and straightening of any bony projections often produces a surgical wound cavity or compartment of a defined extent. Anterior-to-posterior ethmoidectomy performed with an operating microscope is a good example of this kind of "functional compartment surgery." The advantages of this technique are a certain degree of standardization of the procedure and greater clarity of the postoperative endoscopic findings, which makes it easier to evaluate the outcome of the operation and compare results in different cases. A disadvantage is that the trauma sustained by the tissue is sometimes greater, since the compartments can only be created by quite extensive removal of intercellular septa.

The aim is to develop a universal treatment procedure for all forms of circumscribed and diffuse sinusitis by proceeding with the individual steps of the operation in a consecutive fashion. On this basis, further extension of the indications for endonasal surgery, particularly in the region of the anterior skull base, has become possible.

In this technique it is regarded as important to clear the entire nose of disease, and thus adjunctive measures such as correction of septal deformities or turbinate reduction are always integrated in the treatment plan. Similarly, peripheral areas of the sinus system are also explored. Care is taken not to exclude areas of disease that are difficult to access or presumed to have no functional significance. The limits are set by technical limitations alone. Where necessary, gross pathological changes in the mucosa of the maxillary, sphenoid or frontal sinuses are also treated as aggressively by the endonasal approach as those in the adjoining ethmoid complex. In the case of circumscribed bottlenecks or mucosal foci, the principle of "isthmus surgery" is followed [991, 992]. However, diffuse inflammation of the mucosa inevitably requires a more radical approach which is achieved by systematically including intensive endoscopic postoperative therapy in the treatment plan.

Anatomic Principles and Significance of Mucosal Reactions in the CT Scans of Adults and Children

The ethmoid bone is shaped like a sawn-off pyramid with the base situated posteriorly. The pyramid is 4–5 cm long, 2.5–3 cm high, 0.7 cm wide anteriorly, and 1.5 cm wide posteriorly [478, 641]. It is approximately 1 cm wider caudally than cranially [1028].

The ethmoid bone is composed of 2–10 anterior cells and 2–6 posterior cells per side [31, 160, 907, 933]. The two cell compartments are separated anatomically and functionally by the basal lamella of the middle turbinate. The other lamellae or their rudiments (uncinate process, bulla ethmoidalis, basal lamella of the superior turbinate) are comparatively less significant (Fig. 2.**3**). The anteroposterior position and even the shape of the basal lamella of the middle turbinate are determined by the variations in shape and size of the anterior and posterior ethmoidal cells [892]. Several systems of classifying the ethmoid cells have been described in the literature [3, 31, 323, 933]. Each ethmoid cell is classified on the basis of its origin, which can be determined by the location of the cell ostium [933]. However, the individual ostia are not usually visible on CT scans or endoscopically, especially in the presence of disease. The basal lamella of

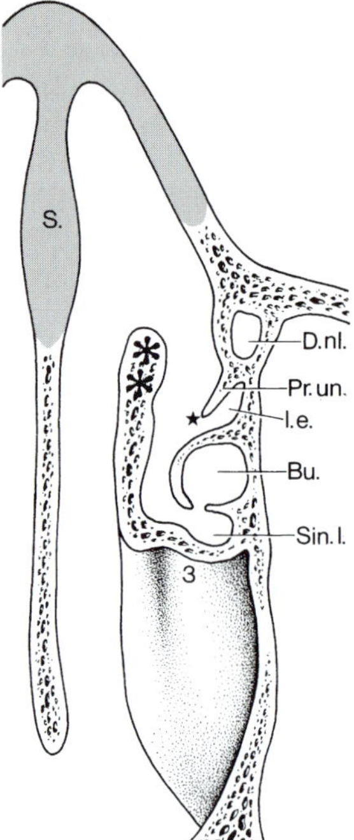

Fig. 2.**3** **Axial section through the ethmoid bone**, illustrating the most important structures of the anterior ethmoid (after Stammberger [860]). The uncinate process forms the first basal lamella, the bulla ethmoidalis the second. The most important lamella is the third, i.e., the basal lamella of the middle turbinate (3): this lamella separates the anterior and posterior ethmoid both functionally and anatomically. The inferior hiatus semilunaris corresponds to the opening to the ethmoid infundibulum. It is formed by the shortest imagined connection between the edge of the uncinate process (★) and the adjacent bulla. The ethmoid infundibulum appears as a V-shape in axial sections. Analogously the opening of the sinus lateralis (recessus suprabullaris et retrobullaris) is termed the superior hiatus semilunaris. ★★, Vertical lamella of the middle turbinate; D.nl., nasolacrimal duct; Pr.un., uncinate process; I.e., ethmoid infundibulum; Bu., bulla ethmoidalis; Sin.l., sinus lateralis; S., nasal septum

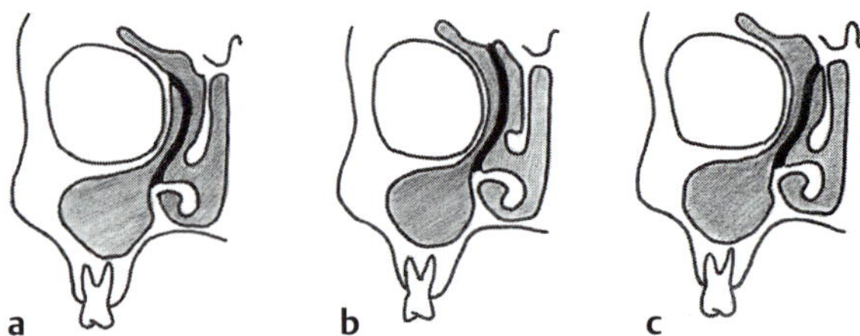

Fig. 2.**4a-c** **Schematic of the anatomic variations of the uncinate process** (outlined in black) according to Stammberger and Hawke 1993 [866]
(**a**) The uncinate process inserts into the lamina papyracea. As a consequence, the ethmoidal infundibulum ends blindly and the frontal sinus drains medial to the ethmoidal infundibulum. (**b**) The uncinate process inserts on the roof of the ethmoid. The frontal recess merges in the ethmoidal infundibulum. The frontal sinus drains directly into the ethmoidal infundibulum. (**c**) The uncinate process inserts on the upper middle turbinate. The frontal recess and frontal sinus drainage are similar to example (**b**).

the middle turbinate is also frequently difficult to visualize well in vivo [909]. Unfortunately, these drawbacks substantially reduce the practical clinical usefulness of the above classification systems, e.g. as a basis for standardizing surgical techniques.

Surgeons should take into consideration the following functional aspects of ethmoid anatomy.

- The uncinate process is 14–22 mm long and usually not more than 5 mm wide. It is rudimentary in 9% of persons and is reported to be absent in 3% [651]. The ostium of the maxillary sinus is accessed via the hiatus semilunaris, in most cases in the region of the posteroinferior half of the uncinate process [478].
- Accessory ostia in the middle meatus are found in about 40% of cases [160]. They are rarer in adolescents. These secondary ostia can lead to pathological mucociliary flow patterns [860].
- The superior-anterior attachment of the uncinate process reveals a series of clinically important variations (Fig. 2.**4**) determining the local microanatomy and the relationship of the frontal recess and the ethmoidal infundibulum [866]. As a consequence, the frontal sinus most frequently drains directly into the frontal recess. Drainage directly into the ethmoid infundibulum is comparatively rare (14%) [417, 935].
- Several distinct cell types of the anterior ethmoid may interfere with the frontal sinus drainage or may cause misorientation during endonasal frontal sinusotomy: Agger nasi cells, frontal cells or "frontal bullae," intersinus septal cells, and supraorbital cells [51, 474, 597, 687, 709]. If the surgeon has opened up a large anterior-superior ethmoidal cell from below, the remaining shell-like dome of the cell adjacent to the skull base may be mistaken for the cleared frontal recess. This cell remnant may persistently impede the frontal sinus drainage. It resembles the cap of an egg—the surgeon is advised to introduce a curved spoon medially and "uncap the egg" by pulling the cell wall away from the skull base, preserving the frontobasal mucosa (Fig. 2.**5**) [863].
- Encroachment of ethmoid cells into the frontal sinus, referred to as frontal bulla, frontal cells or intersinus septal cells occurs in about 10% of cases. Conceptually the distinction between these and accessory frontal sinuses is blurred [478]. Duplication of the drainage channels can lead to false judgments in surgical reventilation. The same applies to some posterior ethmoid cells, which can extend lateral superior to the sphenoid sinus in about 14% of cases [33].
- In one in five patients ethmoid cells grow into the roof of the orbit as supraorbital cells [399, 687]. These cells vary in size. The supraorbital cells have an independent drainage pathway into the frontal recess. Exact surgical exploration of the cell lumina

Instrumente und Endoskope für die Oto-Rhino-Laryngologie

Mit der Entwicklung einer sechsfach vergrößernden Binokularlupe für die Otoskopie konnte KARL STORZ vor mehr als 5 Jahrzehnten einen ersten bedeutenden Beitrag zum Fortschritt der HNO-Medizin leisten.
Auch in den folgenden Jahren haben Entwicklungen der Firma KARL STORZ immer wieder dazu beigetragen, der Oto-Rhino-Laryngologie neue Untersuchungs- und Operationsverfahren zu eröffnen. Heute umfaßt das Angebot Instrumente und Endoskope für den gesamten Bereich der HNO-Heilkunde. Von der Grundausstattung für eine HNO-Praxis bis zum modernen System für computerunterstütztes Operieren erhält der Mediziner alles aus einer Hand: Perfekt aufeinander abgestimmte Endoskope und Instrumente, in denen sich beste handwerkliche Tradition mit der weltweit anerkannten Innovationskraft des schwäbischen Unternehmens verbindet.

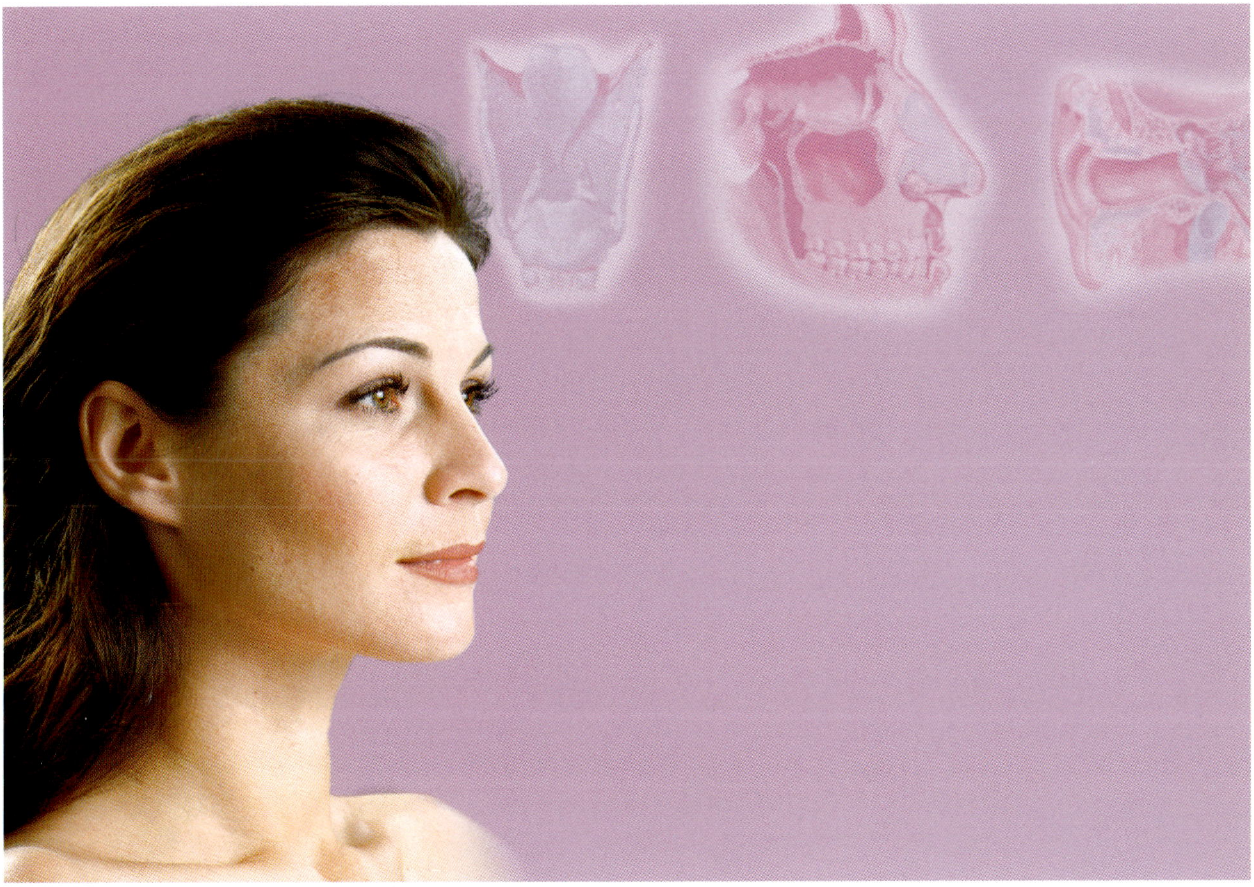

via an endonasal route can be difficult in some cases. The canal of the anterior ethmoidal artery may be separated from the skull base by the expansion of supraorbital cells [831].

Risks for the surgeon can be minimized by attention to the following anatomic details.

- Ohnishi [674] describes five points at which the roof of the ethmoid sinus can exhibit dehiscences or weaknesses of the bony structure.
  1) The medial wall of the ethmoid sinus (continuation of the middle turbinate beyond the level of the cribriform plate)
  2) Along the course of the anterior ethmoid nerve and artery
  3) About the origin of the middle turbinate
  4) At the anterolateral roof of the ethmoid cells
  5) In the vicinity of the foramen of the posterior ethmoid nerve/ artery
- Dehiscences in the region of the anterior ethmoid artery occur more frequently in persons with pronounced pneumatization of the frontal sinus and supraorbital ethmoid cells [625]. The region of the anterior roof of the ethmoid sinus at the medial point of entry of the anterior ethmoid artery has special significance [401]. Keros [445] distinguishes different types based on the different levels between the cribriform plate and the roof of the ethmoid sinus (Fig. 2.**6**): type 1 with 1–3 mm difference (incidence 12%), type 2 with 4–7 mm difference (incidence 70%), and type 3 in which the cribriform plate is located 8–16 mm below the roof of the ethmoid sinus (incidence 18%). The medial lamella of the middle turbinate serves as the medial boundary for resection in ethmoidectomies on which furrows for olfactory fibers are frequently seen superiorly. Identification of these furrows may be a useful aid to orientation [433].
- The intimacy of the relationship between the posterosuperior ethmoid cells and the optic nerve can vary: they can more or less encase it medially, superiorly, and inferiorly as so-called Onodi cells (better termed "sphenoethmoidal cells"). A pyramid-shaped sphenoethmoid cell with the apex of the pyramid pointing toward the optic nerve is characteristic [402]. Depending on how exactly the term is defined, an Onodi cell (sphenoethmoidal cell) is to be found in 40% of cases (12–51%) [402, 1014]. The bone over the optic nerve is often thin and in 3–12% of cases there are dehiscences [402, 550, 814]
- In the lateral wall of the sphenoid sinus, the prominence of the optic nerve parallels that of internal carotid artery. In 22% of cases the covering bone does not present any appreciable mechanical resistance [441]. Both structures can protrude substantially into the sinus. When indentation of the lateral wall by the maxillary nerve is seen, indentation by the vidian nerve is usually also present. De-

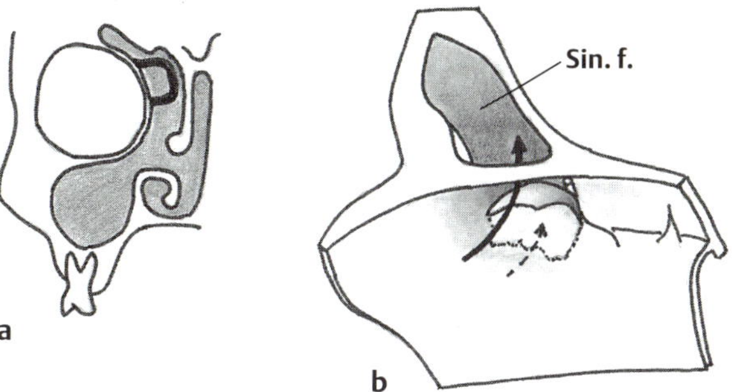

Fig. 2.**5a,b** **Microanatomic constriction of the frontal recess** according to Stammberger [863]
(**a**) Scheme of a frontal section of the paranasal sinuses revealing a large agger nasi cell (outlined in black) that impedes the frontal sinus drainage. Drainage of the frontal sinus is sustained by a narrow cleft only between the middle turbinate and the cell wall. (**b**) Scheme of a right sided anatomic specimen of the anterior ethmoidal cavity seen from medially-inferiorly (middle turbinate not shown). Removal of the inferior parts of a large agger nasi cell leaves a bony "cap" near the skull base that may be mistaken for the cleared up frontal sinus but still may impede frontal sinus drainage. Directly perforating this cell remnant for frontal sinusotomy (dotted line) endangers the local frontobasal mucosa. The frontal sinus may best be entered by introducing a slender, sharp spoon cautiously between the middle turbinate (not shown) and the cell remnant (black arrow), followed by pulling the bony cap inferiorly. Sin. f. = frontal sinus.

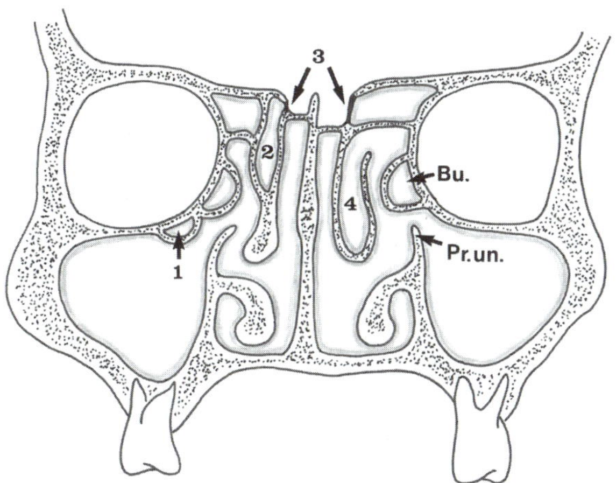

Fig. 2.**6** **Coronal section through the ethmoid bone** showing the most important structures of the anterior ethmoid (after Stammberger et al. [867]). The uncinate process (Pr.un.) is a residual portion of the first basal lamella. Anteriorly the process is in contact with the lacrimal bone, the base of the skull or the lamina papyracea. The bulla ethmoidalis (Bu.) is formed by pneumatization of the second basal lamella. Between the two structures lies the hiatus semilunaris (see Fig. 2.**3**). (1): Infraorbital ethmoid cell (Haller's cell). (2): Interlamellar cell. (3): Different shapes of the roof of the ethmoid sinus as described by Keros. (4): Concha bullosa

hiscences of the bone covering the internal carotid artery are observed in about 5% (0.3–8%) of cases [250, 402, 680, 814]. The roof of the sphenoid sinus is about 3 mm higher than the roof of the ethmoid sinus [934].

- The lamina papyracea is not a flat surface, but is usually idiosyncratically bent in the sagittal and axial planes [752]. The convexity is always medial. In axial sections the contour of the ethmoid and sphenoid sinus at the level of the optic nerve can be classified according to shape. A barrel-shaped outline is the most frequent (66%). In these cases the greatest width is measured in the posterior third of the ethmoid bone [471].
- Medial to the anterior middle turbinate the cribriform plate is relatively thick. Dorsally it becomes thinner [757]. In contrast, the roof of the ethmoid sinus becomes thicker dorsally [677].
- The anterior ethmoid artery is not always a reliable anatomic structure [480]. At the base of the skull it lies 1–2 mm dorsal to the junction between the posterior wall of the frontal sinus and the roof of the ethmoid sinus [175]. It can also be found in the cranial continuation of the anterior border of the bulla ethmoidalis [401]. Where there is extensive supraorbital pneumatization, the artery is "suspended" 1 mm below the level of the base of the skull [178, 636]. This artery is an important landmark when one is opening the frontal sinus. The anterior ethmoid artery lies in the frontal plane dorsal to the eyeball. The orbital fat is relatively thick anterior and inferior to the artery, but is thin posterior and inferior to it [757].
  The posterior ethmoid artery is often embedded in the bone. It can help to identify the base of the skull [433]. It is thicker than the anterior artery [677]. Accessory ethmoid arteries are observed in one-third of cases [480].
- The location of the sphenopalatine foramen varies; it is mostly to be found immediately posterior to the dorsal attachment of the middle turbinate [478].
- Hypoplasia of the maxillary sinus can lead to lateral excavation of the middle nasal meatus and partial fusion with the facies orbitalis maxillae. Fenestration of the middle turbinate can represent a risk to the orbit in such cases [299].
- It is rare for the pneumatization of the entire ethmoid to be symmetrical on both sides [160]. Symmetry of the two sides of the posterior ethmoid bone is common [33], whereas the middle turbinate [96, 190] and sphenoid sinus are only rarely symmetrical [303, 814]. The choana is not affected by asymmetry [357]. This is an important landmark when one is opening the sphenoid sinus and estimating the depth and height of the dorsal sections of the nose.

There are no official anatomic terms for many parts of the ethmoid bone structure. An attempt has been made to introduce a uniform nomenclature [867]. Under this nomenclature the ethmoid infundibulum, for example, must be distinguished from the frontal infundibulum and the maxillary infundibulum, both anatomically and terminologically. Proper names should be avoided. Haller cells should thus be referred to as infraorbital ethmoid cells and Onodi cells in general terms as sphenoethmoid cells (Fig. 2.**6**). No specific definition of the Onodi cell based on the extent of the prominence of the optic nerve is given.

Location of Mucosal Changes in Chronic Sinusitis

The distribution of the mucosal change across the individual compartments of the paranasal sinuses naturally reflects the differences in the pathophysiology of the various forms of sinusitis. Thus, in more diffuse nasal polyposis the anterior ethmoid is affected in 100% of cases, the maxillary sinus in 96%, the posterior ethmoid in 91%, the frontal sinus in 87% and the sphenoid sinus in 74% [957]. Table 2.**3** gives an overview of the distribution of mucositis in patients with sinus complaints, while Table 2.**4** shows a comparison between the figures reported by different authors. In all cases the anterior ethmoid and maxillary sinus were most frequently involved [115, 513, 1024]. It is possible to discern certain patterns of sinus opacification that coincide with the mucociliary transport pathways (Table 2.**5**)

Significance of Mucosal Changes in Imaging Procedures

Studies using CT or MRI scans of the sinuses performed for evaluation of other underlying diseases reveal a relatively high rate of clinically silent mucosal reactions: 20% (11–63%) of the "patients without sinus disease" show widely varying degrees of opacification [127, 187, 223, 309, 376, 512, 728]. In adults, no correlation between the patterns of opacification or their incidence and the age of the patients was found [187, 309]. These areas of mucosal swelling are most frequently found in the region of the ethmoid bone, followed by the maxillary sinus, sphenoid sinus, and frontal sinus [512]. Other investigators have found both higher [127] and distinctly lower rates [223] for the maxillary sinus.

The rate of demonstrated opacification is clearly elevated in "healthy" patients with a history of sinusitis [94, 309]. The time of year is reported to have no influence [127]. Ongoing complaints usually indicate the presence of relatively large areas of mucosal swelling: areas with a thickness greater than 3 mm are significant in this regard and are frequently associated with subjective complaints. Peripheral mucosal swelling measuring less than 3 mm is usually clinically silent. The incidence of retention cysts is the same for both patients with and patients without complaints [728].

These results cast some doubt on the clinical significance of low-grade opacifications of the paranasal

Table **2.3** CT-study of patients with sinusitis complaints. Topographic distribution of mucosal reactions (Kennedy and Zinreich [437])

Location of mucosal swelling	Percentage of all patients with complaints (%)	Percentage of patients with complaints and positive radiographic findings (%)
Anterior ethmoid	78	93
Maxillary sinus	66	79
Frontal sinus	34	41
Posterior ethmoid	31	38
Sphenoid sinus	16	22
(No mucosal swelling)	16	

Table 2.**4** Topography of inflammatory changes (%) in the mucosa of the paranasal sinuses in patients with chronic paranasal sinusitis (P), in children (C), and after unsuccessful operations (R)

	Stoney et al. [890]	Weber et al. [957]	April et al. [15]	King et al. [453]
Anterior ethmoid	58 (P)	83 (P)	85 (C)	81[a] (R)
Maxillary sinus	78 (P)	64 (P)	89 (C)	98 (R)
Frontal sinus	35 (P)	24 (P)	63 (C)	37 (R)
Posterior ethmoid	37.5 (P)	44 (P)	57 (C)	81[a] (R)
Sphenoid sinus	21.5 (P)	21 (P)	39 (C)	51 (R)

[a] Anterior and posterior ethmoid not distinguished

Table 2.**5** Patterns of opacification in CT scans of the paranasal sinuses in patients with suspected chronic sinusitis (Babbel et al. [23])

Pattern of opacification	Relative frequency[a] (%)	Description
Infundibular type	26	Involvement of the ethmoid infundibulum and ipsilateral maxillary sinus
Ostiomeatal type	25	Involvement of the middle nasal meatus and adjacent sinuses (anterior ethmoid, maxillary, and frontal sinuses)
Recessus-spheno-ethmoidalis type	6	Involvement of the posterior ethmoid cell and/or sphenoid sinus
Polyposis type	10	Irregular opacification of the entire paranasal sinus system
Unclassifiable type	24	-

[a] 27% no opacification; individual types may be included more than once

sinuses. This support the approach that patients with transient and minor changes of the mucosa should undergo appropriate pharmacological treatment before radiological evaluation of the sinuses is performed (see below).

Radiology in Children

The rate of incidental opacification of the paranasal sinuses is even higher in healthy children than in adults. The percentage for children under 13 years is 50% [156] and that for children under one year is 72% [270]. After the age of 13 years opacifications become less frequent [156]. When symptoms occur, the radiological findings usually show a distinctly worse mucosal reaction than in adults [15]. Half of the children between six and nine years with sinus complaints have significant radiological findings [376]. The rate of incidental mucosal reactions in healthy children is roughly the same in the maxillary (32%) and ethmoid sinuses (31%) but lower in the sphenoid sinus (17%) [156, 501]. Bronchial asthma probably has no direct influence on the incidence of mucositis [15, 501]. However, previous infections lead to an increase in the degree of opacification, even after clinical resolution [270]. In the light of these observations it would seem advisable in children to evaluate CT scans only in conjunction with the clinical findings.

The incidence of microanatomic variants is the same for children as for adults, with the exception of septal deviations, which are observed less frequently in children [15]. The incidence of concha bullosa also reportedly only rises with increasing age [936]. In principle, in children a pneumatized middle turbinate is associated with sinus opacifications in 63% of cases, and with a paradoxical middle turbinate in 71% [616].

In the growing skull there is a special relationship between lateral deviation of the uncinate process and pneumatization of the maxillary sinus. Such a deviation is found in 55% of young patients with hypoplasia of the maxillary sinus [616]. Bolger et al. [63] distinguish three types of maxillary sinus hypoplasia:

1. Normally developed uncinate process, fully developed ethmoid infundibulum, mild hypoplasia of the maxillary sinus
2. Hypoplastic or missing uncinate process, missing or hypoplastic infundibulum, and marked hypoplasia of the maxillary sinus with complete opacification of the remaining lumen
3. Missing uncinate process, massive hypoplasia of the maxillary sinus

Chronic sinusitis as such does not affect the growth of the maxillary sinus [15] but in cystic fibrosis frontal sinus pneumatization is reduced, possibly in association with infection.

Preoperative Evaluation of the Patient

Physical Examination and Endoscopy

Before every operation on the paranasal sinuses the patient undergoes a general examination by an otolaryngologist. This complements the endoscopic examination of the nasal cavity [882] that is performed routinely before and after decongestion of the mucosa using scopes with various viewing angles. Documentation of the endoscopy results is standard procedure and special forms have been designed for this purpose [396].

In the patient population of a specialized department, 28% of sinusitis patients can be expected to show bilateral diffuse polyposis at preoperative endoscopy. Circumscribed polyposis of the middle meatus is observed in 31%. A large proportion of the patients (41%) do not show endoscopic evidence of obvious polyposis. Thus, endoscopy usually does not provide reliable evidence of the extent of disease [433] and in a number of cases the results can be disappointing, even in patients with advanced inflammation of the sinuses [993]. The extent of disease can only be determined on the basis of preoperative imaging studies and the intraoperative findings [433]. In other cases, however, the endoscopic results can be used to analyze the microanatomic abnormalities or, for example, the soft tissue that obstructs the middle meatus. The endoscopic findings can provide confirmation of the pathology seen on a CT scan and permit its classification in terms of pathogenesis. It is rare to find a significant pathological endoscopic finding that is not evident on CT [652, 940].

Effective diagnosis and establishment of the indication for surgery can only be achieved by a combined evaluation of imaging studies and endoscopic results. Not every area of pathological mucosal contact will necessarily have led to radiologically detectable mucosal reactions [104]. It is very important to take a thorough history [838]. In one in twenty patients the indication for sinus surgery is established mainly on the basis of the patient's sinusitis history and the history of medical therapy, despite normal radiographic (CT) findings and normal findings on endoscopy [125, 491].

Some authors also routinely conduct an allergy test, determine IgE and IgA titers and obtain a nasal smear before sinus operations [370]. Lowered titers of IgG2–4 are found in some cases [531]. In children with chronic recurrent sinusitis or chronic sinusitis, allergy testing is supplemented by a sweat test to rule out cystic fibrosis, and determination of immunoglobulins and immunoglobulin classes and examination of a mucosal biopsy to establish whether the patient has ciliary dyskinesia [948].

Radiological Examination and CT Scans

It is standard procedure to perform a preoperative CT scan before conducting extensive ethmoid surgery. The CT is intended to demonstrate extent and distribution of the disease and to identify anatomic landmarks, variants and danger zones. The surgeon must personally evaluate the scans and they must be available for consultation in the operating room [390]. However, there is no conclusive evidence that the rate of complications can be reduced by routinely performing preoperative CT scans [442, 515].

Shankar et al. [820] have published a monograph on the techniques and findings of computed tomography of the paranasal sinuses. Opinions in the literature on the protocol for the roentgenographic examinations vary widely. Axial scans have advantages for the visualization of the anterior and posterior walls of the frontal sinus, infundibulum frontale, and the relationship of the carotid artery and optic nerves to the posterior ethmoid and sphenoid [190, 358]. Scans in the coronal plane offer optimal visualization of the ostiomeatal complex and the skull base in a way that is immediately familiar to the surgeon [437]. However, in 5% of adults and 10% of children difficulties are encountered with the positioning required of the patient. Only in a few cases do artifacts caused by dental fillings interfere with the assessment of the most important anatomic structures in the anterior ethmoid [15, 56]. Coronal CT scanning is performed from the frontal sinus to the sphenoid sinus; axial scanning

Table 2.**6** Recommendations for CT examination in sinus surgery

Author	Plane	Section thickness	Table incre-mentation	Window width (bone)	Center	Window width (soft tissue)	Center
Wigand [996]	Coronal (axial)	2 mm	5 mm	-	-	-	-
Simmen and Schuknecht [831]	Coronal	3 mm / 2 mm	3 mm / 2 mm	4000 HU	800 HU	300 HU	80 HU
Kösling et al. [467]	Coronal (axial)	3–4 mm	3–4 mm	3200 HU	700 HU	-	-
Zinreich et al. [1027]	Coronal	4 mm	3 mm	2000 HU	-200 HU	-	-
Evans and Shankar [209]	Coronal (axial)	4 mm	3–4 mm	2000-HU	-250 HU	300 HU	65 HU

from the teeth of the upper jaw to the suprasellar region. Contrast is not given routinely and is reserved for when operative or inflammatory complications are suspected, vascular anomalies or tumors in particular, to define intracranial extension [1018].

A number of authors advise preoperative scanning in both the axial and coronal planes [183, 363, 957]. The increased radiation dose can be reduced by performing axial scanning with three-dimensional reconstruction [175]. The same objective can be achieved by limiting the complementary axial scans performed after coronal sectioning to a few sections through the frontal and sphenoid sinuses [190, 191]. The conventional procedure is a high-resolution technique in combination with thin sections [711, 820]. The preferred section thickness is usually 2(-4) mm [175, 289, 865, 1023]. Some authors select a greater section thickness for coronal CTs of the frontal sinus and posterior ethmoid than for those of the anterior ethmoid [22, 190, 191, 1018]. Sections are usually obtained at 3- or 4-mm intervals. Depending on the section thickness selected, overlapping sections may be obtained for 3D-reconstruction. The window width for routine imaging of the sinuses is 1500–2000 (4000) HU (Hounsfield units), with a center of +100 to +300 HU (-250 to +700 HU) [209, 289, 467, 542, 849, 1018, 1023, 1024]. Table 2.**6** summarizes some of the recommendations given in the literature.

Duvoisin et al. [186] describe a special technique that provides exact visualization of the ostium of the frontal sinus on CT scans. Its use is limited to the clarification of certain specific issues.

A complete CT examination in a single plane consists of up to 30 sectional images [467]. The dose of radiation received by the lens of the eye should not be underestimated, particularly in scans performed in the axial plane [513, 828]. A conventional CT examination delivers roughly 4% of the acute radiation dose required to cause a cataract [828]. The so-called "low-dose CT" reduces the dose by varying the physical parameters without leading to an appreciable loss of information [563]. The dose, examination time, and costs are reduced by screening sinus CTs or CT miniseries [22, 105, 191, 849, 982, 983]. About 80% of the disease foci can be demonstrated with limited-slice CT scanning. However, changes in the microanatomy of the bone or isolated air-fluid levels are often missed and such limited-slice CTs are therefore more suitable for repeat examinations [290].

➤ Computerized tomography miniseries according to White et al. [982]
Three coronal sections:
1. Frontal sinus and frontonasal duct
2. Anterior ethmoid and middle meatus
3. Posterior ethmoid and spheno-ethmoid recess
   One axial section: sphenoid and ethmoid sinuses midway between their caudal and cephalad extents.

Prompted by the frequently observed minor opacifications in the sinus systems of healthy subjects, a course of medical preliminary treatment is recommended prior to scanning. In patients with suspected chronic sinusitis, systemic antibiotics in combination with decongestant nasal drops, topical corticosteroids, and possibly mucolytics are given before performing CT scans in order to suppress the reversible mucosal changes. This pretreatment usually takes at least 2–4 weeks. An oral broad-spectrum antibiotic, often a cephalosporin or macrolide, is preferred. Antihistamines and decongestants are given concomitantly, in oral or spray form. Some authors also give 20 mg oral prednisone daily for four days. Topical treatment takes the form of a corticosteroid spray. Mucolytics are considered mandatory by some authors, optional by others [197, 244, 493, 711]. Similar pretreatment with antibiotics and a topical steroid spray and topical decongestant is also recommended for children [289, 536, 923]. The recommended duration of antibiotic treatment is between two and four weeks and in some cases low-dose corticosteroids are also given systemically [536, 923].

Immediately before the CT examination, some authors give a decongestant nasal spray and ask the patient to clear the nose by blowing it [22].

Computed tomographic evaluation of chronic sinusitis:
Preparatory pharmacotherapy in children (after [536])

- Oral antibiotic, e.g. amoxicillin-clavulanic acid, cefaclor, erythromycin, clarithromycin.
- Topical corticosteroid, e.g. beclomethasone spray (children over seven years), fluticasone, budesonide
- Duration of pretreatment: four weeks
- Scheduling of the CT: in patients with a long history of sinusitis after the end of the pretreatment; in patients without a history of sinusitis conclude treatment and observe, perform CT if complaints recur and after renewed pretreatment

The pretreatment described above suppresses false-positive mucosal reactions. The symptoms and clinical findings of up to half of the patients are reported to respond so well to this therapy that surgery can be deferred [214, 923]. However, in other patients this treatment probably leads to a temporary regression of significant mucosal reactions, thus obscuring evidence of the pathogenesis of the complaints [125].

Evaluation of the preoperative CT scans should always be carried out by the operating surgeon themselves [390]. Special reporting schemes have been developed to aid evaluation, the most important points of which are given in the following overview [831, 890].

Main points of the radiological evaluation of preoperative CT scans in suspected chronic sinusitis [890]

- Sinuses: changes in the mucosa?
- Drainage pathways: retained secretions?
- Lateral nasal wall: structural changes?
- Nasal septum, bony midface: structural changes?
- Evidence of previous operations: accessory ostia, partial resections, scars?
- Surgical risks: prominence and concealment of optic nerve and internal carotid artery, position of the cribriform plate, shape and thickness of the lamina papyracea

Several authors report a lack of agreement between radiological and intraoperative findings [140, 191, 491, 545, 553]. Discrepancies have been found in between 18% and 60% of cases. In the majority of cases (13–85%) the findings are underestimated in the CT. This applies particularly to diseased areas in the posterior ethmoid. In children, disease in the frontal recess is more often overlooked [491]. According to the literature, in many cases these differences cannot be explained by the interval between the radiological evaluation and the operation.

After operations on the sinus system, radiologically demonstrable scars are formed, depending on the extent of the trauma to the tissue. In contrast to the mucosa, 4–6 weeks postoperatively these scars do not absorb any contrast media. Exposed bone, for example, in the region of the lamina papyracea, reacts by becoming thicker [844, 845]. Difficulties in distinguishing scars, mucosal swelling and areas of reinfection in radiological studies are not unusual. False-positive evaluations are frequent [56, 420].

Special Radiodiagnostic Cases

Special problems may arise in the diagnostic differentiation of tumors from chronic inflammation. Nasal polyposis may produce a typical radiological pattern on CT scans, consisting of a mucosal border covered with a layer of low-density (10–15 HU) mucus with sections through the polyp stroma appearing as arch-shaped strips of soft-tissue density [846]. In cystic fibrosis, an expanding "pseudomucocele" is frequently visualized, especially in the maxillary sinus, appearing as hypodense mucosa surrounding a hyperdense center of highly viscous mucus [131]. These criteria are not reliable, however. The purpose of CT is the visualization of the bony architecture and possibly also areas of destruction [469]. Without evidence of bone destruction, diagnosis of a tumor is difficult [844]. However, bone erosion can be caused not only by tumors but also by polyps, mucoceles and mycoses [844, 848]. In these cases, MRI is an important additional source of information. It is used to visualize the orbit, dura mater, brain, cavernous sinus, and carotid artery [469]. A tumor can often be differentiated from associated soft-tissue swelling and retained secretions. Bony or cartilaginous tumors are less well visualized owing to signal void of calcification [105, 106]. Imaging does not usually allow one to differentiate inverted papillomas from malignant epithelial tumors [1020].

MRI is not the technique of choice for the routine evaluation of inflammatory paranasal sinus disease. However, for patients with suspected regional or intracranial inflammatory complications, MRI with gadolinium-DPTA contrast enhancement also provides valuable additional information. There is a risk of false interpretations in the evaluation of protein-rich secretions such as those associated with fungal sinusitis, for example. Highly protein-rich secretions lead to low signal intensity in T1- and T2-weighted images and can be missed on account of their hypointensity [847, 1018].

In emergencies, for example impaired vision in connection with a sinus operation, the first step should be to perform a CT without delay. These scans can be performed rapidly and reliably. Artifacts from eye movements are rare. The same applies to iatrogenic injuries to the base of the skull [1018].

Olfactory Testing

In chronic hyperplastic sinusitis 14–76% of patients have an impaired sense of smell, especially patients with aspirin intolerance [913]. Opacification of the left-sided sinuses seems to have an overproportional influence on olfaction [340]. Disturbances of olfaction are more common than one would suspect from patients' reports of their subjective symptoms. Impaired discrimination is often already demonstrable when the olfactory threshold is still unaffected [152, 865].

Preoperative olfactory testing is therefore expedient for diagnostic reasons and is also advisable for medicolegal reasons [129, 150, 370, 872, 996]. It is strongly recommended for patients in particular occupations (cooks, perfumers).

Wigand [996] and Yamagishi et al. [1011] have presented special olfactograms. The University of Pennsylvania Smell Identification Test and olfactory threshold measurement are commercially available and are useful in the evaluation of chronic rhinosinusitis [529]. The same holds true for the "Sniffin' Sticks" screening test [457].

Provisions for Blood Replacement and Autologous Blood Transfusion

The issue of the usual loss of blood during endonasal sinus operations is discussed in Chapter 7 (p. 91). In the case of more extensive surgery, preparations for a blood transfusion should be made on account of the possibility of relevant blood loss. Some authors recommend having red cell concentrate available [166, 175, 993]. At all events, blood replacement products should be readily available for use in emergencies.

The organizational and legal questions relating to autologous blood transfusion cannot currently be answered conclusively. According to provisional criteria announced by the relevant medical societies, preoperative donation of autologous blood is indicated when the likelihood of its being required perioperatively is greater than 5%. Moreover, there are certain cases in which autologous transfusion is not to be recommended, for instance, when the patient is suffering from a suppurative infection and there is therefore a risk that the banked blood will be contaminated [265]. Even in extensive operations on the paranasal sinuses the likelihood of autologous blood being used is less than 5% and purulent sinusitis can be considered to be a suppurative infection. Hence, patients with chronic sinusitis need not necessarily be offered the option of preoperative autologous blood donation.

Preoperative Medical Treatment

The indication for surgical treatment of chronic sinusitis was discussed on p. 5. Before performing a CT as a basis for establishing the indication, preparatory pharmacotherapy is frequently carried out to suppress transient reactions of the sinus mucosa (see p. 12).

Immediately before the operation, a further course of medication is often carried out. Where the sinusitis has a purulent component antibiotics are given. Corticosteroids reduce marked mucosal hyperplasia and polyps, which facilitates surgery. Polyposis patients are also reported to benefit postoperatively from a longer period of freedom from recurrences [455] when combined therapy is used. The recommended dose of corticosteroids in polyposis is between 40 and 100 mg prednisone over a period of 1–2 weeks [455, 503]. Lower doses are given for perioperative treatment of asthmatic complaints or to reduce allergic swelling of the mucosa.

Preoperative medication in preparation for sinus surgery for chronic sinusitis

- Patients with evidence of suppurative sinusitis: an oral antibiotic for 1–3 weeks (amoxicillin/clavulanic acid, trimethoprim-sulfamethoxazole, clarithromycin)
- Patients with evidence of allergy: prednisone (20–30 mg)
- Patients with nasal polyposis: prednisone (60 mg for five days; 30 mg for five days; 15 mg for five days)
- Patients with steroid-treated bronchial asthma: increase dose of steroid for a few days [184, 214, 433, 455, 568]

Ophthalmological Examination

A preoperative ophthalmological examination is to be recommended before any major operations on the paranasal sinuses, particularly if there is an existing visual problem [129, 452, 872]. Pelausa et al. [703] describe a law case on the subjective reduction of visual acuity following ethmoid surgery and stress the forensic importance of a preoperative ophthalmological examination, including determination of visual acuity with glasses or lenses, color vision and the visual field. The importance of this approach is emphasized by our own experience of expert opinion for medicolegal cases in that patients frequently offer either insufficient information or no information at all regarding serious existing ophthalmological disease [351]. It is imperative that the possible circumstance of having to operate in the vicinity of a single remaining seeing eye is taken into consideration in the planning and execution of an operation. In certain eye conditions, such as glaucoma or status post lens implantation, for example, conventional manipulations such as ocular massage for the treatment of orbital hematoma carry a high ophthalmological risk [452].

Informing the Patient

General aspects about informing patients (appropriate time, documentation, language problems, terminology, doctor's manner) will not be discussed here.

The delicate anatomic relationships of the paranasal sinus region are a special problem of endonasal sinus surgery. They can lead to numerous serious surgical complications or side effects. The main indication for endonasal sinus surgery is chronic rhinosinusitis which has proved resistant to medical therapy, a condition that is rarely life-threatening. In the light of this and the possible sequelae of an operation, the information provided by the doctor must satisfy particularly strict criteria. Devastating complications such as total loss of sight, for example, must be unambiguously addressed [872]. For the indication to be established, conservative treatment should have been tried and documented. Points to be covered in the interview at which the patient is informed are given below. Draf and Weber [175] and Hosemann and Kühnel [356] have developed special forms for documenting the information given to the patient though it is recognized that practices differ from country to country.

The patient is informed about emergency procedures that may be undertaken via an external approach should complications occur. In the advanced indications for extended endonasal surgery, for example when there is a tumor, the patient must be informed that during the operation it may become expedient to continue the operation via an external approach, and must give his or her prior consent.

Points it is recommended to address when informing patients before endonasal sinus surgery [356]

- Failure, revision surgery
- Alternative forms of treatment
- Hemorrhage, postoperative bleeding
- Injury to the ocular muscles or optic nerve
- Cerebrospinal fluid leaks
- Epiphora
- Meningitis
- Intracranial or intracerebral hemorrhage
- Disturbances of wound healing, adhesions
- Olfactory disturbances
- Pain or changes in sensation in the palate, teeth, or face, rarely in most ESS
- Infection from blood transfusions (hepatitis, AIDS)
- Increase in or first occurrence of asthmatic complaints (extremely rare, usually the opposite)
- Osteomyelitis (extremely rare)

3 Technique of Endoscopic Endonasal Surgery

Anesthetic Technique and Positioning

Selection of the anesthetic technique depends on the planned extent of the procedure, the characteristics of the patient, the basic preferences of the surgeon and anesthesist and the general conditions.

General anesthesia is to be preferred in children or anxious patients. This is combined with local anesthetics and decongestants.

Procedures under local anesthesia require shorter operating times and are generally associated with less bleeding than those under general anesthetic, but many surgeons prefer general anesthesia for most cases. Whether there are differences in the rate of complications is unproven (see Chapter 7).

Local Anesthesia

In the paranasal sinus area, local anesthesia is used particularly for limited procedures which may sometimes be performed on a day case basis. In principle, however, more extensive procedures can also be carried out under local anesthetic with intravenous sedation and monitoring of blood pressure, pulse, cardiac rhythm and oxygen saturation. Patient satisfaction with local anesthesia is usually excellent [912]. Administration of atropine is not generally recommended [866].

A summary of the local anesthetics normally used is given below. The most common combination is 10% cocaine or 2% tetracaine for topical application, and 1% lidocaine with 1:100 000 epinephrine for injections.

Local anesthetics most commonly used in endonasal sinus surgery

Topical application
- 5% cocaine [866]
- 10% cocaine [866]
- 25% cocaine paste containing 0.01% epinephrine [496]
- 2% tetracaine with epinephrine 1:1000 (mixed in the ratio 5:1) [856, 866]
- 4% lidocaine with epinephrine 1:25 000 [503]
- 10% lidocaine with epinephrine 1:100 000 [205]

Injection
- 1% lidocaine with 1:100 000 epinephrine [433, 856]
- 2% lidocaine with 1:100 000 epinephrine [205, 238]

Oral/i.m. medication
- Diazepam, fentanyl, midazolam, pethidine/promethazine, etc.

A number of comparative investigations have been carried out. In combination with epinephrine, cocaine (5%) is regarded by patients as more effective than lidocaine (5%) for procedures carried out under local anesthesia [394]. Basically, cocaine (10%) has a less pronounced decongestant effect than oxymetazoline (0.1%) [998]. Lidocaine (4%) with oxymetazoline (0.05%) proved superior to cocaine (4%) with regard to anesthesia and vasoconstriction [901]. In combination with oxymetazoline, tetracaine (1%) is more effective than lidocaine (2%) [668]. The administration of longer-lasting bupivacaine (0.25%; 0.5%) instead of lidocaine (1%; 2%) does not offer benefits for the patients [235].

The formula for a 10% cocaine hydrochloride solution is: cocaine hydrochloride 0.5; aqua conservans to 5.0. Cocaine is applied topically with moist cotton pledgets. The dose must be limited to 100–150 mg for each side of the nose [394, 433]. The rate of absorption is about 30% [286]. The pledgets should remain in place for at least 10 minutes. In addition, an injection of 1% lidocaine with epinephrine (1:100 000) may be given [433]. The number of injections should be kept low to avoid the inconvenience of bleeding from injection sites. Injections are given into the anterior middle meatus below the attachment of the uncinate process down to the upper border of the inferior turbinate and the attachment of the anterior middle turbinate. The sphenopalatine foramen and the greater palatine canal may also be included [433, 632, 866]. Transfacial infiltration of the anterior and posterior ethmoidal foramina is reported by Ohnishi et al. [675]. In more than 2000 procedures, local reactions observed have included ptosis and occasionally ecchymosis, temporary diplopia or edema. Although no further complications have been reported, this method of supplementing local anesthesia cannot in general be recommended. In the cases described above, the quantities injected were generally below 1.5 mL [866]. Other authors used up to 6mL with additional injections at the septum [238, 676]. After injections of dilute epinephrine solution, the plasma epinephrine level rises to a greater or lesser extent after approximately four minutes without clinical signs of appreciable circulatory reactions [393].

Under local anesthesia, endoscopic rather than microscopic methods are generally used [162]. The use of self-retaining specula also appears to be possible in principle under local anesthetic [39, 693], but it is unusual. The pressure of the speculum blades and the fixation of the instrument usually necessitate a general anesthetic.

When operating under local anesthesia, attention must be paid to the postnasal drainage of blood and secretions. To avoid aspiration, special balloon catheters may be installed in the nasopharynx [574].

General Anesthesia

Major operations such as complete sphenoethmoidectomy or procedures in children are usually performed under general anesthesia. A number of measures are recommended to achieve decongestion of the nasal mucosa and to reduce blood loss. A summary of these measures is shown below. Hypopharyngeal packing should be provided in the anesthetized patient [175, 993]. Selection of the method of anesthesia should take into account the use of epinephrine in the operative field [166].

In adults, for example, 2 mL of a 10% cocaine solution is applied inside the nose using gauze strips. A maximum of 2 mL = 200 mg is given [173]. In addition, injections of 1% lidocaine with 1:120 000 epinephrine are given [175]. The injection sites are the same as for local anesthesia. Infiltration of the infraorbital and nasopalatine nerves at the foramen incisivum may also be carried out [178]. Some authors give no additional local injections [9].

Supplementary local treatment in paranasal sinus operations under general anesthesia

Adults

- Epinephrine 1:1000 (squeeze out pledget before application; never inject epinephrine undiluted) [194, 996]
- 10% cocaine (gauze strips) [178]
- 4% cocaine (gauze strips) [58, 829]
- 1% lidocaine with epinephrine 1:120 000 (injection) [175, 178]
- 1% prilocaine with epinephrine 1:200 000 (injection) [763]

Children

- 2% lidocaine with 1:100 000 epinephrine (injection) [493]
- 1% lidocaine with 1:100 000 epinephrine (injection) [86, 536]
- 0.05% oxymetazoline (gauze strips) [751]
- 4% cocaine (neuropads) [493]
- 2% cocaine (neuropads) [86]

For children, a 2% or 4% cocaine solution is used depending on age. The maximum dose is 4 mg/kg body weight [289]. In a comparative investigation, local administration of 0.05% oxymetazoline showed a better ratio of effect to side effects than 4% cocaine or 0.25% phenylephrine [751]. Some authors also inject 0.3–1 mL lidocaine with 1:100 000 epinephrine [536].

General use of hypotensive anesthesia is advocated by some authors [317, 989, 993] but not by others [370]. Where this method is used, a mean arterial pressure of 60–80 mmHg is the target. Attention must be paid to the relevant contraindications, such as heart failure, coronary insufficiency, hypertension, arteriosclerosis of the cerebral vessels, pronounced anemia, and severely impaired lung function. Adequate monitoring of the ECG, mean arterial pressure, body temperature, blood gases, hemoglobin/hematocrit is necessary [9, 166, 317].

Positioning

Patient positioning, the layout of instruments and optical aids, and the positioning of the patient, surgeon, anesthetist, and scrub nurse are handled in a wide variety of ways in paranasal sinus surgery.

Some authors prefer to raise the head end by anything from 10°–40° up to the semi-seated position [9, 30, 39, 238, 240, 317, 534, 989]. This position allows blood and secretions to drain away from the operating area and is thought to help to reduce blood pressure. Other operators do not raise the patient's head, preferring the almost horizontal position so that optical monitoring of the cranial and caudal areas of the nasal cavity is equally possible in a comfortable position [701, 866, 996]. The patient's head may even be hyperextended and turned toward the operator for a period, as necessary. Heermann uses a special head support that can be turned and fixed in all directions [989]. In most cases, the operator stands or sits near the patient's right shoulder. Left-handed surgeons sit or stand on the opposite side [506]. For endoscopic procedures, Stammberger uses an instrument table placed above the patient's upper body. This is used for placing instruments and also as an arm rest for the operator (Fig. 3.**1a**). When operating with a monitor, a video device is placed at the head of the patient. The position and direction of the monitor are selected so that the surgeon can work in a comfortable position. For procedures under general anesthesia without televisual aids, the scrub nurse is in this position (Fig. 3.**1b**) [860]. Wigand uses no scrub nurse and places the instruments within easy reach above the head of the patient (Fig. 3.**1c**) [996]. When using microscopic methods, the microscope stand must always be positioned opposite the operator (Fig. 3.**1d**) [701]. A changeover during the operation, with the surgeon and microscope always being on the side opposite the working area, is time consuming [370, 956].

The patient's eyes should never be covered. Bleeding into the lids, exophthalmos, changes in the pupils, or any movement of soft tissues during intranasal manipulations must be visible at all times to the surgeon and assistants. At the same time, appropriate measures (e.g., plasters on the upper lids, transparent ointment) must be taken to prevent lagophthalmic

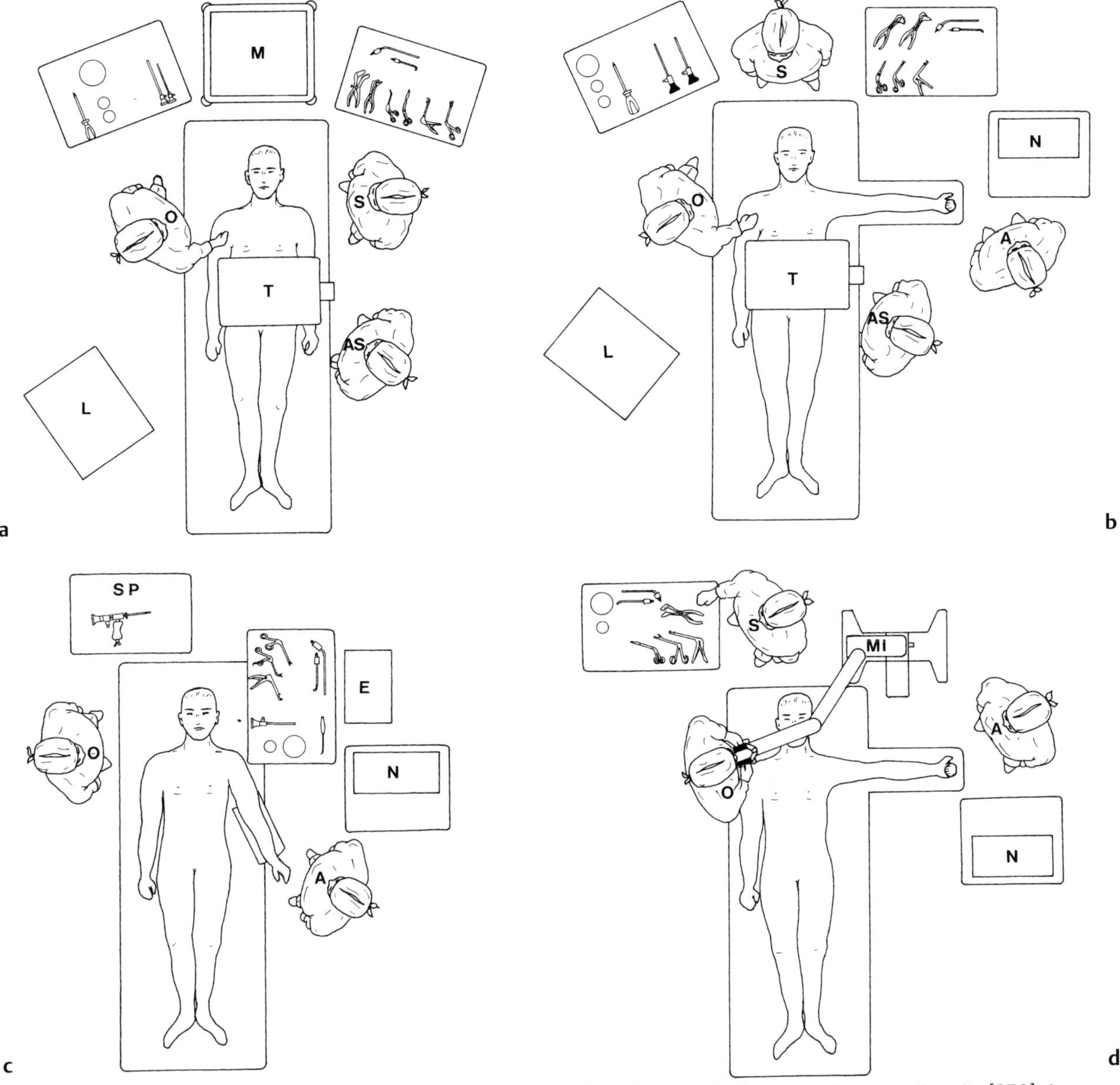

Fig. 3.**1a-d** **Layout for paranasal sinus operations** (**a**) Endoscopic procedures under local anesthesia (Stammberger [860]). (**b**) Endoscopic procedures under general anesthesia (Stammberger [860]). (**c**) Endoscopic procedures using suction-irrigation optics (Wigand [996]). (**d**) Microscopic procedures (Paulsen [701]). A minority of operators change sides and position the microscope on the side opposite the respective operating site [370]. A, anesthetist; AS, assistant; E, basic equipment for bipolar coagulation; L, light source; M, monitor; MI, microscope; N, anesthetic equipment; O, operator; S, nurse; SP, suction-irrigation optics (light source and water supply not shown); T, additional table for arm support

keratitis. If necessary, converting to an external approach must also be possible. The patient's ventilating tube must be firmly fixed and should not obstruct the surgeon during instrumentation [166, 996].

The patient's nasal hair is often trimmed before the operation [173, 996], though some surgeons do not regard this as necessary [866].

General Points on Operating Technique, Adjunctive Measures, and Duration of Operation

Endonasal sinus surgery is made up of a wide variety of individual surgical steps. These are combined depending on the nature and extent of the disease present and on the objective of the operation.

Resection of the uncinate process with a sickle knife, a double-ended elevator or a curved knife has long been recognized as the first stage in opening the anterior ethmoid [451]. For an anterior ethmoidectomy *re-*

moval of the bulla ethmoidalis is the next step. First, a small opening is generally made in the anterior wall of the bulla. The bulge of the bulla is then removed, usually exposing the lamina papyracea and the anterior base of the skull. Dorsally, the *basal lamella of the middle nasal turbinate* can then be *penetrated carefully on the medial and inferior aspects*. Here again the principle of anterior-to-posterior dissection applies: the next layer of ethmoid cells is opened in a safe location and the cavity thus exposed then incorporated in stages into the operative field by controlled removal of clearly identifiable cell septa. In this way, more or less inevitably and without risk, important marginal structures will be encountered such as the lamina papyracea and the base of the skull with the anterior ethmoidal artery. A *concha bullosa is divided vertically* and the lateral section is carefully removed without breaking the remaining vertical lamella. Introductory opening of the concha bullosa with a sharp biting instrument is helpful in this aspect and may be followed by the introduction of a pair of scissors. Both instruments avoid undue forces on the head of the turbinate. Anteriorly, it is often necessary to *punch out the agger nasi* to gain a better view into the ethmoid or frontal sinus and for ventilation of diseased cells [238]. The possibility of further destabilization of the middle nasal turbinate and sometimes problematic scar formation must be borne in mind here [516, 636, 866].

In extensive ethmoid procedures, generous *partial resection of the middle nasal turbinate* or even subtotal excision is often advocated [238, 421, 829, 919, 993]. A concha bullosa or interlamellar cells can hide chronic foci of infection as the origin of recurrent polyps [450, 615]; the rate of postoperative adhesions is reduced by the appropriate resections [477]. The extent of the resection appears to have no effect on the sense of smell [353], but increased crust formation is a potential problem [218]. An important landmark is lost for any revision procedures that may be necessary [317]. Other surgeons therefore resect only the posterior third or half with its attachment to the lateral nasal wall [9, 996]. Yet other authors advocate sparing as much of the turbinate tissue as possible [195, 437]. A preserved but fractured vertical lamella of the middle turbinate following ethmoidectomy tends to lateralize postoperatively, with adhesions and secondary drainage problems [746]. This disadvantage must be borne in mind when recommending routine intraoperative medial displacement of the nasal turbinates, for example using a self-retaining speculum [9, 173, 175, 632]. Particularly in extensive procedures, it is advisable to spare the middle turbinate as far as possible initially and use it as a landmark and then finally to shorten it if required, depending on the intraoperative findings and structures [744, 919]. In this way the turbinate will be lost only in approximately 10% of the most advanced cases of disease [959].

Adjunctive measures in endonasal surgery for chronic sinusitis relate to the correction of septal deviation and reduction of the enlarged inferior turbinates. In individual cases rhinoplasty can also be carried out at the same session [917]. In some centers, sinus surgery aimed at global removal of disease is combined with anterior inferior turbinoplasty and cauterization of posterior ends [9, 663, 956, 990]. The same objective is served by the performance of adjunctive septoplasty in approximately 40% (17–61%) of patients [10, 218, 335, 493, 959]. This removes a potential contributory factor in sinusitis [21, 238, 453, 632, 763, 993]. Since this also provides room for surgical manipulations, even nondeviating septa are frequently "mobilized" [763, 906, 996] by some surgeons. Others rarely regard either procedure as necessary. The immediate postoperative healing process is favored by leaving the septum intact [459]. Septoplasty is therefore indicated only where freedom of movement with the 4-mm endoscope is considerably restricted [860].

For intraoperative orientation, a number of surgeons employ a measuring scale that uses the anterior nasal spine as a reference point [580, 892]. At an angle of 30° to the floor of the nose, the anterior wall of the sphenoid sinus should lie at a depth of 7 cm [196, 238, 580]. Hajek [299] gave a value of 6–7 cm as early as 1926.

The wide variety of surgical procedures reported in the literature are matched by correspondingly varying *operating times*. Experienced surgeons estimate that complete and meticulous dissection of all sinuses on both sides together with adjunctive surgical measures takes barely two (1–3) hours [9, 139, 162, 238, 269, 564, 675, 873, 883, 993]. The figures are correspondingly lower for functional endonasal sinus surgery. Even with massive polyposis, operating times of only 25 minutes per side have been reported [856]. In principle, procedures under local anesthesia can be kept shorter or require less time in the operating room [269]. Depending on the nature and extent of the procedure, revisions are generally shorter [490] but sometimes require the same time as or even considerably longer operating times than the complete dissections mentioned.

The figures reported for procedures in children are essentially the same [183, 289, 492, 751].

Endoscopic Ethmoid Surgery (Anterior-to-Posterior Technique)

In the anterior-to-posterior technique, an "infundibulotomy" is first performed with resection of the uncinate process (Figs. **3.2a-c**). This procedure opens the ethmoid sinus, and is then extended step by step as dictated by the pathological findings and the anatomy of the patient. The ostium of the maxillary sinus is explored and widened if necessary, preferably at the cost of the anterior fontanelle. The bulla ethmoidalis is then opened and excised and the base of the skull is identified. The frontal recess is explored and the

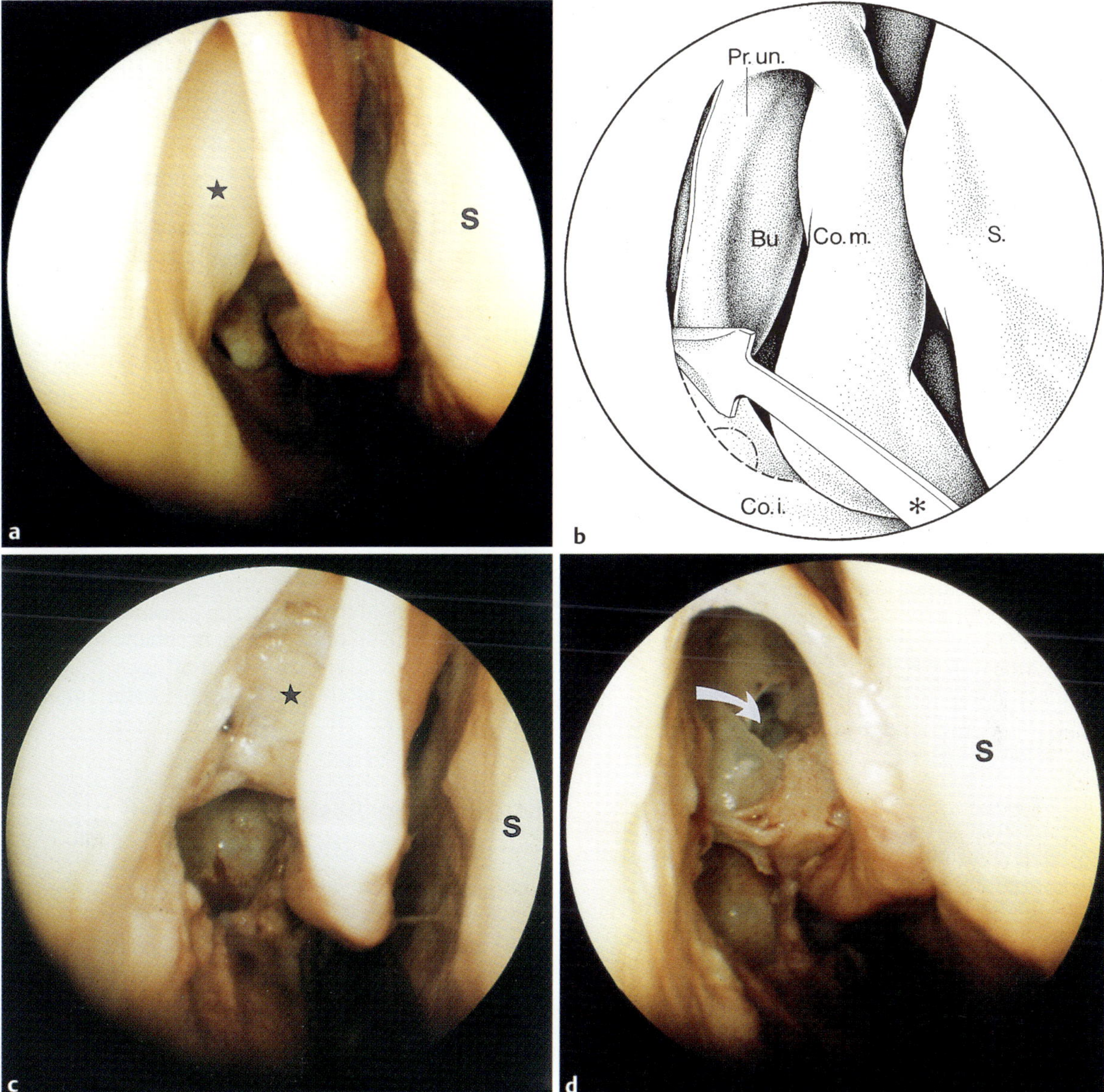

Fig. 3.**2a-d** **Steps in anterior-to-posterior endonasal ethmoid surgery** (cadaver specimen, right side)
(**a**) Initial findings. Right nasal cavity with septum, middle turbinate, and uncinate process (★). S, nasal septum. (**b**) Using a curved nasal knife (★) (or a sickle knife) the uncinate process is resected and removed. The continuing line of the incision is shown with a broken line and the concealed maxillary ostium with a dotted line. The anterior attachment of the uncinate process may be located by palpation or by careful traction on its free edge. Co.i., lower turbinate; Co.m., middle turbinate; Pr.un., uncinate process. (**c**) After removing the uncinate process and wide fenestration of the maxillary sinus in the middle meatus, the view of the bulla ethmoidalis (★) is unobstructed. (**d**) The bulla ethmoidalis is removed, the basal lamella of the middle turbinate is exposed. By perforation of the basal lamella (arrow) inspection of the posterior ethmoid is carried out

access to the frontal sinus is examined. Wide opening of the frontal sinus access is carried out only in advanced disease of the frontal mucosa or other diseases of the frontal sinuses. The posterior ethmoid is opened through the basal lamella of the middle turbinate (Fig. 3.**2d**) and resected if necessary. The vertical lamella of the middle turbinate is spared. The sphenoid sinus is opened if necessary, as for the frontal sinus. It is fenestrated through the ethmoid or directly via the sphenoethmoidal recess. Septoplasty is necessary only if the septal deviation prevents manipulation of the endoscope. Isolated septal spurs may be removed endoscopically. Major manipulations in the maxillary sinuses can be undertaken via an additional transoral puncture of the anterior wall of the maxillary sinuses. The procedure may be extended step by

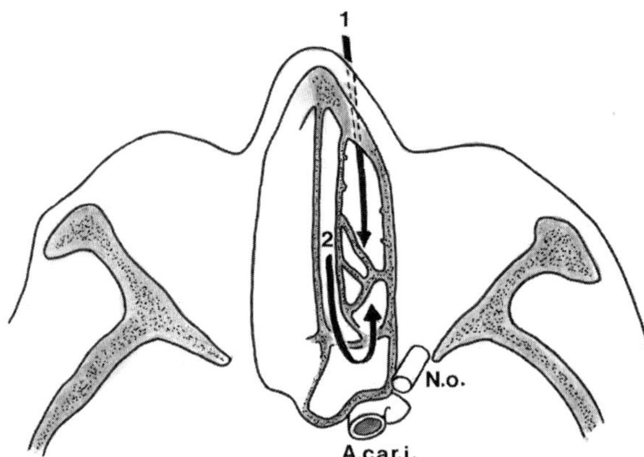

Fig. 3.3 **Axial cross-section through the ethmoid bone**
Principle of anterior-to-posterior (1) and posterior-to-anterior (2) operating technique in ethmoidectomy. For diagnostic reasons and to improve access, in diffuse rhinosinusitis an anterior ethmoidectomy (1) is generally performed to begin with. If the decision to remove the posterior ethmoid is taken after perforation of the third basal lamella, a change in the operating direction is advisable. The widely exposed anterior wall of the sphenoid sinus is opened medially. In the case of posterior-to-anterior completion of the procedure, the direction of dissection (2) is away from the optic nerve and the internal carotid artery
A. car. i. = internal carotid artery
N. o. = optic nerve

step to complete clearance of the maxillary, ethmoid and sphenoid sinuses with fenestration of the frontal sinus (pansinus operation).

The medial wall of the orbit is used as an important landmark. It is exposed at a relatively early stage. The second landmark is the base of the skull, which is sought at the cranial bulla or in the posterior ethmoid cell system. From here, the base of the skull can also be explored step by step in a posterior-to-anterior direction [432, 433, 866].

Ethmoid Surgery Using the Suction-Irrigation Endoscope (Posterior-to-Anterior Technique)

A suction-irrigation endoscope for endonasal sinus surgery was described by Wigand [990]. Irrigation at the tip of the endoscope keeps the lens free from blood and secretions. Uninterrupted vision is particularly important when using the 70° endoscope and for manipulations in the far reaches of the operating field. The main domains of the suction-irrigation endoscope are operations for polypoid pansinusitis and procedures in the maxillary sinuses and in the approaches to or inside the frontal sinuses [993].

Pansinus procedures are performed under general anesthesia. The first stage is polypectomy, the second a still limited anterior-to-posterior removal of the ethmoid cells with excision of the uncinate process (Fig. 3.**3**). After resection of the posterior attachment of the middle turbinate, the anterior wall of the sphenoid sinus can be broadly exposed. The sphenoid sinus is then opened transnasally via the sphenoethmoidal recess, with exposure of the ethmoid roof from posterior to anterior (Fig. 3.**4a, b**). The lateral groups of cells over the lamina papyracea are then removed and the access to the frontal sinus is exposed and widely opened under optical guidance (Fig. 3.**4c**). The maxillary sinus is broadly fenestrated in the middle meatus by removing the anterior and posterior fontanelle. Accurate endoscopically aided manipulations in the maxillary and frontal sinuses require special instruments such as slim and long-handled upturned cupped forceps. The vertical lamella of the middle turbinate is increasingly spared [993, 996].

Dissection in the posterior-to-anterior direction is part of a number of procedures involving the ethmoid, including exploration of the frontal sinus access. Frequently, the anterior base of the skull is also located retrogradely by opening larger and undiseased posterior ethmoid cells. During procedures on the posterior ethmoid bone, as in the pansinus operation, preference is given to early median sphenoidotomy in the more favorable working direction away from delicate structures of the lateral wall of the sphenoid sinuses (Fig. 3.**3**).

Microscope-Assisted Ethmoid Surgery

Compared with the endoscope, the microscope offers the advantage of stereoscopic vision and the ability to work bimanually. The microscope is positioned outside the operative field and vision is not appreciably disrupted by secretions and blood. The disadvantage is that the operator can only look straight ahead. This affects procedures in the maxillary and frontal sinuses. In these cases, endoscopes with the appropriate viewing angles are also used. An observer arm (or a video camera) can be used at all times without obstructing the operator and is an important aid to teaching.

As long ago as 1958, H. Heermann [312] reported two years' experience of use of a binocular microscope in endonasal surgery, in operations on the lacrimal sac, in clearance of the ethmoid sinus, in frontal sinus procedures and in ligation of the ethmoidal arteries. The technique was subsequently developed further, particularly by Prades [721] and also by J. Heermann [314] and Dixon [161]. The spectrum of procedures was soon extended to include decompression of the optic nerve [39].

The microscope is fitted with a lens with a focal length of 300 mm or occasionally 250 mm. Heermann and Neues [317] advocate a balanced suspension, so that the operator can control the microscope by means of head movements. The view of the operative field is provided by a series of self-retaining specula. A

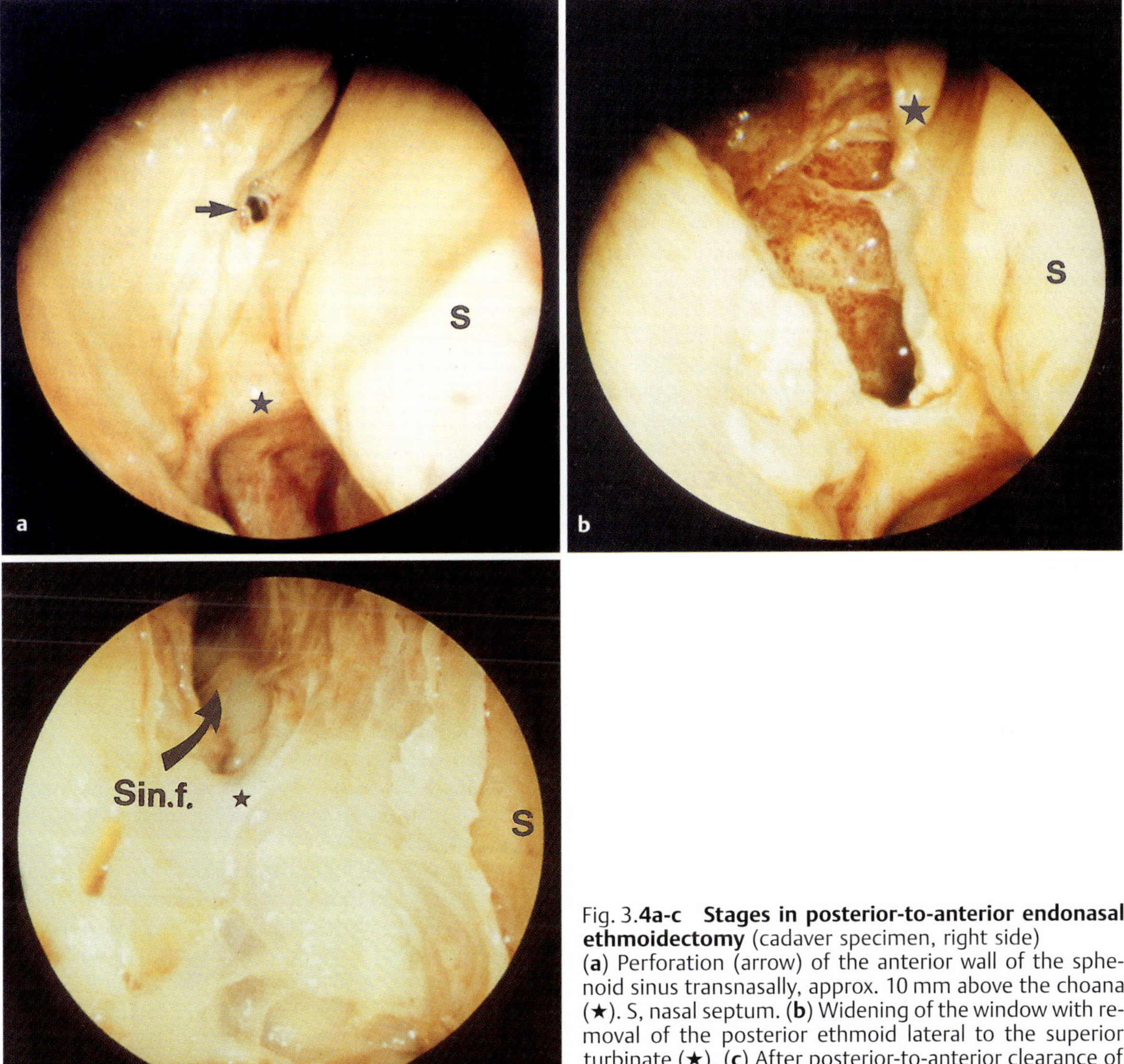

Fig. 3.**4a-c** **Stages in posterior-to-anterior endonasal ethmoidectomy** (cadaver specimen, right side)
(**a**) Perforation (arrow) of the anterior wall of the sphenoid sinus transnasally, approx. 10 mm above the choana (★). S, nasal septum. (**b**) Widening of the window with removal of the posterior ethmoid lateral to the superior turbinate (★). (**c**) After posterior-to-anterior clearance of the base of the skull, broad access is provided to the frontal sinus (Sin.f.). ★, anterior ethmoidal artery

number of specula have unequal branches, some with serrations to allow fixing in the lateral nasal wall [30, 39, 161, 162, 177, 763]. The position of the instruments is fixed on the patient's head by various retaining systems [30] or preferably by an articulated arm [173, 763, 829]. The speculum may also be held by the assistant [370] or sometimes by the operator [173].

The surgeon generally operates in a seated position. The indication for septoplasty is generally broadly established. The middle turbinate is then displaced medially and the nasal speculum is put in place. The preferred operating direction under the microscope is initially anterior-to-posterior. The anterior ethmoid cells are opened, and dissection is carried along the middle turbinate as far as the sphenoid sinus. The overview can be improved by using a 4 mm diamond burr to reduce the agger nasi and the frontal process of the maxilla to the level of the lamina papyracea and by exposure of the lacrimal ducts [175]. After opening the sphenoid sinus it is possible to dissect the posterior ethmoid roof from posterior to anterior. Additional use of the endoscope (suction-irrigation endoscope; preferably 25°/30°, 70° viewing angle) allows visualization and dissection of areas of the lateral ethmoid bone, lamina papyracea, maxillary sinus access, or the lumina of the frontal and maxillary sinuses, which can be seen less clearly or not at all in the direct line of vision of the microscope. In one-third of cases, the view obtained through the microscope alone is reported to be sufficient [9]. To complete the procedure, the ethmoid shaft can be polished using the diamond burr [32, 162, 173, 175, 370, 763, 906].

Technical Modifications

Operation Using the Monitor

If the microscope is used, a video system may be installed routinely. This allows the scrub nurse, assistants and doctors observing the procedure to follow the surgical procedure in detail. The same advantage can be achieved during endoscopic procedures by fitting a camera. However, the camera, cable and sheathing can make the equipment combination heavier and more cumbersome to handle and the poorer maneuverability can lead to increased tissue trauma [437]. In principle, the surgeon can perform endoscopic procedures via an intercalated beam splitter or directly via the monitor [97]. The operating position is more relaxed when using the monitor, so that the surgeon tires less easily. The video image can be optically modified or enlarged as required [606, 676]. The patient's face with its "external landmarks" remains constantly in view. When the lights are lowered, the light shining through the skull provides an external impression of the position of the endoscope tip, as with transillumination [1005, 1006]. May [579] has the endoscope and camera held by an assistant so that bimanual operating is possible. The younger assistant at the same time obtains a step-by-step introduction to the operating technique. In 10% of cases, however, the procedure has to be supplemented or continued in the conventional manner using a headlight because of restricted visibility due, for example, to bleeding [578]. The monitor image is currently still optically inferior to direct vision through the eyepiece [578]. To compensate for this, Moriyama uses stronger optics with an external diameter of 5–6 mm [632]. Notwithstanding this, surgical task performance using the monitor proved to be excellent in a surgical training model [984]. Other investigators have had different experience [904].

Surgery with Headlight and (Suction-Irrigation) Endoscope

Even the recent literature contains reports from a number of authors who use the endonasal technique without optical aids [240, 380, 839, 884]. The advantages of optical aids are indisputable, however. They have a diagnostic function and contribute to the safety of the procedure. They allow accurate assessment of the microanatomy and the execution of manipulations in obscure areas. This can help to limit or specifically extend the procedure on the basis of the findings obtained. The endoscope and/or microscope have now become indispensable aids in endonasal surgery.

On the other hand, vision with the naked eye can have certain advantages under some circumstances: optical distortion in the endoscope can result in incorrect assessment of individual anatomic details such as a concha bullosa or interlamellar cells [861] (Fig. 2.**6**). The endoscope allows only limited perception of depth because of unaccustomed or absent shadow formation [102]. The simultaneous view of spatially separate landmarks and their relationship is also lost in the endoscope, as is that of the external face [672]. A number of manipulations such as specific hemostasis of branches of the sphenopalatine artery using a bipolar coagulation forceps are often easier to perform using a headlight [578, 903].

The above considerations lead some specialists to perform endoscopic procedures on the ethmoid with simultaneous use of a headlight [421, 486, 919, 1006]. By alternating endoscopic vision with that of the naked eye, an attempt is made to achieve a rational, safe, and thorough working method. Special investigations using a surgical training system give support to this surgical concept [903]. Other authors also use loupes with a magnification of 2 to 3-fold as an aid [444, 920].

Instruments

The selection of instruments is very much dictated by the personal preferences of the operator. In recent years there has been a trend toward sharp, cutting instruments and away from grasping forceps with their less controllable, rather clumsy removal of tissue [632]. Further new developments have related to instruments with combined functions or slim instruments for manipulations in distal or inaccessible areas of the operative field.

Optical aids include the microscope and endoscopes, usually with a diameter of 4 mm and various viewing angles (commonly 25°/30° and 70°, recently 45°) or an optional video camera with or without a beam splitter or articulated arm. For children, endoscopes with a diameter of 2.7 mm are used. Various irrigation or suction-irrigation shafts are available for larger endoscopes [990]. Suction devices of various curvatures and lengths can be used to keep the operating area free from secretions and blood. A sickle knife is generally used for resection of the uncinate process. Partial removal of turbinate tissue requires nasal scissors. Further removal of tissue is carried out with variously angled forceps (e.g. Blakesley-Wilde, Takahashi, Wigand), bone punches (e.g. Hajek or Kerrison), or a conchotome (e.g. Grünwald, Hartmann, or Moriyama). For manipulations in the area of the sphenoid sinus, instruments fitted with a graduated measuring scale are thought by some to be useful. For opening the maxillary sinus, back-biting punch forceps (e.g. Ostrom or Stammberger) are available. The natural ostium can be identified using a special ostium seeker. Manipulations in the maxillary sinus can only be carried out adequately using special, slim grasping forceps or forceps with cupped jaws. Similar instruments are also used for surgery in the frontal recess or frontal sinuses. Further reference will be made to other instruments for opening the frontal sinuses (curettes, rasps and probes, recently even bent

Nasal irrigation –
well tolerated & easy to handle
RhinoCare®
Nasal Douche
& Ems Salt®
a successful system for nasal irrigation in postoperative care: easy to handle, effective, safe, inexpensive
EMSER SALZ®
Wirkstoff: Natürliches Emser Salz
Zur Anwendung im Bereich der oberen Atemwege (Nase und Nebenhöhlen, Rachen und Kehlkopf)
EMS

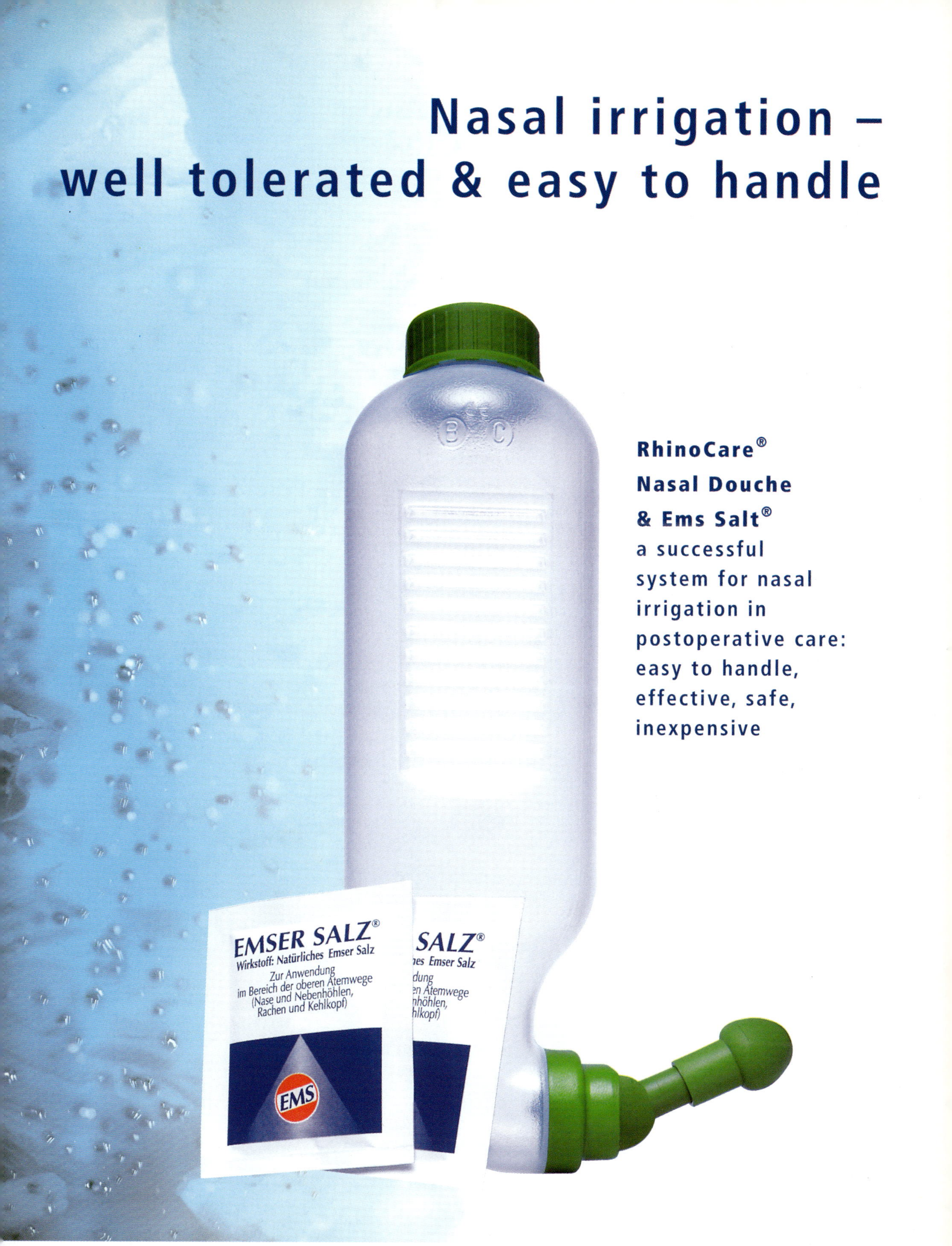

A simple and effective principle

- for loosening crusts after endonasal surgery
- for moistening in cases of sicca syndrome
- for treating chronic cases of rhinosinusitis and sinusitis
- for prophylaxis and adjuvant treatment of allergic rhinitis

RhinoCare® Nasal Douche

- easy to handle
- unbreakable
- variable irrigation pressure
- easy to clean

Ems Mineral Salt

Natural salt with a complex composition

- Contains bicarbonate:
  an anti-inflammatory buffer
- more than 20 essential minerals
  and trace elements

Broad efficacy

- neutralizes acid and acts as a decongestant
- reactivates ciliary epitheleum
- regenerates mucous membrane

Excellent safety profile

- safe to use on regular basis
- single unit bags for exact dosage

punches). A combination of forceps with suction makes operating with one hand easier [437, 661]. It is questionable whether special miniature drills, e.g. for opening a bulla ethmoidalis, are advantageous [261]. Cushions of edema in the maxillary sinus can be removed with rotating nylon threads fitted to the drill [669], a procedure that might threaten the infraorbital nerve. An abundance of technical advice is available to facilitate handling of the various instruments [389]. For example, endoscopes may be fitted with supports [1011] and special irrigating devices have been designed using disposable items [146, 465, 772].

The shaver systems adopted from orthopedic surgery (287, 815, 816) suck tissues into the working channel where they are then removed by rotating blades. Shaver systems, also known as microdebrider or microresector systems, are available from several companies (Karl Storz, Xomed, Smith & Nephew, Stryker). Some even have bent tips permitting work in the frontal recess and inside the maxillary sinus. The development of shaver systems was paralleled by the introduction of new bone drills for intranasal use [538].

Endonasal Laser Surgery

For technical and physical reasons, the use of lasers in endonasal surgery is currently limited mostly to the treatment of hereditary hemorrhagic telangiectasia (Rendu-Osler-Weber disease), "vasomotor rhinitis," the reduction of hyperplastic turbinates, and choanal atresia. No details will be given here of procedures in the area of the nasal cavity. Laser surgery of the lacrimal ducts will be discussed separately.

In principle, the use of lasers in the nose offers the advantages of minimal intraoperative bleeding, little reactive edema, limited postoperative problems and a short stay in hospital. The laser may also allow procedures to be carried out in patients with coagulation disorders. Argon, holmium:YAG, neodymium (Nd):YAG and potassium titanyl phosphate lasers in particular are used in paranasal sinus surgery. They are fitted with flexible light conductors. Procedures include sphenoidotomy, excision of a concha bullosa, maxillary sinus fenestration and polyp removal. Scar tissue can be excised, smaller tumors are removed. In treating nasal polyps, longer operating times must always be allowed. There is no tactile feedback for the operator, who thus has little control over possible deep effects in delicate areas. The first devastating complications have been reported [745]. Under the current technical conditions, wider use of laser surgery in diffuse polyposis cannot be recommended.

Considerable experience is available with the carbon dioxide laser in the removal of polyps or readily accessible papillomas and in division of adhesions. However, the rate of recurrence reported for papillomas appears unacceptable [832].

The argon laser can be used to fenestrate the maxillary sinuses by excision or vaporization [498]. In animal studies there was considerable delay in healing [943]. The argon laser has proved useful in mild to moderate epistaxis.

The Nd:YAG laser has been used in the postoperative treatment of mucosal hyperplasia, for example, in the maxillary sinus area [633]. Tissue removal in animal studies proved comparatively less precise [418]. The specific deep tissue penetration represents a special problem for procedures near the skull base.

Depending on the power, duration, and area of action, the potassium titanyl phosphate laser can be used for cutting, coagulation or vaporization. This laser can be used for clean division or ablation of adhesions resulting from previous interventions and for fenestration of the maxillary sinus [499, 502, 883]. Smaller and solid polyps can be carbonized, larger polyps or choanal polyps can be removed bloodlessly [437, 499, 503]. In individual cases inverted papillomas can also be removed as well as intranasal hemangiomas [502]. The potassium titanyl phosphate laser is not suitable for hemostasis [437]. A concha bullosa can be divided using a no-touch technique. The fiberoptic cables are incorporated in an aspirator or a special endoscope sleeving [437, 502].

The particular advantage of the holmium:YAG laser lies in the ablation of sufficient volume of bone with simultaneous coagulation of soft tissue. Explosive vaporization or flaming must be prevented by constant irrigation. Scattering within the nasal cavity of blood and debris collecting on the tip of the endoscope should be prevented by an irrigation system. Thermal necrosis extends up to 1 mm beyond the laser-cut edge of tissue, restricting use of the laser near delicate anatomic structures (skull base, optic nerve, lamina papyracea) [607]. Early reactive mucosal edema may be increased, but wound healing in general is only slightly delayed. The holmium:YAG laser is used for the reduction of large polyps, for removal of the uncinate process and bony ridges, for opening the bulla, and for widening the maxillary ostium. Another indication may be choanal atresia [690]. Major surgery of the sinuses may be performed using conventional instrumentarium in addition. Blood loss is reduced, but total surgical time is increased. The holmium:YAG laser is not able to control active bleeding [273, 424, 433, 607, 821, 822].

Special Partial Ethmoidectomy Procedures, the Endonasal Pansinus Operation

The step-by-step system of surgical procedures to the ethmoid bone has already been described (p. 19). Only a few reports in the literature describe further specific surgical procedures.

Less than 2% of cases of sinusitis are caused by localized mucositis in a concha bullosa. The principle of treatment by conservative endonasal surgery has been described by Hajek [299]. Bouton et al. [74] report eight cases of a diseased concha bullosa treated in endoscopic surgery by partial removal of the lateral wall of the concha. A concha bullosa can assume monstrous proportions [1013]. Even in these cases, careful removal under endoscopic control can achieve a cure. Cannon [98] identified four distinct procedures in concha bullosa ranging from lateral marsupialization to simple crushing.

Only the recommendation to perform sagittal division with excision of the lateral portion can be recommended unreservedly. Care must be taken to use suitable instruments for the incision to exclude the possibility of fracturing the vertical lamella. The bite of a conchotome may open up the concha bullosa, easing the introduction of a pair of scissors. Treatment by partial horizontal resection of the turbinate may also be considered if ventilation of the lateral middle meatus is ensured [746].

Agger nasi cells are extremely common. Depending on their size they may restrict drainage of the frontal sinuses. Removal of the caudal cell walls alone (marsupialization) is insufficient in these cases. The residual "dome" of these cells compromises the frontal recess and can remain the cause of persistent frontal sinusitis. Kuhn et al. [474] described the removal of this type of agger cell, preserving the mucosa of the frontal recess and frontal ostium. A slim, curved curette is introduced between the base of the skull and the dome of the agger cell and compresses the cell wall caudally. This procedure is popularized as "uncapping the egg" (see Fig. 2.**5**). Cell septa are removed under direct vision using small biopsy forceps with cupped jaws.

Complete ethmoidectomy with opening of the sphenoid, frontal, and maxillary sinuses is described as the pansinus operation. The procedure is necessary where diffuse chronic sinusitis is present with the involvement of all paranasal sinuses. The operation consists of a combination of all the operative steps described earlier (p. 19).

Maxillary Sinus Procedures

Endoscopic procedures on the maxillary sinus have a long tradition, their various variants and outcomes having been described by Draf [172]. The following comments represent merely a few updates.

Endonasal Maxillary Sinus Fenestration

Fenestration in the middle meatus generally starts with excision of the uncinate process. Incomplete removal of the inferior-posterior process may present special difficulties [686]. Applying microsurgical techniques, the natural ostium of the maxillary sinus may be palpated using a fine bent suction catheter or even a special curved olive-tip probe ("maxillary ostium seeker"). The anatomy of the maxillary ostium is variable, landmarks being the superior attachment of the inferior turbinate, the anterior and caudal resection edges of the uncinate process, and the bulge of the nasolacrimal duct. The appearance of air bubbles or secretions from the ostium when the fontanelles are palpated can indicate the direction [866]. Separate puncture of the maxillary sinus with irrigation is rarely necessary to identify the natural ostium [55]. If the surgeon intends to widen the maxillary ostium and maintain its mucociliary transport function and if extensive endoscopic monitoring or manipulation in the maxillary sinus are not required, the natural ostium may be widened anteriorly and inferiorly using a curette or back-biting punch at the cost of the anterior fontanelle. The lacrimal duct must be spared. The mucosa of the postero-superior edge of the ostium is preserved and functional neo-ostia of 4–6 mm diameter are created [433, 536]. These ostia remain patent in up to 98% of cases [436, 865]. In principle, maintenance of function can be expected where the diameter is more than 2.5–3 mm [20, 865]. As an additional measure to prevent stenosis due to scarring, mucosa from the maxillary sinus may be drawn over the resulting wound [439]. In 17% of cases, difficulties are encountered in widening the natural ostium as described: the ostium may be difficult to locate, there may be scarring from previous procedures, the bone may be locally thickened, or bleeding may obscure visibility [436].

If there is an accessory ostium in the middle meatus, the creation of a common larger neo-ostium during fenestration connecting the ostium primum and the ostium secundum is recommended. Unproductive, circular mucociliary currents through two ostia into and out of the maxillary sinus can be prevented in this way [866]. Pathological recirculation of mucus may occur in several conditions related to middle meatal primary ostia, accessory ostia, and neo-ostia. Even inferior antrostomies may be involved. The underlying pathophysiology is not fully understood. Sometimes during prior surgery a middle meatal antrostomy has been created too far posteriorly following failure to identify the natural ostium, which is hidden by the uncinate process. The resulting condition of recirculation and infection has been coined "missed ostium sequence" [697]. Patients revealing mucus recirculation may present with therapy-refractory recurrent infection, mostly of the maxillary sinus. Nasal endoscopy detects the exact pattern of recirculation. The surgical concept in any case consists in joining the inflow and the outflow ostium [99, 121, 413, 571].

Small neo-ostia allow neither complete endoscopic inspection of the maxillary sinus nor targeted tissue removal within the maxillary sinus. For this reason, other surgeons mostly produce neo-ostia of around 1 × 2 cm at the cost of both the anterior and posterior fontanelles [175, 406, 503, 744, 891, 996]. The 45° upturned, pointed ethmoid forceps are introduced posteriorly immediately above the inferior turbinate and laterally through the fontanelle [996]. Alternatively, the incision may be extended inferoposteriorly to an infundibulotomy so that the uncinate process together with parts of the natural ostium and the posterior fontanelle can be displaced medially, detached caudally, and removed under direct vision [495]. Extensive detachment or stripping of the maxillary mucosa must be avoided [534, 866]. Superiorly the orbit must be respected, and anteriorly the lacrimal duct. Great care is necessary where there is partial fusion of the middle meatus with the orbital process of the maxilla [299]. Widening of the initial opening is primarily achieved with the anterograde sharp instruments and back-biting punch, though caution must be exercised to avoid damage to the nasolacrimal duct. For maximum fenestration, parts of the vertical lamella of the palatine bone must also be removed up to the sphenopalatine foramen [243]. Widening at the cost of neighboring portions of the inferior turbinate is another option, as is incorporating a lower window through the turbinate body [267, 908]. In a reduced fenestration, two flaps of mucosa may be formed by means of a horizontal scissor-cut from the posterior fontanelle and are then reflected cranially and caudally [436]. A slightly more elaborate mucosal repair is occasionally undertaken by Wigand. After removal of the nasal mucosal layer and a star-shaped incision of the basally exposed maxillary mucosa in the region of the posterior fontanelle, the maxillary sinus mucosa can be placed in the direction of the nasal cavity, preserving its mucociliary transport pathways.

Larger neo-ostia remain structurally preserved in up to 97% of cases [144, 145, 343, 406]. Recovery of the maxillary mucosa is reported in almost the same percentage [406]. Stenoses of the neo-ostia develop slowly over a period of more than two years [144, 145]. There is a relationship between the remaining size of the neo-ostium and the patient's symptoms [770]. In patients over 40 years of age, in pronounced and purulent sinusitis or nasal polyposis, and in respiratory allergy, the outcome of the operation is said to be less favorable [144, 145, 726].

The effects of fenestration surgery on mucociliary clearance of the maxillary sinuses have been analyzed in a number of animal studies. No uniform picture emerges. Hilding [325] showed that placing a window near the natural ostium was functionally disadvantageous with regard to overall drainage. Fenestration distant from the natural ostium did not compromise the physiological cleansing mechanism in this way [234, 325, 439]. Even later secondary closure of a distant window in the lower meatus often remained without sequelae [234]. Other investigators have achieved similar outcomes in maxillary sinusitis with an antrostomy in the inferior nasal meatus and fenestration near the natural ostium [49]. The mucociliary apparatus of mucosal flaps retains its direction of ciliary beating even after displacement of the mucosa [679]. Surgical widening of the natural ostium itself can upset the delicate balance of ciliary drainage of the maxillary sinuses [439, 707].

Hosemann et al. [359] showed that on both sides of the medial maxillary sinus wall there is a superficial and deep network of lymph capillaries directed along the surface of the mucosa toward the ostium. The density of the capillaries increases from cranial to caudal and from posterior to anterior and in the vicinity of the ostium primum. The network of maxillary and nasal lymph vessels communicates not only via the ostium but also through the natural bony dehiscences of the middle meatus. Unusually pronounced postoperative swelling following fenestration in the middle meatus may be explained by the ablation of the additional transmural drainage pathways. Widening of the window should be undertaken in a posterosuperior direction.

Fenestration in the Inferior Meatus

Fenestration of the maxillary sinus in the inferior meatus alone ignores the fact that most inflammations of the maxillary sinuses arise from the nose via a pathological focus in the area of the adjoining ostiomeatal unit. Inferior meatal antrostomy is comparably unfavorable from the point of view of mucociliary flow patterns [649]. Neo-ostia in the inferior meatus play only a limited part in mucociliary drainage of the maxillary sinuses [83, 245, 248, 343]. On the other hand, minor inflammation of the middle meatus can certainly arise secondarily from the maxillary sinuses [82, 864]. Only the removal of the focus in the maxillary sinus would lead to resolution of the problems in the ostiomeatal unit. Accordingly, there are clinical reports in adults and children of good subjective results of inferior meatal antrostomy [16, 343, 689].

Additional fenestration in the inferior meatus may be indicated if foci of disease in the maxillary sinuses cannot be reached by surgical instruments in any other way. Where there is ciliary dyskinesia or where some other form of mucociliary insufficiency is suspected, inferior meatal antrostomy is justified as passive "overflow drainage" [865, 906, 919]. The same applies following orbital decompression with obstruction of the middle meatus [749]. For processes in the maxillary sinuses that cannot be interpreted as secondary to disease of the middle meatus, fenestration in the inferior meatus can contribute to preservation of the ostiomeatal unit [82]. The target size for the window is 1 × 0.5 to 1 × 2 cm [520]. Temporary windows may also be created in specific individual cases with isolated foci of infection in the maxillary sinuses [740]. Windows in the inferior meatus are known to have a greater tendency to form adhesions or stenoses due to scarring [172, 341]. Within the first five weeks postoperatively, there is a mean reduction in the size of the ostium of around one-quarter [522]. Closure is observed in 5–23% of cases [520, 689, 735]. This must be taken into consideration in younger patients with local infections and where the initial window size is inadequate [520, 523]. Stenting for about six weeks or reduction of the adjacent inferior turbinate may prevent stenosis [84, 176, 959]. However, patients often benefit from this fenestration despite occlusion due to scarring [523].

Endonasal Maxillary Sinus Surgery

After the creation of a small maxillary sinus neo-ostium, the diagnostic and therapeutic measures in the maxillary sinus itself are very limited. The vast majority of cases of maxillary sinusitis result from disease of the adjacent ethmoid complex. A number of authors therefore refrain from performing specific manipulations within the maxillary sinus and wait for spontaneous healing of mucosal hyperplasia or allow areas of clinically and functionally insignificant mucosal disease to remain [406, 433]. Others, if it is necessary, perform additional transoral endoscopy of the maxillary sinus with simultaneous transnasal instrumentation [434, 436, 578]. Any more extensive combination of optically aided endonasal procedures with transoral surgery of the maxillary sinuses [829, 838] in uncomplicated chronic sinusitis contravenes all the principles of functional sinus surgery.

The creation of larger neo-ostia allows the surgeon using optical aids with suitable viewing angles (70° or 25°/30°) to illuminate almost all recesses of the maxillary sinuses and to reach them with curved grasping forceps and curettes. The only exceptions are large palatine recesses and the prelacrimal recess. Here, it may be necessary to widen the window or create a second neo-ostium [632, 763, 992]. This also allows removal of larger granulomas and foci of inflammation [562]. Extensive areas of hyperplastic mucosa can be scarified with a rotating nylon thread ("sinus abrasion" as described by Herberhold) [669]. Damage to the infraorbital nerve must be avoided during this process.

If foci of disease or predisposing factors in the middle meatus are also attended to and treated at the same time, the endonasal maxillary sinus operation offers a good overall rate of success [842, 992]. After adequate imaging and when the corresponding symptoms are present, revision surgery may be worthwhile even after previous radical, transoral procedures [995]. However, the postoperative endoscopic findings do not always agree with the subjective assessment by the patient [384]. In some cases the fenestration even induces secondary changes in the maxillary sinus mucosa [341].

Antro-Choanal Polyps

The first step in the case of choanal polyps is endoscopic visualization of the pedicle in the middle meatus. The reported sites of origin of the polyp vary. The pedicle can generally be traced back through an accessory ostium and less often through the natural ostium. A better view may be obtained via anterior ethmoidectomy with creation of a larger window in the middle meatus. The natural ostium and accessory ostia are united to form a common window. Sooner or later the pedicle of the polyp is divided in the nose and the polyp extracted through the nose or pharynx depending on size. The stump of the polyp in the maxillary sinus must then be precisely located via the middle meatus using suitable optical aids (70° endoscope). It generally lies in the area of the posterior or medial maxillary sinus wall [407, 866]. The procedure ends with circumscribed excision of the polyp pedicle. If this cannot be undertaken via the medial meatotomy, an additional window is created in the inferior meatus. In one-quarter of patients, concomitant chronic sinusitis requires extension of the endonasal ethmoid procedure [407].

Recurrences should be the exception when optically guided surgical techniques are used. The overall rate is 7% (0–25%) [124, 203, 407, 517]. Some authors recommend transoral follow-up endoscopy after completion of the procedure and report that this frequently reveals a small residual polyp pedicle or covered maxillary sinus cysts, which should be carefully removed. Other authors always remove the polyp pedicle transorally and attempt to preserve the structures of the middle meatus irrespective of accurate polyp extraction [866]. After removal, small cysts sometimes form at the original base of the polyp [517].

Endonasal Sphenoid Sinus Surgery

For the anatomic background, operating principles, and specific hazards of sphenoid sinus fenestration, we refer to the publication by Draf [172]. The sphenoid sinus can in principle be reached via the septum, ethmoid, nose, antrum, or palate. However, for routine endonasal procedures, sphenoidotomy is generally performed by a transethmoidal (through the ethmoid portion of the anterior wall, i.e., laterally) or transnasal approach (through the nasal portion of the anterior wall, i.e., medially). A transseptal approach is indicated only in exceptional cases. The comments below relate to the routine procedures mentioned. The possibility of endoscopic procedures on the pituitary [385, 812] should also be mentioned.

Anatomically, depending on the extent of pneumatization, a distinction is drawn between conchal, presellar, and sellar types of sphenoid sinus. Rudimentary pneumatization (conchal type) is encountered in around 3% (0–8%) of cases, extensive pneumatization in 14%. Pneumatization is usually similar on both sides; a deviated sphenoid sinus septum results in asymmetry of size and the dominance of one side in the majority of cases [33, 303, 813]. With increasing pneumatization, the bone becomes thinned over vital structures of the lateral sphenoid sinus wall [102]. The bony covering is less than 0.5 mm thick over the carotid artery in 90% of cases and over the optic nerve in 80% [250]. The consequences of this are of clinical significance: in one case out of five a probing instrument will meet no appreciable resistance [441]. Dehiscences have been reported over the course of the optic nerve in 3–12% of cases and over the carotid artery in around 5% (0.3–8%) [402, 657, 680, 814].

According to Kainz et al. [404], the course of the carotid artery in the wall of the sphenoid sinus, can be divided into five different anatomic forms. In 78% of cases the artery causes an anterior bulge in the wall and in 25% a second posterior bulge is also seen. More tortuous courses of the artery are more common with advancing years and inevitably associated with greater deformation of the wall by the vessel, which can project anteriorly up to 4 mm and posteriorly up to 7 mm. Similar deformations of the wall by the optic nerve are observed in 8–50% of cases [33, 155].

In 14%, a posterior ethmoid cell projects superiorly into the sphenoid sinus [33]. Cells of this kind may lead to incorrect assessment during attempted transethmoidal fenestration.

In view of the anatomic variability described and the delicate relationships with neighboring structures, adequate radiographic diagnosis (CT) must be completed before any procedure in the sphenoid sinus is attempted. Axial scans optimally demonstrate the relationship of sphenoid sinus surgery [102].

Polyps arising from on the sphenoid sinus mucosa are found in around half (19–74%) of all cases of chronic pansinusitis [258, 341, 957]. Sphenoidotomy forms an integral part of the therapeutic procedure in these cases. In view of the known inconsistencies between imaging and intraoperative findings, opening of the sphenoid sinus in chronic pansinusitis also has a diagnostic function. Other surgeons employ a more restricted indication for sphenoidotomy and regard sphenoid sinus procedures as justified in only one-third of cases in the same patient population [404, 632]. In the course of posterior-to-anterior ethmoid or skull base procedures, according to Wigand [996], even a nondiseased sphenoid sinus may be opened. This part of the procedure provides the operator with a view of the face of the sphenoid and the lateral wall of the sphenoid sinus as important landmarks for the further steps of the operation.

Comparatively rare indications for interventions in the sphenoid sinus are mucopyoceles, cerebrospinal fluid fistulas, fungal infections, the extraction of foreign bodies, biopsies and the excision of tumors, or decompression of the optic nerve.

Sphenoidotomy may be undertaken under optical guidance through the ethmoid after an anterior-to-posterior ethmoidectomy . For safety reasons, perforation of the median and inferior ethmoidal part of the anterior wall is carried out. The route along the lamina papyracea leads in the direction of the optic nerve and must be avoided. This dangerous craniolateral orientation often appears to be dictated by the configuration of the pyramidal sphenoethmoidal cells [9, 433, 860, 866].

Other rhinological surgeons prefer the transnasal approach and attempt first of all to probe the sphenoid ostium in the upper third of the anterior nasal wall. The bone here is relatively thin, and widening of the ostium is correspondingly easy [101]. If probing fails, perforation of the pars nasalis is undertaken by the paramedian and inferior approach [172, 874]. The bone becomes thicker in the vicinity of the choana [101]. Bearing in mind these conditions, a simple and safe paramedian perforation can be performed 10–12 mm above the choana [996] (Fig. 3.**5**).

The anatomy of the anterior wall of the sphenoid sinus is variable. The width of the ethmoidal portion and nasal portion and the thickness of the bone are subject to variations [357]. For these reasons, some surgeons decide their surgical approach on the basis of the local anatomy or CT findings. Large sphenoid sinuses can be approached relatively safely via a transethmoidal approach. Small sinuses are better opened transnasally [460]. A median opening via the rostrum of the sphenoid sinus should be necessary only in exceptional cases [776, 803]. Where the anatomic conditions are unclear, the fullest possible visualization of the nasal and ethmoidal portions of the anterior wall and transnasal fenestration is advisable. Neo-ostia should be made as large as possible. These considerations apply equally to adults and children.

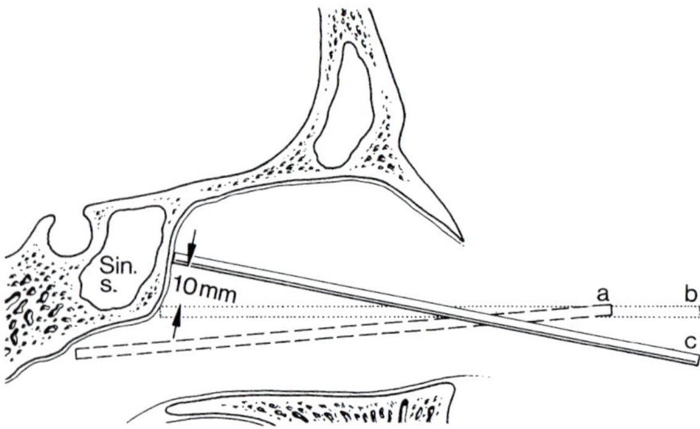

Fig. 3.5 **Fenestration of the anterior wall of the sphenoid sinus** by the method of Wigand [996]. Using a blunt instrument (e.g. straight suction tip) the anterior wall of the sphenoid sinus is palpated and identified from the direction of the nasopharynx (a-c). At 10 mm cranial to the choana, an opening is made by exertion of controlled pressure. Sin.s., sphenoid sinus

To assist with orientation in sphenoidotomy, Mosher [640] undertook a series of specific measurements as early as 1902. If an instrument is placed at an angle of 30° to the anterior floor of the nose, the anterior wall of the sphenoid sinus with the ostium should lie at a depth of 7 cm [196, 237, 750, 874]. These measurements are not without their problems [357]: the distance from the nasal aperture to the anterior wall and posterior wall of the sphenoid sinus gives partly overlapping series of measurements [93]. After accurate measurement, Lucente and Schoenfeld [518] report a value of 5.5 cm and an angle of 41° for the distance from the bony aperture to the sphenoid ostium. If there is a 10° deviation in the angle, the skull base is already threatened when the usual measurements are applied [580]. For this reason, reference to regional landmarks is preferable. The most reliable landmark in the posterior section of the main nasal cavity is the choana [175, 357]. To begin with, the surgeon must ensure good visibility, if necessary by means of partial removal of the ethmoid bone or septal correction [622]. Fracturing of the middle and superior turbinates laterally can be avoided in this way. The posterior attachment of the middle turbinate is divided. The punch can then be introduced into the sphenoethmoidal recess and the posterior ethmoid cautiously opened. Having thus created sufficient space, the sphenoid sinus can be opened safely 10 mm above the choana under optical guidance or using the headlight. This target can easily be identified by probing the anterior wall, approaching from the nasopharynx (Fig. 3.**5**). The sphenoidotomy is performed using a probe, closed forceps or a suction tip [996]. The blunt ended circumferential punch (Stammberger's "mushroom" punch) is ideal for enlarging the natural ostium. If greater force is required, the blunt end of the double-ended elevator may be useful. While applying pressure to the anterior wall of the sphenoid sinus, its slightly angled end is held in the direction of the nasal septum to control possible deviation at the septum. If there are problems of orientation, the diamond burr allows relatively risk-free opening of the sphenoid sinus [162, 163, 175]. Use of the operating technique described makes lateral radiographs for the purpose of intraoperative orientation superfluous [93]. After the opening of the sinus, the necessary manipulations may be carried out within the sphenoid sinus under direct vision using a microscope or endoscope. Manipulations in extensive lateral recesses require the use of endoscopes with adequate and appropriate viewing angles [507]. For mucoceles the procedure is terminated with a wide fenestration (marsupialization) [875, 908]. Endoscopic follow-up investigations show that the sphenoid sinus mucosa generally has a markedly better tendency to heal than the maxillary sinus mucosa [511].

The specific risk of transethmoidal sphenoid sinus fenestration lies particularly in the threat of damage to the optic nerve and the internal carotid artery. Bleeding from branches of the sphenopalatine artery (medial posterior nasal artery, nasal septal artery) can be troublesome. Hemostasis can be achieved with a bipolar coagulation forceps, though in rare cases use of a monopolar suction coagulator or diamond burr may be necessary [175, 996].

Revision Surgery in Chronic Sinusitis

Differences in the length and nature of follow-up, in the definitions of successful outcome and recurrent polyposis, in the distinction between outpatient and revision procedures, and in the indications for further surgery are reflected in the divergent figures given in the literature concerning revision surgery in chronic paranasal sinusitis.

Patients in need of revision surgery manifest a combination of systemic, mucosal, and anatomic problems [110]. Revisions are mostly considered one year after the initial operation [238, 490, 660]. In other cases, however, intervals of three (2–4) years are usual [660, 784, 884, 906]. The differences in surgical technique are of no significance in this connection [660]. The main reasons for revision surgery are unwanted scar formation, particularly between the turbinate and the lateral nasal wall, new flare-ups of sinusitis, and frontal sinus complaints. As would be expected, recurrent polyposis is seen generally in the area of the ethmoid sinuses, the preferred site for persistent or recurrent disease being the frontal recess [437, 474, 838, 913]. The maxillary sinus can also become the starting point for new symptoms despite adequate ventilation [241].

Before revision surgery is carried out, a further thorough attempt at conservative treatment should be made unless the findings indicate from the outset that this type of therapy will be of no avail. The recommendations are similar to those for first procedures, with 2–4 weeks of antibiotic treatment and short-term administration of systemic steroids [128]. The usual recommendations also apply with regard to preparatory treatment immediately prior to surgery (see pp. 12 and 15). Intensive postoperative care is of particular importance. Treatment of allergy, gastroesophageal reflux, and strict restraining from smoking should be included in the therapy concept [99].

Adequate diagnostic radiology (CT) is a prerequisite for the revision operation (see p. 12). The postoperative scans frequently show false positive findings as a result of scarring [420].

Sometimes the technical performance of revision surgery is relatively simple. In other cases, however, tricky and time-consuming manipulations may be necessary. Key points for the assessment of preoperative anatomy and intraoperative landmarks are listed below.

Anatomic aspects to be considered in revision surgery for chronic sinusitis [128]

- Extent and completeness of previous interventions
- Presence of remnants of the middle/superior turbinates
- Location and condition of anatomic approaches to the maxillary, sphenoid and frontal sinuses
- Location and condition of endangered anatomic structures (olfactory fossa, lamina papyracea, lateral wall of sphenoid sinus and optic nerve)

Landmarks for endonasal revision surgery [584]

- *Posterior lacrimal crest*: arch-shaped transition to a possible rudiment of the anterior middle turbinate
- *Anterior superior attachment of the middle turbinate*: medial limit of the operative field
- *Middle meatal antrostomy:* aids in locating the lamina papyracea.
- *Lamina papyracea:* lateral limit of the operative field
- *Nasal septum*
- *Arch of choana:* together with the nasal septum, aids in fenestration of the sphenoid sinus through the medial and inferior anterior wall

The actual technical procedure and instrumentation do not differ basically from those used in the initial operation. The plan of action should be definite [72]. For dissection in the posterior ethmoid, it is advisable first to locate the sphenoid sinus and then, after identifying further landmarks, to undertake dissection in a posterior-to-anterior direction. The fate of the middle turbinate will depend on its structure: polypoid degeneration can force the surgeon to reduce it radically. A remnant of the turbinate should be left as an important landmark.

The complication rates for revision procedures are the same overall as for initial operations. The percentage of complications does, however, rise significantly if the middle turbinate has already been removed [942].

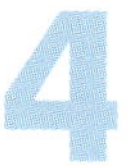 Results of Endonasal Sinus Surgery for Chronic Rhinosinusitis

It is difficult to compare the reported results of surgery for chronic rhinosinusitis for a number of reasons. These reviews include heterogeneous cohorts in terms of age, sex, etiology, extent, and site. It is not unusual for studies to include patients with different underlying diseases (e.g., asthma, allergy, aspirin intolerance, cystic fibrosis), whose influence on the outcome of surgery is not yet well enough understood. Furthermore, neither the operations described nor any previous surgery and its findings are standardized or comparable. The same applies to the techniques and planning of the respective follow-up studies. Widely varying percentages of patients participate in follow-up studies, and after several years the number is often reduced to half or less [841]. It is reportedly those with mild complaints or none at all who are lost to follow-up [839], though this is supposition.

Credit must be given to a number of authors who, often after many years of specialization, have demonstrated the efficacy of endonasal ethmoid surgery on the basis of their own personal case statistics. On the other hand, statistics arising from the routine work of different surgeons at a single teaching hospital, and thus based on different degrees of training and specialization, also merit special attention [959, 972].

The patients‘ individual symptoms respond differently to surgery. The longer the duration of the complaints, the poorer the subjective outcome of the operation [334]. There is no correlation between the extent of disease in the preoperative CT and the subjective improvement [276, 570], but probably a negative correlation exists with the chances of cure [433]. Thus, involvement of the sphenoid sinus, for example, is reported to be associated with less favorable chances of cure in diffuse rhinosinusitis [570]. However, it is not possible to predict the success of an operation on the basis of the extent of inflammation alone [503]. Diffuse, hyperplastic inflammation appears to have a poorer prognosis than simple polyposis. In the description of postoperative findings in which a frequently arbitrary distinction is made between mucosal hyperplasia and (recurrences of) polyps, it should be borne in mind that in general pathology a polyp is defined as “any excrescence of tissue that extends beyond the surface” [60]. Patients with aspirin intolerance also have a lower rate of subjective cure [341]. Other investigators have observed neither an effect of aspirin intolerance on subjective outcome nor any difference between polyposis and chronic rhinosinusitis [528]. In many cases the subjective assessments of the outcome of surgery by the patients are not in agreement with the postoperative endoscopic appearance [341, 436, 633, 784, 865]. They also often bear no relationship to the specific type of sinus inflammation [184] or the extent of surgery [433]. As the time since the operation increases, the subjective success of the operation gradually diminishes [784], although this experience is not shared by all surgeons [341]. Nevertheless, observations of this kind have led some authors to call for longer follow-up periods of about 3(–7) years [784, 829]. Whatever the case may be, there is certainly no point in evaluating outcome sooner than 6 months after the operation [575].

Subjective Results

Seen in the light of the current state of the art, it may come as a surprise that, according to the literature, surgery of the paranasal sinus system without optical aids produces highly respectable results in patients with chronic rhinosinusitis. In many cases surgery with a headlight reportedly had comparable subjective results to those of endoscopic surgery [230] (Table 4.**1**)

Subjective Results of Endoscopic Surgery and Improvement of Individual Symptoms

Larger reviews usually show success rates of over 80% for endoscopic sinus surgery [742, 913] (Table 4.**2**). However, more exact analyses add the following observations to these favorable figures. In one study, although up to 91% of patients described the operation as successful, fewer than 50% reported that they no longer had any symptoms [570]. In another study, 88% of the patients described their operations as successful, but 42% of these simultaneously required further sinus treatment [838].

The individual symptoms of patients with chronic rhinosinusitis show different responses to the surgical treatment. According to a number of studies, preoperative *nasal airway obstruction* is improved in about 90% of cases [341, 370, 633]. This percentage is based on various surgical procedures and, above all,

Table 4.1 Subjective results of sinus surgery without optical aids

Author(s)	No. of patients (age) No. of operations	Operation	Postoperative follow-up (y: years; mo: months)	Subjective results	Recurrences
Reusch [741]	275 patients	ethmoidectomy	?	84% cure	
Dixon [159]	125 patients (14–70 y)	total ethmoidectomy	3.5 y	94% completely satisfied 4% satisfied 2% not satisfied	27% recurrences
Friedman et al. [238]	50 patients	total ethmoidectomy	4 y 6 mo		8% recurrences
Eichel [195]	46 patients	mostly total ethmoidectomy	3.8 y	83% cure or improvement	
Stevens and Blair [884]	87 patients 230 operations	mostly total ethmoidectomy	11 y 6 mo	75% success	25% recurrences
Friedman and Katsantonis [239]	1178 operations	total ethmoidectomy	?		15% recurrences
Sogg [839]	146 patients 276 operations	various ethmoid operations	6–13 y	73% cure nonpolypoid rhinosinusitis 66% cure polypoid rhinosinusitis	16 % recurrences
Friedman and Katsantonis [241]	14 patients	total ethmoidectomy	?	?	29% recurrences
Lawson [485]	90 patients (21–81 y) 166 operations	total ethmoidectomy	3.5 y	73% success	

varying rates of concomitant surgery on the turbinates and septum such as partial resection of the middle turbinate [126]. In some cases, preoperative and postoperative evaluation by active anterior rhinomanometry reveals no difference despite a subjective improvement in nasal breathing [526]. A comparison of patients with fenestration of the inferior meatus alone and patients after ethmoidectomy suggests that the sensation of nasal obstruction can be triggered by pathological processes in the middle meatus and may consequently resolve after removal of this pathology, although the geometry of the nose remains essentially unchanged [528].

Headache and facial pain respond well to surgery. The percentages with improvement are about 80% (69–93%) [258, 335, 341, 370, 528], though headache often takes 3–6 weeks to resolve after sinus surgery [458]. Similarly, a sensation of pressure in the face has an excellent prognosis (over 90% improvement) [335].

A number of other complaints that patients report have received less attention in the literature. None the less, a positive effect on *sore throat*, *susceptibility to infections* or symptoms in the region of the eyes and ears, for example, has been observed in 70–80% of patients [996].

About 23% of patients with chronic rhinosinusitis suffer from an impaired *sense of smell* [865]. This symptom responds relatively well to sinus surgery and an improvement may be expected in about 75% of cases [152, 247, 335, 353, 370, 528, 805, 865, 992]. A deterioration in the sense of smell occurs in roughly 8% of patients; however, the majority of these patients were hyposmic prior to surgery. Anosmia occurs postoperatively for the first time in 1% [152, 353]. Significant improvement in olfaction is reported after various operations by different surgical schools. However, not all authors have obtained the same good results: in a few reports the success rate was only about 25% (17–41%) [32, 258, 633, 676].

To maintain the recovered sense of smell, postoperative administration of at least topical corticosteroids may become necessary [381]. This medication is not always effective [199] in the longer term and postoperative deterioration of the sense of smell has been attributed to synechiae, mucosal edema or recurrent/residual polyps [152]. The size of the remaining middle turbinate has no direct influence on postoperative olfaction in patients with chronic rhinosinusitis, whereas the postoperative accessibility of the olfactory groove does play a role. This is further

Table 4.2 Subjective results of sinus surgery with optical aids

Author(s)	Patients (P) Sides (S)	Operation	Postoperative follow-up	Results	Remarks
Kennedy and Zinreich [437]	95 (S)	endoscop. operation (extent?)	9 months	92% symptom-free or improved	
Schaefer et al. [782]	100 (P)	endoscop. operation (extent?)	5 months	83% improved 10% rec. chron rhinosinusitis 7% same	
Levine [503]	221 (P)	endoscop. operation (extent?)	17 months	88% success in polyposis 80% success in chron. rhinosinusitis	
Stammberger and Posawetz [865]	500 (P)	endoscop. operation (extent?)	8 months to 10 years	85% success 6% improved 4.2% slight improvement 4.6% no improvement (worse)	
Moriyama et al. [633]	62 (P), 102 (S)	endoscop. operation (extent?)	?	73% success	
Schaitkin et al. [784]	91 (P)	endoscop. operation (extent?)	36–52 months	91% improved	
Lund and Mackay [528]	650 (P)	endoscop. operation (extent?)	6 months	9% cure 87% improved 11% same 2% worse	
Kennedy [433]	120 (P)	endoscop. 108 sphen. 74 eth. 42 ant. eth.	18 months	85% marked improvement 12.5% slight improvement 2.5% same/worse	
Wigand [993]	84 (P)	endoscop. pansinus operation	12 months	83% symptom-free	
Gammert [258]	37 (P)	endoscop. pansinus operation	up to 5 years	65% symptom-free 19% improved 16% same	
Hosemann et al. [341] (Wigand [996])	220 (P)	endoscop. pansinus operation	4.3 years	48.6% cure 33.2% improved 12.3% same 5.9 % worse	
Weber et al. [972]	170 (N)	micro-endoscop. pansinus operation	20–120 months	89% symptom-free or improved Mixed classification:* Grade 1: 40% Grade 2: 52% Grade 3: 8%	15 different surgeons

[a] Abbreviations: endoscop.: endoscopic operation; extent?: operations of varying extents; same: no change in symptoms; rec.: recurrent; sphen.: total sphenoidectomy; eth.: total ethmoidectomy; ant. eth.: anterior ethmoidectomy;* classification acc. to [972]

supported by the observation that patients with a history of one or several polypectomies and associated scarring have a less favorable prognosis for recovery of olfaction [353]. The prognosis for patients with aspirin intolerance is also poorer [913].

In routine operations the olfactory groove is not usually directly affected. However, Yamagishi et al. [1011] carried out special manipulations in the olfactory groove under the guidance of an endoscope with a diameter of 1.5 mm. Impaired olfaction is reported to respond especially well to the removal of small polyps. Septoturbinal synechiae can be prevented by insertion of a silastic stent. However, the results after 6 months (subjective improvement of 70%, and 80% improvement in the olfactory test) are approximately the same as those reported by other authors.

Postnasal discharge carries a less satisfactory prognosis [21, 179, 526]. The percentage of patients with postoperative improvement reported in the literature fluctuates between 25% and 92% [258, 334, 335, 341, 370, 633, 838]. The very fact that this symptom is reported by 72% of the patients who do not feel better after undergoing sinus surgery speaks for itself [503]. The number of patients who complain of a runny nose is often only marginally influenced by further surgery [179]. About 14% of patients have strikingly thick nasal secretions postoperatively [660]. The persistence of such findings and complaints can be the outward manifestation of a permanent remodeling of the nasal mucosa, particularly with respect to the glands and mucociliary apparatus. This assumption is supported by the fact that postoperative improvement becomes increasingly less likely in patients with a long history of sinus disease [334], although transient improvement may be seen immediately after the operation [784, 919]. Immunological and allergy tests are usually negative [523, 660]. Long-term postoperative administration of erythromycin is reported to lead to an improvement in the findings [637].

Objective Results in Nasal Polyposis

The results of postoperative endoscopic follow-up of the operative site in patients with chronic rhinosinusitis are summarized in Table 4.**3**.

The postoperative endoscopic findings are normal in about 77% of patients after a circumscribed operation on the paranasal sinuses. However, after surgery for polypoid rhinosinusitis, complete cure is observed in only about 24% (see Figs. 4.**1**, 8.**1**). Moreover, postoperative stenoses of the maxillary ostium (7%) or frontal recess (27%) are also seen more frequently in these patients with advanced mucosal disease [433]. In larger series, a recurrence of polyposis in the ethmoid sinus is observed in about 20% [913]. In patients with aspirin intolerance this percentage increases to up to 50% [369]. The rate of recurrences is related to the preoperative extent (stage) of the disease [421]. Normal endoscopic findings for the mucosa of the maxillary sinus occur in 60% (56–72%) of cases after a pansinus operation. Usually extensive hyperplasia and cysts or less often fully fledged polyps are observed [341, 959]. If infected foci in the anterior ethmoid are treated surgically together with middle meatal antrostomy, spontaneous resolution of severe hyperplasia of the maxillary mucosa can be expected only in a minority of cases [384, 511]. The difficulties involved in postoperative imaging have already been discussed (see p. 12).

Despite the fact that patients often report a subjective improvement in their general condition, postoperative radiographic examinations frequently de-

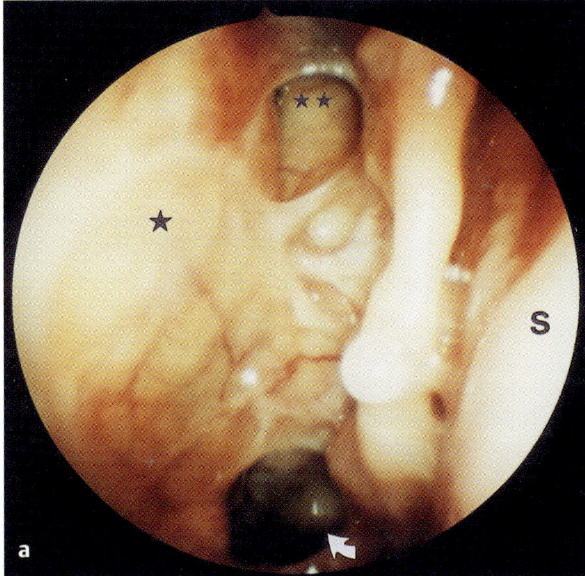

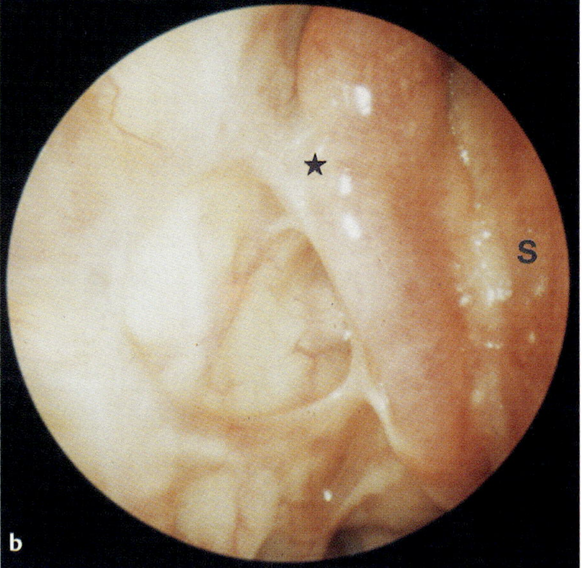

Fig. 4.**1a,b** **Endoscopic findings after a pansinus operation in chronic diffuse rhinosinusitis** (right side in both cases)
(**a**) Good healing within sphenoid sinus (arrow) and frontal sinus (★★) visible after four months. ★, lamina papyracea; S, nasal septum. (**b**) Poor healing: lateralization and scarring (★) of the vertical lamella of the middle turbinate narrows the access to the anterior frontal recess and frontal sinus

Table 4.3 Objective (endoscopic) results of sinus surgery in chronic rhinosinusitis

Author(s)	Patients (n)	Operation[a]	Postoperative follow-up (y: years; mo: months)	Results (endoscopy)
Bagatella and Mazzoni [30]	30	microscop. ethmoid-ectomy	3 y	86% normal mucosa 14% hyperplasia no recurrent polyps
Bagatella and Mazzoni [32]	155	microscop. ethmoid-ectomy	1–10 y	59% cure 22% small polyps 19% large polyps
Silverstein and McDaniel [829]	31	microscop. ethmoid-ectomy	2.4 y	90% no polyps
Amedee et al. [10]	325	microscop. ethmoid-ectomy	2 y	22.5% recurrent polyps
Teatini et al. [906]	78	microscop. ethmoid-ectomy	> 2 y	60% no polyps 25% medically treatable recurrent polyps 14% mucositis or recurrence with revision surgery
	22	microscop. ethmoid-ectomy	1 y	86% polyp-free 14% recurrences
Weber et al. [972]	170	microendoscop. ethmoidectomy	20–120 mo	ethmoid mucosa: 56% normal 19% hyperplasia 25% polyps
Kennedy [433]	120	endoscop. ethmoid-ectomy or partial operations	18 mo	44.9% signs of remaining areas of disease (22.7% of patients without polyposis, 42.3% of patients with poly-posis, 76.5% of pat. with dif-fuse polyposis)
Gammert [258]	37	endoscop. ethmoid-ectomy	up to 5 y	73% cure 11% small polyps 16% large polyps
Friedrich and Terrier [249]	22	endoscop. ethmoid-ectomy	20 mo	52% cure 32% small/few polyps 16% circumscribed polyposis
Hosemann et al. [341] (Wigand [996])	90	endoscop. ethmoid-ectomy	4.3 y	52% cure 30% hyperplasia 18% recurrent polyps
Jankowski et al. [384]	50	endoscop. ethmoid-ectomy	18 mo	ethmoid mucosa: 40% normal 38% local edema 11% asymptomatic recurrence 11% symptomatic recurrence

[a] Abbreviations: microscop./endoscop./microendosc.: microscopic/endoscopic/microendoscopic guided operation

monstrate some persistent opacification in the individual sinus systems. This applies to both the maxillary sinus and the frontal sinus. After circumscribed surgery on the ethmoid complex, persistent mucosal swelling in the adjoining frontal sinus is observed in about 8% of cases [230, 384, 931]. On the other hand, in a different patient series with diffuse rhinosinusitis, the frontal sinus still showed more or less marked opacification in 71% postoperatively, despite specific intraoperative drainage [358]. In up to 70% of cases residual ethmoid cells are found postoperatively even after "total" ethmoidectomy [384]. The postoperative radiological findings must be assessed individually for each patient in conjunction with the clinical and endoscopic findings. Repeated CT-scans should be performed only in "symptomatic" cases as a rule.

The analysis of the causes of recurrences of chronic rhinosinusitis is controversial. While various authors stress that painstaking removal of bony ridges and septa should not be undertaken intraoperatively [866], others attribute new inflammatory lesions in the mucosa to a failure to open the operative cavity sufficiently [474]. Incomplete healing of the mucosa of the maxillary sinus is attributed to missed disease in the anterior ethmoid, particularly after partial ethmoidectomy [842]. Conversely, purulent mucosal inflammation throughout the entire operative area after total ethmoidectomy may be the result of inadequate removal of disease from the maxillary sinus [906].

Recurrences are usually observed after one year, but may also be seen up to seven years after the operation [421, 829]. Fortunately, once mucosal normalization does occur, the majority of patients remain stable over several years [529] and, conversely, not every recurrence of polyposis requires revision surgery. Depending on the extent of the disease and the anatomic conditions, in up to 84% of cases the polyps can be successfully resected or cauterized on an outpatient basis [10] in addition to medical therapy, which usually provides the mainstay of treatment.

It has been demonstrated that the mucociliary apparatus can recover after ethmoid surgery, with postoperative measurements revealing an increase in ciliary beat frequency [526, 529].

Problems of Quality Assurance, Standardization, and Documentation of Results

Chronic inflammation of the paranasal sinuses can manifest itself in a number of different ways. Little is known to date about the natural history and pathogenesis of and the distinctions between the different forms of rhinosinusitis. Without a generally accepted method of classifying findings, surgical procedures, and outcomes, comparison of the different surgical approaches will continue to be difficult in the future. In view of these problems in the analysis of reported results, the development of a system for classification of surgical procedures, findings, and complaints is fundamentally desirable.

Several criteria should be met by a classification system. For clinical purposes it must be precise, clear, and simple. It must be clinically relevant and permit a reproducible assignment to categories. It should none the less be comprehensive and complete, i.e., the number of unclassifiable cases should be small. A staging system for CT findings should be such that it can be used by radiologists and ENT specialists. A number of currently discussed proposals for classification are presented in the following sections.

Classification of Preoperative Findings and Concomitant Factors

The classification systems presented here were devised for chronic and acute recurrent rhinosinusitis. Criteria for the clinical definition of chronic rhinosinusitis and important underlying diseases and concomitant factors of the patients are summarized in the overview listings below. Together with the patient's age, sex, and surgical history, they form the basis for a standardized analysis of the results.

Criteria for chronic rhinosinusitis (Lund et al. [530])

In adults

- Symptoms and findings persisting for eight weeks, or
- Four episodes of recurrent, acute rhinosinusitis annually, each lasting at least 10 days associated with
- Persistent CT changes four weeks after preparatory pharmacotherapy, with no intervening infection

In children

- Symptoms and findings persisting for 12 weeks or
- Six episodes of recurrent, acute chronic rhinosinusitis annually, each lasting at least 10 days associated with
- Persistent CT changes four weeks after preparatory pharmacotherapy with no intervening infection

Important underlying diseases and concomitant factors in patients with chronic and recurrent acute rhinosinusitis (after Lund et al. [530])

- Disturbed mucociliary clearance (e.g., primary ciliary dyskinesia, Young syndrome)
- Asthma
- Aspirin intolerance
- Cystic fibrosis
- Immune disorders
- Atopy
- Special forms of local inflammation (e.g., mycosis, allergic fungal chronic rhinosinusitis, Churg-Strauss syndrome)
- Diabetes mellitus
- Other severe underlying diseases (e.g., generalized or local tumors, specific inflammations)
- Others: nicotine abuse

A number of *radiological classification systems* for staging chronic rhinosinusitis on the basis of the preoperative CT have been published in the literature [115, 184, 230, 242, 274, 530, 659]. An example is given in the list below. The systems presented by Friedman et al. [242] and von Eichel [197] are similar. They were devised for CT scans performed after appropriate preparatory drug treatment and take into account the reversibility of the mucosal changes. Friedman et al. [242] describe a good correlation between the stage and the probability of a posttreatment recurrence. The classification system developed by Kennedy [433] differs only in minor points and combines the radiological findings with the intraoperative endoscopic findings. The radiological classifications are based on the assumption that the extent of chronic rhinosinusitis is currently the only prognostic parameter for the disease [433]. In these classifications, important clinical parameters such as aspirin intolerance can only be expressed in terms of an advanced disease stage.

Staging of chronic rhinosinusitis in the CT (Gliklich and Metson [274])

Stage 0: Normal findings (mucosa always less than 2 mm thick)
Stage 1: All unilateral disease and anatomic abnormalities
Stage 2: Bilateral disease, limited to the ethmoid or maxillary sinus
Stage 3: Bilateral disease, involvement of at least one sphenoid or frontal sinus
Stage 4: Pan-rhinosinusitis

A simple system of *classifying endoscopic findings* has been presented by Kennedy [433]. It distinguishes only between nonpolypoid disease, polyposis of the middle nasal meatus, and diffuse polyposis. More complex systems that distinguish between advanced forms of polyposis have been developed by Levine [503] and Lund et al. [530].

Gliklich and Metson [275] attempted to classify the patient's subjective well-being before and after surgical therapy. Questioning the patient about symptoms and the time course (duration of complaints and treatment during the previous eight weeks) proved to be superior to simply entering symptoms on a graduated scale. Lund et al. [530] have published a 0–10 visual analogue points system for symptoms. For surgery in children, Rosenfeld [759] employs a points system that combines the parents' evaluation with changes in general subjective well-being and improvement in cardinal symptoms.

Complex classification systems include radiological, endoscopic, and clinical findings. An example is given below. Although the authors find agreement between the staging and prognosis of the disease [784], the multiplicity of the parameters is likely to stand in the way of large-scale use of this classification. The same applies for other, similarly complex systems [262, 527, 575]. In systems with a simple structure, the parameters are extent of disease (circumscribed, diffuse), type of disease (infection, polyposis), and concurrent factors (asthma, no asthma) [485].

Classification of chronic rhinosinusitis (according to Schaitkin et al. [784])

I *Anatomic variations*

- Turbinoseptal deformity (determined by pre- or intraoperative endoscopy after decongestion):
  TS1: medial and lateral aspect of middle turbinate visible
  TS2: anterior attachment of middle turbinate partially obscured by septum
  TS3: anterior attachment of middle turbinate completely obscured by septum
  TS4: septum impacted into lateral nasal wall
- Narrowed ethmoid infundibulum associated with the following variations:
  Paradoxical middle turbinate
  Concha bullosa
  Lateralized uncinate process
  Bulla ethmoidalis
  Haller cell
  Agger nasi cell (narrow nasofrontal recess)
  Other or combinations of the above.

II *Hyperplastic disease of the mucosa* (endoscopy and/or CT) with thickening of the mucosa and retained secretions

III *Chronic purulent infection* (history, endoscopy, CT and intraoperative findings)

IV *Polyps*

Classification and Standardization of the Surgical Treatment

A fixed system of surgical procedures would be valuable for documentation, quality assurance, and comparative reporting of results, particularly after partial ethmoidectomies. However, there are basic problems involved in this kind of classification of endonasal interventions. It is the fundamental and express aim of functional endoscopic sinus surgery to reestablish ventilation and drainage of the paranasal sinuses using procedures that are individualized and tissue-preserving. This therapeutic principle is not compatible with the rigid stipulation of operative steps.

In principle, as "functional compartment surgery," operations that leave defined anatomic cavities in the ethmoid cell system would also permit classification of the individual surgical steps. These would apply to paranasal sinus surgery according to Wigand and microscope-assisted operations, rather than other procedures. The procedures listed below can be distinguished. Leaving aside the difficulties mentioned above, Lund et al. [530] presented a simple scoring system of 0 or 1 for the various surgical maneuvers.

Surgical procedures for clearing disease from the paranasal sinuses

A Infundibulotomy
B Anterior ethmoidectomy
  (a) with/without fenestration of the frontal sinus
  (b) with/without fenestration of the maxillary sinus
C Posterior ethmoidectomy
  (a) with/without surgery on the sphenoid sinus
D Total ethmoidectomy
  (a) with/without fenestration of the frontal sinus
  (b) with/without fenestration of the maxillary sinus
  (c) with/without surgery on the sphenoid sinus

From the anatomic and functional standpoints, anterior ethmoidectomy as classified above leaves a defined operative cavity, the anatomic limits of which are set by the vertical lamella of the middle turbinate, the lamina papyracea, the anterior cranial fossa and the basal lamella of the middle turbinate. Unfortunately, such definitions are not compatible with individual anatomy. In 14% of cases, for example, posterior ethmoid cells can lead to an anterior deflection of the basal lamella of the middle turbinate into the bulla. Entry into the bulla ethmoidalis could then, unwittingly, lead to entry into the to posterior ethmoid exploration [355].

For the methodological reasons mentioned above, a practicable system of classifying ethmoid operations across all the different schools of surgery is not currently feasible.

Classification of Outcome

In the *analysis of subjective outcome*, different authors distinguish different degrees of improvement in the findings, in addition to no change in well-being and usually also a group with increased complaints. Kennedy [433] gives three classes of subjective improvement in well-being: no improvement (less than 25%), slight improvement (25–50%), and marked improvement (over 50%). In the grading system presented by Schaitkin et al. [784], measures that may become necessary postoperatively to achieve the treatment objective are also taken into account in the overall assessment (see below).

In their *classification of endoscopic findings*, Uchida and Sugita [927] differentiate between normal wound healing and healing with increased inflammation, increased scarring, or both. In their comprehensive analysis, Lund and Mackay [527] give scores of 0 to 2 points for the presence or absence of polyps, secretion, edema and scars or adhesions, and crusting.

Grading of outcome after operations on the paranasal sinuses in chronic rhinosinusitis (Schaitkin et al. [784])

Postoperative symptoms (minimum follow-up period three years)

- I Symptom-free (best possible outcome)
- II Symptom-free after additional therapy (second-best outcome)
  - A Medical treatment
  - B Revision surgery
- III Improved (improvement in 3 major symptoms) without additional treatment
- IV Improved with additional treatment
  - A Medical treatment
  - B Revision surgery
- V Same or worse (no response to further treatment)
- VI Lost to follow-up

In 1992 and 1997 Weber and Draf [959, 972] presented a classification of results after operations on the paranasal sinuses that is based on a combination of the endoscopic and clinical findings. This objective/subjective grading was improved in 1995 [179] and is presented below.

Subjective/objective grading of outcome after operations on the paranasal sinuses (Draf et al. [179])

- Grade 1a: No complaints/symptoms, local findings normal
- Grade 1b: No complaints, local findings pathological
- Grade 2a: Mild complaints, local findings normal
- Grade 2b: Mild complaints, local findings pathological
- Grade 3a: Marked complaints, local findings normal
- Grade 3b: Marked complaints, local findings pathological

5 Results in Defined Patient Groups

Revision Surgery

Overall, a second procedure is necessary in around 10% (3–15%) of cases of chronic rhinosinusitis [72, 120, 241, 335, 341, 370, 490, 528, 838, 994, 996]. The percentage depends on the particular patient group with its specific risk factors, the length of follow-up, the willingness of the patient and surgeon, and finally on a differential definition of outpatient "tidy up" procedures compared with genuine revisions that may be performed on an outpatient basis [196]. In nasal polyposis combined with aspirin intolerance, a recurrence within three years must be expected in almost half of all cases [369]. In children the percentage requiring further surgery is 8% [490].

Up to one-third (6–49%) of patients have already undergone other procedures involving the paranasal sinuses before their referral to specialized departments [341, 433, 493, 503], although the number of prior Caldwell-Luc operations is currently declining.

The subjective outcome of revision procedures, with improvement in around 80%, does not differ essentially in some reports from that of initial operations [195, 335, 490]. In other investigations, results were comparatively less favorable, at 72% improvement in adults and 66% in children [493]. Special attention must be given to a subgroup of patients who still complained of headache postoperatively in spite of normal local findings. Patient in this specific group cannot necessarily be identified before the operation, but in one study were apparently mostly women [660]. With regard to a cure, the prognosis for the revision operation is reported to be less favorable [433, 784, 865].

Recurrences of diffuse, chronic hyperplastic rhinosinusitis present a special problem. The likelihood of recurrence depends on the particular underlying disease, and also on the length of the history of the illness and the age of the patient at onset. The prospect of a cure for young patients with this type of diffuse rhinosinusitis is poor [196] and patients with aspirin intolerance are particularly prone to recurrence [181, 196]. The same is reported also to be particularly true for asthmatics [196, 238, 240, 485] with up to 80% of patients undergoing revision surgery having asthma and 60% showing aspirin intolerance [196]. Other factors reported to be associated with recurrence are atopic dermatitis and inspissated secretions in the paranasal sinuses [181, 196].

Patients with Type I Allergy

A respiratory allergy in itself is obviously not an indication for surgery on the paranasal sinuses. However, allergy is more common in patients with rhinosinusitis and may predispose to its development by the adverse effect it has upon mucociliary clearance [777]. The best results are reportedly obtained in patients with anatomic obstructions and allergy who responded well preoperatively to antiallergic drug treatment [865].

An allergy has no effect on the subjective results of sinus surgery in patients with more extensive rhinosinusitis [341, 865]. Perennial allergy is, however, held responsible for a higher rate of postoperative adhesions. The rate of recurrence of polyposis is said to be higher in atopic individuals [382, 726, 818, 819, 839], although this view is not shared by all authors [433]. The effect of perioperative hyposensitization on relief of rhinosinusitis is controversial [837]. At all events, patients should be offered a combination of medical and surgical treatment [44].

Surgical clearance of the paranasal sinuses may have a favorable effect on an existing allergy. One in five allergic children with rhinosinusitis required no specific antiallergic treatment after appropriate surgery [695] and the percentage for adults has been reported to be as high as 40% [662, 784].

Patients with Bronchial Asthma

Around 30% of patients with bronchial asthma suffer from chronic rhinosinusitis [628, 725]. Conventional radiographic investigations reveal abnormal findings in the paranasal sinuses in up to one-half of asthmatics [53]. The percentage increases with the precision of diagnostic evaluation. Even in asthmatics with few or no nasal problems, CT scans of the paranasal sinuses show opacities in over two-thirds of cases [710].

On the other hand, a varying group (8–60%) of our patients with nasal polyposis have a hyperreactive bronchial system, even without clinically manifest bronchial asthma [170, 344, 378, 617]. Twenty percent of patients with nasal polyposis also suffer from bronchial asthma [181, 628]. In a selected patient population in specialized departments, the percentage can be even higher [433]. Patients with chronic polypoid rhinosinusitis generally suffer from nonallergic adult bronchial asthma [181]. In almost half of cases they show a positive skin test to perennial allergens, though a clinical correlate of this test is often absent [78, 378].

Rhinosinusitis in patients with asthma is often associated with relatively few symptoms and in almost half of cases no specific complaints are reported [834]. Nasal operations with a view to improving lung function are still frowned upon by our neighboring disciplines [798]. ENT treatment of patients with bronchial asthma is therefore undertaken primarily for the rhinological symptoms. The indication for surgical treatment and the operating procedures follow the recommendations already described.

Rhinological and Pneumonological Results of Surgery in Asthmatics

In discussing the results of treatment of asthmatics, a distinction must be drawn between children and adults, between patients with acute and chronic sinonasal infections, and between patients with purely extrinsic asthma and those with intrinsic or mixed forms. The following comments relate to adults with chronic rhinosinusitis and intrinsic or mixed bronchial asthma.

Overall assessments of the outcome of the operation by patients relate mainly to the effects on nasal symptoms. These subjective data on the success of surgery should be considered alongside the findings of endoscopy of the operative field. Changes in the pulmonary situation of the asthmatic patient following the operation require separate investigation. The rhinological outcome does not always match the pulmonary changes [78]. Precise analysis of the asthma symptoms themselves is time consuming and the use of differentiated lung function tests requires a prospective series of investigations with standardization of asthma treatment and repeated testing over a long postoperative period. In addition, the setting up of treatment control groups is methodologically impracticable.

Endoscopic follow-up investigations in asthmatic patients show no special features with regard to local findings. Asthma patients often suffer from advanced forms of chronic hyperplastic rhinosinusitis, so that the local curative prospects are often limited [433]. Whether bronchial asthma is also characteristic of patients with a poor healing tendency of the nasal mucosa is a controversial issue but seems rather doubtful [433, 485]. There is no constant relationship postoperatively between the appearance of the operative field and the pulmonary situation [344].

Assessments of changes in the lung function of asthmatic patients following sinus surgery are often based on statements concerning subjective findings, on the frequency of treatment by a chest specialist or on changes in the use of medication. However, there is only a limited degree of agreement between patients' subjective statements and the results of lung function tests [624]. Investigations of this type with systematic standardization of drug use and repeated investigation of lung function are rare, however. Recent reports in the literature are summarized in Tables 5.**1** and 5.**2**. Varying degrees of improvement in bronchial asthma following paranasal sinus clearance are seen in around 70% of patients [865]. Patients with a general hyperreactivity of the bronchi without manifest asthma also respond favorably. Reports indicate that between 25% and 100% of patients may show normalization of bronchial reactivity postoperatively [170, 344, 617].

A precise analysis and quantification of the effects of paranasal sinus surgery in asthmatic patients is complicated by difficulties in the standardization of treatment over a long period and by the additional nasal medication following surgery. It is impossible to form control groups for comparison with the surgical treatment. Classification of local findings and standardization of surgical treatment is not yet the norm. The nose and sinuses must be considered separately in asthmatic patients in some cases: the vast majority of asthmatic patients with chronic rhinosinusitis complain of nasal obstruction that may be secondary to inflammation and/or due to mechanical obstruction to air flow. Without doubt, restoration of the nasal air passage for asthmatic patients is of great importance. This is achieved in the context of sinus surgery, sometimes with adjunctive operative measures. The specific contribution of the operation on the paranasal sinus system is then difficult to determine in these patients. Procedures solely designed to restore breathing through the nose, such as septoplasty [671], turbinectomy [681] or polypectomy (Table 5.**1**), can produce respectable improvements in lung function; however, their effects are surpassed by combined clearance of inflammation in the nose and paranasal sinuses (Table 5.**1**). From the rhinological viewpoint, in asthmatic patients with chronic rhinosinusitis resistant to medical treatment, endonasal sinus surgery with restoration of nasal breathing is therefore indicated.

In some cases, paranasal sinus surgery may be associated with unfavorable changes in lung function. The figures in the literature vary widely [218]. In our own patient population we have observed a deterioration in lung function in 8% of cases on accurate lung function testing one year postoperatively [344]. However, on the basis of overall questioning of patients at various postoperative intervals, a considerably higher rate of 20% was obtained [341]. An annual

Table 5.**1.** Chronic rhinosinusitis and bronchial asthma: Effects of various paranasal sinus procedures on lung function

Author	Patients (age)	Procedure	Post-operative interval	Results	Comments
Brown et al. [78]	101 patients with ASA triad[a] (10–74 y)	Polypectomy[b]	12 mo	Clinically:[c] 32% better, 53% unchanged, 15% worse	60% nasal passages free postoperatively
Drake-Lee et al. [181]	58 patients (14–81 y)	Polypectomy	?	Clinically: 37% better, 60% unchanged, 3% worse	
Settipane et al. [818]	8 patients	Polypectomy	3 mo	Lung fuction unchanged	
Jäntti-Alanko et al. [387]	34 patients	Polypectomy	48 mo	Clinically: 59% better, 29% unchanged, 12% worse	
Juntunen et al. [400]	15 children (9 y)	Caldwell–Luc	97 mo	Clinically: 100% better	FEV_1 post-op.[d] average 80%
Werth [980]	22 patients	Caldwell–Luc	24 mo	Clinically: 100% better	Steroids "markedly reduced or discontinued." Emergency treatment less frequent.
English [207]	205 patients with ASA triad[a] (91% adults)	Caldwell–Luc[b]	6–156 mo	Lung function: 98% better, 2% unchanged, 0% worse	Steroids reduced in 84%
Slavin et al. [835]	33 patients (17–72 y)	Variable, ethmoidectomy	?	Clinically: 85% better	10/33 patients post-op. without steroids
Howland et al. [360]	44 patients	Variable[e] ethmoidectomy	12 mo	Clinically: 57% better, 38% unchanged, 5% worse	3/4 of patients: post.-op. reduction of drugs/ treatment

[a] ASA triad: asthma + chronic rhinosinusitis + aspirin intolerance.
[b] Additional endonasal procedures to the ethmoid.
[c] Clinically: clinical investigation (assessment based on questioning of patient, consumption of medication, admissions to hospital etc.).
[d] FEV_1: forced expiratory volume (1/s).
[e] Variable: various procedures, operating technique unclear. mo: months, y: years.

reduction in pulmonary performance must always be considered in the context of the natural history of bronchial asthma [928].

The success of an operation probably cannot be predicted on the basis of the various preoperative signs and symptoms of asthma [78]. The risk of an unfavorable course is thought to be higher in patients over 40 years of age, in patients with no respiratory allergy, and particularly in patients with aspirin intolerance or a history of several previous operations [514, 627, 790].

If the bronchial asthma deteriorates after paranasal sinus surgery, an accompanying recurrence of rhinosinusitis must be excluded. In some cases a relationship can be demonstrated between recurrent rhinosinusitis and worsening of asthma [207]. A relationship of this type is supported by the rough overall match between the frequency of recurrent polyps and postoperative deterioration of lung function values. Apart from deterioration of existing signs and symptoms, bronchial asthma may also develop after paranasal sinus surgery. In our patients, the onset of asthma was seen in 4% of cases 1–4 years after the operation [218]. Can this asthma be attributed to the operation? The natural history of the two diseases suggests that it cannot and has been best investigated for the ASA triad. In this condition, the clinical onset of asthma usually, but not always, precedes rhinosinusitis [699]. Around 60% of patients first suffer from asthma and then from rhinosinusitis. In 20% rhinosinusitis appears before asthma or both diseases are diagnosed at the same time [482, 485]. According to the literature, nasal polyps are diagnosed 2–13 years later than the asthma [181, 482]. In general it should be assumed that around 7% of patients with polyposis will develop asthma later in the course of

Table 5.**2.** Chronic rhinosinusitis and bronchial asthma: Effects of endonasal sinus surgery on lung function

Author	Patient (age)	Procedure	Post-operative interval	Results	Comments
Parsons and Phillips [695]	24 children	Partial endonasal ethmoidectomy	22 mo	Clinically: 88% better, 12% unchanged	Emergeny treatment reduced in 79% post-op.
Nishioka et al. [663]	20 patients (16–72 y)	Partial endonasal ethmoidectomy	12 mo	Clinically: 95% better	90% nasal obstruction preop.
Friedman et al. [238]	50 patients	Endonasal ethmoidectomy	6–36 mo	Clinically: 93% cortisone reduced	100% nasal obstruction preop.
Slavin et al. [836]	31 patients (21–71 y) 18/31 ASA triad	Endonasal ethmoidectomy	3–60 mo	Clinically: 66% better, 66% steroids discontinued, 19% recurrence of polyposis	
Mings et al. [624]	31 patients	Endonasal ethmoidectomy	2 y	Clinically: 65% better	100% nasal obstruction preop.; 38% recurrence of polyposis after 5 years
Hosemann et al. [341] (Wigand [886])	51 patients	Endonasal ethmoidectomy	4.3 y	Clinically: 18% cured, 39% better, 23% unchanged, 20% worse	
Hosemann et al. [344]	13 patients (27–75 y)	Endonasal ethmoidectomy	12 mo	Lung function/medication: 77% better, 15% unchanged, 8% worse	
v. Ilberg [369]	32 patients	Endonasal ethmoidectomy	36 mo	Clinically: 50% better	
Jankowski et al. [386]	30 patients	Endonasal ethmoidectomy	18 mo	Lung function/Clinically: 91% better, 9% unchanged	
Korchia et al. [464]	25 patients	Endonasal ethmoidectomy	1 y	Clinically: 66% unchanged, 29% better, 5% worse	Lung function 100% unchanged
Manning et al. [558]	14 children (3.5–13 y)	Endonasal ethmoidectomy	12 mo	Lung function 100% the same. Medication: 86% better, 14% unchanged	5/14 children discontinued steroids post-op.

For abbreviations/notes: See Table 5.1.

their disease [627]. If this rhinosinusitis underwent early surgical treatment, the postoperative occurrence of asthma would correspond to the natural course of the disease and bear no causal relationship to the operation. Nevertheless, in any case where bronchial asthma develops, the nose and paranasal sinuses should always be subjected to thorough investigation with regard to the recurrence of chronic rhinosinusitis.

Relationship between Upper and Lower Airways

The pathophysiology of the relationship between chronic rhinosinusitis and bronchial asthma is currently still insufficiently understood. Of particular importance is the sinobronchial reflex, which is thought to be activated by the stimulation of trigeminal nerve receptors in the nose and sinuses [422, 423, 667, 670, 671, 799]. Pharyngeal reflexes may also play a role [755]. A further factor in many cases is certainly mouth-breathing by an asthmatic patient with chronic rhinosinusitis. The nasal filtering and moisturizing function is lost and the bronchial mucosa is subject to an abnormal burden [826]. A third possible factor comprises bacterial, descending infection, activated inflammatory cells, or mediators in the form of postnasal drip in the rhinosinusitis patient [7, 54, 236, 373, 645]. Less common theories are the reabsorption of mediators from the inflamed sinuses with an effect on the bronchi via the bloodstream [53] or intensified β-adrenergic receptor blockade in the bronchial system in rhinosinusitis [827, 895].

A number of investigations may be employed in attempting to explain the sinobronchial pathophysiology. There are a number of references to the importance of nasal breathing for pulmonary physiology [670]. Covert aspiration of fluid from the nose or mouth into the tracheobronchial tree has been demonstrated in many cases [7, 368]. In others, however, no evidence of bronchial aspiration of sinus secretions was found [34]. Swabs taken from the upper airways or material obtained by aspiration of the trachea failed to show unambiguous evidence of direct bacterial invasion of the lower airways [54, 236]. The paranasal sinuses of the asthmatic patient often show no significant microbial colonization [53]. In a current series of animal studies, attention has nevertheless again been drawn to the importance of craniocaudal spread of pathogenetic factors in sinobronchial syndrome [373]. It is possible that mediators play a role in this process since they are to be found in high concentrations in nasal secretions of chronic rhinosinusitis [373, 888].

Patients with Aspirin Intolerance, "ASA Triad"

A high percentage of patients with the pulmonary form of aspirin intolerance and nasal polyposis also suffer from bronchial asthma, a condition known as the ASA triad or Samter syndrome. These patients represent around 7% of cases within the average population of patients with chronic rhinosinusitis. More than 80% of these patients with aspirin intolerance suffer from advanced, chronic hyperplastic rhinosinusitis [433].

Patients with aspirin intolerance are of particular importance since they suffer from a greatly increased rate of recurrent polyposis [181, 196] (see pp. 32, 35, 40). The high rate of recurrence may be mainly an expression of the advanced"stage" of the disease [433], but complete freedom from symptoms following surgical procedures cannot be expected in these patients [784]. Extensive surgical clearance is, however, more likely to be successful, at least for a time, than are limited procedures [590]. Because of the tendency to recurrence, intensive concomitant treatment or even adaptive desensitization should be considered (see p. 105).

Patients with Cystic Fibrosis

Life expectancy in patients with cystic fibrosis has risen in recent years from less than 10 years to an average of 28 years. Diagnosis of cystic fibrosis in older children and adults is also occasionally made [911, 988]. Conventional diagnosis is based on the sweat test, but DNA analysis may be necessary in individual cases [454].

Radiologically, these patients almost always show opacification of the paranasal sinuses, the frontal sinuses are generally not developed, and anatomic variations such as a concha bullosa are generally absent. Indeed, extensive pneumatization of the paranasal sinuses suggests that cystic fibrosis is not present [15, 541]. The stage of rhinosinusitis is usually advanced and around 50% suffer from nasal polyposis [15, 131, 642].

Although rhinosinusitis is not always associated with serious complaints, generally it considerably impairs the quality of life of these patients. In around one-third of the patients nasal obstruction and purulent rhinorrhea represent a serious health problem [131] even though inflammatory complications are comparatively rare.

Surgical intervention is indicated where nasal symptoms are persistent or infections are recurrent. Opacities on the radiographs alone do not represent an absolute indication for surgery [136, 137] and conservative treatment with steroids or antibiotics may help to gain time [642]. In patients awaiting a lung transplant, clearance of the paranasal sinuses as a reservoir of pseudomonas is regarded as important [141].

Simple polypectomy is only temporarily helpful, since symptomatic recurrence occurs after at most 18 months in 90% of cases [132, 182]. The main emphasis with regard to surgical treatment is now placed on endonasal procedures. Generally an anterior ethmoidectomy is performed in combination with endonasal fenestration of the maxillary sinus. The middle turbinate is shortened to facilitate postoperative irrigation of the maxillary sinus. Septoplasty is often undertaken for the same reason. Acceptance of the procedures is good. Subjectively, high rates of improvement are achieved [136, 137, 141, 664]. In the medium term, significant recurrence of polyposis can be expected in 40% of cases, and patients and their parents should be advised accordingly [132, 664]. However, CT changes will not disappear completely and episodes of rhinosinusitis requiring treatment are still to be expected [136]. A particular problem is presented by immunosuppressed patients following lung transplantation [528]. In general, however, suitably extensive operations can often achieve symptom-free intervals of several years [923]. Radical procedures are apparently associated with fewer recurrences [642]. A summary of the literature is shown in Table 5.**3**.

Adequate inpatient treatment must be given preoperatively to minimize the pulmonary risks of the anesthetic in children. Patients should be screened for

Table 5.**3.** Results of paranasal sinus surgery in chronic rhinosinusitis associated with cystic fibrosis

Author	Patient	Age	Procedure	Post-operative interval	Result	Comments
Crockett et al. [132]	40	8.4 y	(a) polypectomy (b) endonasal ethmoidectomy + Caldwell–Luc	4.3 y	(a) 9% recurrence (b) 5% recurrence	
Duplechain et al. [183]	14 y		Endoscopic partial ethmoidectomy	11,3 y	Fewer sick days, Secretion 75% better, URI 61% better	
Cuyler [136]	7	9 y	Endoscopic partial ethmoidectomy	2.9 y	100% improvement	2/7 revision after 2.5 and 3 years, resp.
Davis et al. [143]	6	6–22 y	Endoscopic marsupialization of mucoceles	3 mo	Nasal breathing improved, olfactory function better	
Jones et al. [395]	17	10 y	Ethmoidectomy	29 mo	Improved: nasal obstruction, secretion 100% of patients satisfied	Headache, cough, halitosis not improved, Hospital treatment postop. no less often
Lund and Mackay [528]	28	?	ESS	6 mo	54% better 46% unchanged	
Thaler et al. [911]	2	36, 39 y	ESS			Adults!
Davidson et al. [141]	37	?	ESS	?	"Majority" subjectively better	
Moss and King [643]	32	23 y (3–33)	ESS, antrostomy, Caldwell-Luc	12 mo	19% revisions	ESSAL
Nishioka et al. [664]	26	12 y	ESS	34 mo	Improvement in individual symptoms in 37–70%	Recurrent polyposis in 46%

Abbreviation: ESS: endoscopic sinus surgery of varying extent; conv. procedures: in particular transoral procedures; URI: upper respiratory tract infections; ESSAL: endoscopic surgery with serial antimicrobial lavage, see text.

secondary coagulatory disorders due to vitamin K deficiency [366]. Prophylactic oral administration of vitamin K on the day before the operation is recommended and perioperative antibiotic treatment (one day preoperatively, two days postoperatively) is advisable. In cystic fibrosis patients, *Pseudomonas aeruginosa*, *Staphylococcus aureus* or *Haemophilus influenzae* are frequently detected in the paranasal sinuses, requiring selection of appropriate antibiotics. Some authors also give prednisone systemically for 10–14 days preoperatively at a dose of 2 mg/kg [695].

The operation is generally carried out under general anesthesia, but operating times must be kept as short as possible for the sake of the lungs [141]. Nasal packing is often avoided or inserted only for one day [137, 141].

Postoperative treatment in children with cystic fibrosis is of particular importance. Usually recolonization of the operative field with Pseudomonas can be expected. Topical antibacterial treatment has been advocated by some authors [642, 643]. The sinuses are irrigated three times daily with antibiotic through an indwelling catheter in the maxillary sinus with 40 mg tobramycin added to the irrigating solution three times daily. The catheter is removed 10 days after the operation. During outpatient follow-up, further irrigations are performed every 2–4 weeks using temporary catheters. In acute episodes of infection, topical treatment is again intensified. This combination treatment (ESSAL: endoscopic surgery with serial antimicrobial lavage) appears to reduce the rate of recurrence of polyposis considerably. For irrigation, dental irrigators (Water Pik with attachment) are also recommended; 20 mg tobramycin is added to the last 50 mL of irrigating fluid. Recurrent polyps may be removed on a day-case basis, e.g., using shaver systems [140].

McArthur et al. [539] reported the case of a patient with Hurler-Scheie syndrome (mucopolysaccharidosis I, H/S) and massive nasal polyposis. Endonasal ethmoidectomy achieved a considerable improvement in the patient's general condition with little perioperative compromise.

Patients with Primary Ciliary Dyskinesia

Patients with confirmed primary ciliary dyskinesia are sometimes included in reports of the outcome of surgery in children [289].

Parsons and Greene [694] reported three children with primary ciliary dyskinesia diagnosed by bronchial biopsy. Limited surgery was performed in one child, the other two being treated more extensively with bilateral sphenoethmoidectomy with fenestration into the inferior meatus. There was considerable improvement in their health, with a reduction in the frequency of medical treatments. The follow-up period was around 30 months. In a series of 650 patients, 14 patients with primary ciliary dyskinesia derived a significant improvement or cure of 79% at 6 months compared with an overall improvement of 87% in the entire group [528]. However, this would not necessarily be borne out in the long term.

Endonasal Sinus Surgery in Children

Chronic inflammation of the paranasal sinuses in children is sometimes based on definable underlying diseases such as cystic fibrosis, primary ciliary dyskinesia, or immunodeficiency. After exhausting conservative management and depending on findings and complaints, surgical treatment is indicated in these cases. The indication for surgical treatment for an antrochoanal polyp is similarly undisputed.

Remaining cases of chronic or recurrent acute rhinosinusitis in children are subject to discussion.

Rhinosinusitis in children is not uncommon and the frequency of clinically silent opacification on the CT or MR scan is high (see p. 11). Childhood rhinosinusitis is generally self-limiting, with the incidence declining after the age of 7–8 years. Up to 95% of cases of chronic purulent rhinitis resolve spontaneously after this time [685, 718]. For this reason, extreme restráint should be exercised with regard to performing sinus surgery in children not suffering from polyposis, mucoceles, or complications of infection. Careful, long-term, and if necessary repeated conservative treatment based on microbiological investigations [536, 718] (see p. 12) is indicated. Even children with *immunodeficiency* should initially be treated medically (see p. 49). Accompanying allergy testing is also recommended, as well as the exclusion of enlarged adenoids, turbinate hypertrophy, or septal deviation [556]. Adenoidectomy and/or inferior turbinectomy alone may improve up to 80% of cases of rhinosinusitis [365, 535, 689, 759], although the pathogenetic importance of the size of the adenoids and the effects of adenoidectomy in individual cases are disputed [254, 535, 596].

Rosenfelt [759] proposes a stepped treatment plan for children with chronic rhinosinusitis. The first stage is antibiotic treatment for up to six weeks (cefuroxime, cefixime, amoxicillin and clavulanate, or clindamycin). Prophylaxis then continues for two months, with half the dose in the evening. If the adenoids are enlarged, adenoidectomy is performed. Only then is endoscopic sinus surgery discussed. Other authors propose similar systems of drug treatment [301, 492, 536]. The stepped treatment plan makes it clear that even in recurrent acute rhinosinusitis without polyposis in children, sinus surgery should only be considered on an individual basis.

A number of anatomic details must be borne in mind for procedures in children. Even in neonates, the uncinate process, hiatus semilunaris, and bulla ethmoidalis are already developed, so they can be used as landmarks. The relative position of these structures does not change with growth. The ethmoid cells are generally complete with regard to number and still show thickened intercellular septa. The width of the ethmoid bone increases linearly with age, having a mean anterior dimension of 4 mm up to the age of one year. At the age of around seven years there is increased pneumatization of the frontal sinus and the floor of the maxillary sinus reaches the middle of the inferior meatus. The inferior meatus abuts inferiorolaterally on cancellous bone. There may be tooth buds in the immediate vicinity, which may be damaged by fenestration of the maxillary sinus and irrigation via the inferior meatus. The biomechanics of the tissue is modified in children and structures are often fragile. Manipulations below the inferior turbinate may dis-

Table 5.4. Results of endonasal sinus surgery in children with chronic rhinosinusitis

Author	Patients (mean age)	Operation	Length of follow-up	Findings	Comments
Gross et al. [289]	54 children (3–15 y)	Partial endoscopic ethmoidectomy	3–13 mo	92% success	
Lusk and Muntz [536]	31 children (6.6 y)	Partial endoscopic ethmoidectomy	12 mo	71% cure, 23% improvement, 6% unchanged, 0% worse	7 children require more than 1 operation
Duplechain et al. [183]	32 children (3.8–16.9 y)	?	?	88% improvement	14 children with cystic fibrosis
Lazar et al. [492]	210 children (14 mo to 16 y)	Various endoscopic procedures	18 mo	79% success, 88% parents satisfied	8% revisions
Halton and Cannon [301]	58 children (4.5 y)	Partial endoscopic ethmoidectomy	7.4 mo	86% improvement, 7% no improvement	
Parsons and Phillips [695]	52 children (7.4 y)	Partial endoscopic ethmoidectomy	21.8 mo	83% parents satisfied, 5% dissatisied, 12% not sure	
Michel [612]	112 children (8.6 y)	Partial endoscopic ethmoidectomy Fenestration of maxillary sinus	48.6 mo	95.9% success	
Wolf et al. [1002]	124 children (12 y)	Partial endoscopic ethmoidectomy	?	41% complete success, 46% success, 13% failure	53 children with nasal polyposis, 4 immunodeficiency, 3 cystic fibrosis, 2 Kartagener's syndrome
Bolt et al. [66]	21 children with polyposis (13.5 y)	Partial endoscopic ethmoidectomy	27 mo	77% subjective success, 52% endoscopic cure	Revisions: endoscopic cure only in 36%
Stankiewicz [878]	77 children (1–18 years)	Various endoscopic procedures	42 mo	38% cure, 55% improvement, 7% no improvement or deterioration	Follow-up: 50% stenosis maxillary ostium; 30% granulation tissue or adhesions

place the turbinate body together with the uncinate process cranially and laterally, resulting in narrowing of the ethmoidal infundibulum. In children, the uncinate process is directly next to the orbit, a relationship that must be borne in mind during infundibulotomy or fenestration of the maxillary sinus via the middle meatus. Pneumatization of the paranasal sinuses is almost complete in children by the age of around 12–14 years.

There are certain differences between the execution of endoscopic procedures in children and in adults. Local anesthesia is unsuitable for children and the extent of the operation is limited as far as possible in children, the posterior ethmoid and sphenoid sinus being approached only in the event of serious lesions [492, 536]. Exploration of the frontal sinus recess is rarely indicated, and only after adequate visualization by CT. Septal surgery is rarely if ever indicated. It is essential to avoid fracture of the vertical lamella of the middle turbinate, which would result in more difficult aftercare when there is postoperative lateralization. For endoscopic procedures where space is limited, a suction-irrigation device should not be used and where the nasal passages are very narrow the 2.7-mm diameter endoscope is available. Nevertheless, in 27% of children dissection presents certain difficulties intraoperatively owing to the combination of limited space and diffuse bleeding [1002]. The operative field should preferably not be packed on completion of the procedure [289]. Some authors spray methylprednisolone onto the inferior turbinate and fill the operative cavity with ointment (antibiotic plus corticosteroid) [289, 492], but this is not recommended because of the risk of myelospherulosis

Topical aftercare in children is considerably more difficult. To prevent adhesions, silastic sheeting may be introduced between the lamina papyracea and the vertical lamella of the middle turbinate. This is fixed to the septum with a suture for 10 days to three weeks [183, 536]. Removal of the sheeting requires a further brief anesthetic. The majority of authors recommend a second anesthetic in any case for thorough cleaning of the operative area 2–3 weeks postoperatively [493]. Concomitant antiallergic treatment should also be given where appropriate.

Sinus surgery in children is successful in more than 85% of cases [183, 289, 759]. Headaches are a frequent symptom in children and improve in up to 96% [695, 1002]. Further assessment of the postoperative condition of the child is generally based on statements from the parents. Complete relief from all complaints and symptoms is rarely achieved [759]. As with adults, there is often a difference between the subjective assessment by the patient (or parents) and the endoscopic findings on follow-up [66]. Table 5.**4** gives a summary of the relevant literature. In general, a greater tendency to heal can be expected in children [612]. However, recurrences can occur shortly after the operation [923]. Windows in the inferior meatus close more quickly in children than in adults [524, 647]. Even in the middle meatus, stenosis of the ostium and formation of granulation tissue are observed relatively frequently [878].

There is essentially no minimum age limit for endonasal surgery [301], but concerns have been expressed that secondary effects may occur on the development of the facial skeleton. In animal studies, surgery during the growth phase resulted postoperatively in retarded growth of the bony structures. Similar changes also occur in individual cases in children without causing any appreciable changes in the external facial contours [544, 878, 929, 1001]. This is also supported by studies on children undergoing major sinonasal surgery for neoplasia without significant facial distortion. [531].

Fungal Rhinosinusitis

Fungal rhinosinusitis can be subdivided as shown in Table 5.**5**. Fungal rhinosinusitis is most often seen in the maxillary sinus, followed by the sphenoid, ethmoid, and frontal sinuses. CT scanning is sufficient for preoperative evaluation where there is no evidence of tissue invasion. In three-quarters of cases the diagnosis may be suspected from the preoperative CT scan and in around 50% hyperdense structures are demonstrated [835, 1025]. On MRI, these produce a reduced signal intensity that appears to be characteristic for mycetoma in T1 images and a very reduced intensity in T2 images. In fungal maxillary sinusitis, endoscopy may reveal pus, polyps, or amorphous material in the middle meatus, although sometimes findings are normal [147].

Depending on the extent of disease, the operation is performed endonasally by the technique described [525]. In maxillary fungal sinusitis, the fungal masses can usually be extracted without problems through wide fenestration in the middle meatus. The window can be extended caudally at the expense of the upper sections of the inferior turbinate, additional fenestration of the inferior meatus rarely being necessary [267]. With the use of curved grasping forceps and suction tips under the guidance of scopes with suitable viewing angles, additional transoral endoscopy of the maxillary sinus or a transoral approach can be avoided [855]. In all cases it is important to remove the fungal masses completely, to avoid recurrence. This also applies to root fillings displaced into the maxillary sinus, which can be the cause of fungal colonization [171 172a]. The tissue samples taken should be investigated for fungal invasion.

Fungal rhinosinusitis is generally caused by *Aspergillus fumigatus*, less often by mixed cultures or by *Cladosporium* or *Penicillium* [855], although many other species have been described such as the Dermataceous fungi (*Alternaria*, *Bipolaris* and *Curvularia*).

Wound healing after the appropriate procedures is reported by some to be better than average [433], while other authors report the contrary [453]. Local aftercare is as for bacterial rhinosinusitis with removal of bacterial crusts and scabs. Topical treatment with antifungal agents is generally unnecessary [41, 861]. Routine radiological follow-up is not required unless patients are symptomatic. Revision operations must be expected in around 13% of cases [855].

A special consideration is *allergic fungal rhinosinusitis*, which accounts for around 2–7% of cases of chronic rhinosinusitis. Mostly younger patients are affected [130, 206]. Clinically, two-thirds of cases show nasal polyposis and atopy with a positive skin test for fungal antigens, while laboratory tests show peripheral eosinophilia and elevated total IgE. There are increased levels of specific IgG and IgE antibodies to fungal antigens in the serum. One-third to one-half of patients suffer from bronchial asthma. Intranasally there is a viscid, greenish mucus full of eosinophils. In the mucus specimens, fungi can be detected directly or by means of culture (often *Aspergillus* or *Alternaria*, *Bipolaris* or *Curvularia*) though often microbiological testing may be inconclusive. The CT scan often shows lesions with bony destruction particularly in the area of the ethmoid septa and the medial wall of the maxillary sinus, and concomitant ophthalmological symptoms may occur. The diagnosis is confirmed by the characteristic histological triad of tissue eosinophilia, Charcot-Leyden crystals and noninvasive mycosis [118, 130, 206, 761, 947].

Treatment consists of total endonasal removal of the allergic mucin together with polyps and should be accompanied by systemic administration of steroids

[118]. The duration and dose for this treatment are still controversial. For example, 0.5 mg/kg prednisone per day may be prescribed for two weeks, followed by alternating administration every other day for 3–6 months. The dose is then tapered off. Others regard a shorter treatment period as sufficient. For more limited lesions, steroids alone are occasionally sufficient even without surgical intervention. In one such case report, 60 mg prednisone was given for two weeks. The surgical treatment is followed by topical therapy with a steroid spray or ointment and the usual aftercare with salt water irrigation, removal of crusts, etc. Systemic administration of antifungal agents is generally unnecessary. Occasionally amphotericin B is administered topically. Recurrences are reported to be common, so close postoperative monitoring is advisable [130, 206, 761] and may relate to residual fungal material in the frontal sinuses. Postoperative immunotherapy has been recommended additionally [219, 225]. Endonasal endoscopic surgery alone is not usually indicated for invasion fungal disease, although it may be used in combination with more radical procedures.

Table 5.5 Classification of Fungal Sinusitis

Noninvasive
Fungal ball (mycetoma)
Allergic fungal sinusitis
Invasive
Chronic
➤ immunocompetent
➤ immunocompromised Acute/fulminate
➤ immunocompromised
Sclerosing
Mycetoma

Other Special Cases

Particularly in younger patients with refractory rhinosinusitis, after careful exclusion of other factors, the possibility of immunodeficiency must be considered. This may be suspected in patients with frequent occurrence of rhinosinusitis, pharyngitis, and pneumonia, and other types of pyogenic infection. Sinus surgery has often already been performed but to no avail. In other cases, in spite of specialist diagnostic investigation, more or less continuous conservative treatment may have been necessary [717, 814]. The pattern of rhinosinusitis in the CT scan in patients with immunodeficiency does not differ from that seen in other patients [537].

A review of supplementary investigations in patients with chronic or chronic recurrent rhinosinusitis and suspected immunodeficiency is shown in the following summary. The possibilities for diagnosis of subtle immunodeficiencies are currently still limited, since standardized provocation tests can only be performed with a limited number of antigens. Specific diagnostic investigations are generally performed by the immunologist.

Supplementary investigations in rhinosinusitis patients with suspected immunodeficiency (After [717, 814])

Baseline investigations

- Allergy testing, test of delayed immune response
- Differential blood count
- Quantitative determination of serum immunoglobulins

Further investigations

- IgG subclasses; C3 and C4 complement, total hemolytic complement
- Granulocyte function test
- B and T lymphocyte populations
- Immune response to specific challenge (protein antigen, polysaccharides) (from the age of three years).

Immunological defects that manifest with rhinosinusitis as the chief complaint are usually based on a humoral immune defect. The most common is IgA deficiency [492, 717]. Other investigators found deficiencies of the IgG subclasses in one-third of patients, mostly with a deficiency of IgG3 [777].

The primary treatment for patients with confirmed immunological defects is drug therapy. If this is unsuccessful, depending on the complaints, findings, and symptoms, an endonasal procedure may be considered. Surgical treatment should always be supplemented by concomitant conservative therapy [717].

Antimicrobial treatment is given on the basis of susceptibility testing and in episodes of rhinosinusitis should be scheduled long-term over four weeks or longer. In some cases antibiotic prophylaxis, for example, with amoxicillin or trimethoprim and sulfamethoxazole, is advised during the winter months or even longer-term. In severe forms, depending on the diagnosis, the administration of intravenous immunoglobulins (400 mg/kg body weight, maintenance dose 200 mg/kg body weight every 3–4 weeks) is recommended.

The most favorable results of treatment are seen in children with transient immunological defects [211, 537, 717]. In general, a marked improvement in findings postoperatively is reported in around 60% (45–83%) of cases [537, 814]. Revision operations have a comparatively poorer prospect of success.

Immune deficiencies in malignant disease or AIDS can lead to particularly severe rhinosinusitis. If, after weighing up all the circumstances, surgical treatment appears unavoidable, the likelihood of being able to control the focus of disease by an endonasal procedure must be assessed in each individual case. In the case of fungal rhinosinusitis, tissue invasion must be expected and radical external procedures are indicated in the majority of cases. Endoscopy can, however, be of great service for frequent and regular postoperative wound care [987].

Churg-Strauss syndrome can present clinically as recurrent chronic rhinosinusitis. Further symptoms and findings include bronchial asthma, eosinophilia with values over 10% in the differential blood count, neuropathy, and pulmonary infiltrations. Foci of disease are characterized by eosinophilic infiltrates. Endonasal surgical treatment of rhinosinusitis forms part of a comprehensive treatment plan [924].

Varney et al. [939] reported endonasal sinus surgery in three patients with *yellow nail syndrome*. The cardinal symptoms are edema of the legs, yellow discoloration of the slowly growing nails and pleural effusions due to hypoplasia of the efferent lymphatics. A number of other complaints may be associated with yellow nail syndrome, including chronic rhinosinusitis. Spontaneous remission of findings can occur. In general, rhinosinusitis in yellow nail syndrome shows an inadequate response to drug treatment. In the three cases reported, sinus surgery led to lasting improvement in local symptoms, while in two of the cases improvement in the other aspects of the syndrome was also seen.

6 Extended Spectrum of Endoscopic Endonasal Surgery

Epistaxis

Many nasal surgeons routinely control bleeding within the nose by means of bipolar electrocoagulation with suitable long, slim forceps [162, 996]. The same surgical techniques can also be used to treat patients with “nosebleeds” as presenting symptom. In the case of profuse bleeding from the posterior nasal cavity, an endonasal procedure is indicated if anatomic anomalies, septal deviation, or the extent and frequency of the bleeding prevent effective treatment by nasal packing. Etiological factors such as coagulopathies must be excluded or treated appropriately.

The source of the bleeding in posterior epistaxis is usually in the region of the proximal branches of the sphenopalatine artery and the venous nasopharyngeal plexus. Topographically this is the region of the posterior middle meatus and the inferior meatus, including the floor of the nose, and the anterior wall of the sphenoid sinus and the nasal septum. The anterior middle turbinate and inferior aspect of the inferior turbinate are also recognized as sources of bleeding [561, 1009].

Severe bleeding hampers treatment by constantly soiling the tip of the endoscope. In such cases it may be advisable to use a microscope, suction-irrigation endoscope or simply a headlight. Cotton pledgets soaked in epinephrine are inserted temporarily to reduce bleeding and improve visibility [996] (see overviews in Chapter 3, pp. 17, 18).

The sphenopalatine artery may be readily located as it enters the lateral nasal wall underneath the horizontal attachment of the middle turbinate. Incision and elevation of the mucosa posteriorly from the posterior fontanelle should bring the vessel into view where it may be liga clipped and/or coagulated. [81, 317, 724, 823]. Endonasal, microscope-guided ligation of the ethmoid arteries was reported as early as 1958 [312]. Following ethmoidectomy, the arteries can be coagulated in their bony canals using a monopolar needle, but great care should exercised in the insertion of the needle to avoid any orbital damage. A septal deviation may also require correction in the presence of epistaxis and this can also be performed endoscopically. Following monopolar coagulation in the region of the posterior lateral nasal wall, patients may experience a temporary sensation of numbness in the palate as a result of damage to the greater palatine nerve.

The use of flexible endoscopes in the management of milder bleeding has been reported. In these cases hemostasis is performed, for example, by cauterizing with silver nitrate, application of hemostatic agents, or injecting lidocaine with epinephrine [67, 591, 722]. A general anesthetic is not necessary. Slightly more vigorous bleeding can be controlled with a suction coagulator using a 2.7-mm or 4-mm, 0° or 25/30° rigid endoscope. The suction tip may be bent slightly as required [561, 678, 1009].

Foreign Bodies

Endoscopic endonasal surgery permits accurate and atraumatic extraction of foreign bodies from the region of the paranasal sinuses on the basis of exact radiographic location. Thus, the technique is indicated, even in patients who are symptom-free, so as to avoid later development of inflammation, infection or rhinoliths.

The foreign body is located and then extracted, taking care to maintain or reestablish ventilation and drainage of the adjacent sinuses. The surgical steps employed are the same as those used in conventional ethmoid surgery. In individual cases, endoscopic location of a bullet may be guided by traces of blood or the track of tissue destruction.

The literature contains isolated reports of endonasal removal of air gun pellets, shell splinters, ectopic teeth, and fly larvae [26, 122, 167, 288, 626, 648, 958].

Endonasal Surgery of the Frontal Sinus

Endonasal opening of the frontal sinus has a long tradition. Operations through the medial floor of the frontal sinus were carried out by Schaeffer [783] as early as 1890 and reports were published in 1899 by Spiess [853], 1905 by Fletcher Ingals [222], 1906 by Halle [300] and 1907/1908 by Good [282, 283]. A wide variety of special instruments have been developed (Fig. 6.**1**); frontal sinus rasps by Good, or, more recently, Schaefer and Wigand; frontal sinus curettes by Schaefer, Wagener, and, more recently, Kuhn-Bolger; frontal sinus drills by Halle, Fletcher Ingals, Spiess, and Watson-Williams; and spacers by Good, Fletcher Ingals, or Rains).

Endonasal surgery of the frontal sinus is indicated when there is significant involvement of the frontal sinus in recurrent, suppurative, or polypoid rhinosinusitis and in cases with orbital complications originating in the frontal sinus. Further indications are mucopyocele of the frontal sinus, less often a small medially placed osteoma (963), duraplasty (Fig. 6.**2**) or for barotrauma. Where the frontonasal recess is involved in midfacial fractures, it may be combined with external approaches, reducing the number of incisions.

Repeated recurrences following appropriate endonasal treatment constitute a relative indication for endonasal frontal sinusotomy, while the procedure is contraindicated in mucopyoceles or osteomas that are located too far laterally or superiorly or in inflammatory osteolysis of the posterior wall of the frontal sinus. A combined endoscopic operation with a "limited external approach" may be employed in borderline cases [173, 178, 335, 994, 996]. Some authors combine an endonasal approach with postoperative frontal irrigation via external trephination [462, 1008]. The following discussion refers to the indication of uncomplicated chronic frontal sinusitis.

Involvement of the frontal sinus mucosa may be expected in roughly 30% of cases of diffuse chronic rhinosinusitis. In 10% of cases the frontal sinus is completely opacified (see p. 10) [606, 997]. Depending on the structure of the frontonasal recess in the individual patient, reactions of the frontal sinus mucosa are also observed in one-third of cases with circumscribed disease of the ostiomeatal complex [949]. In these different forms of frontal rhinosinusitis there is a lack of consensus regarding the indication for endoscopic frontal sinusotomy in each individual case.

Stammberger and Hawke [866] recommended avoidance of opening the frontal sinus if at all possible and limiting the interventions to reventilation of the frontonasal recess in anticipation that the mucosa of the frontal sinus would recover spontaneously. The frontonasal recess is often relatively narrowed by a large anterior ethmoidal cell which has pneumatized superiorly. Removal of this cell, in particular the medial and superior portion, is in many cases more than sufficient to optimize access to the frontal sinus. This has been referred to as "uncapping the egg" and avoids all forms of stenting and more aggressive surgery in this area [473, 474, 866]. Schaefer [779] and Toffel et al. [919] also perform fenestration of the frontal sinus only if the CT scan demonstrates significant mucosal reactions. Jacobs et al. [377] presented 40 patients who underwent endoscopic sinus surgery with conservative dissection within the frontal recess. Postoperative endoscopy 37–60 months (mean 48 months) after surgery revealed mucosal disease within the frontal recess in 97.5%, but only 7.5% were symptomatic. In children, surgery should be minimal and focused [898]. The smaller anatomy increases the inherent difficulties in avoiding iatrogenic stenosis of the nasofrontal outflow tract. Eliminating disease in the ostiomeatal complex often allows the frontal sinus to drain adequately [898]. Wigand [996] recommends routinely opening the frontal sinus as part of total ethmoidectomy.

Three factors determine the need for frontal sinus surgery in chronic rhinosinusitis:

1. Mild secondary involvement of the frontal sinus mucosa in disease of the anterior ethmoid is not an indication for fenestration of the frontal sinus. Significant disease foci require direct surgical treatment.
2. An anatomically narrow frontal sinus recess with a large superior nasal spine makes it difficult to create a sufficiently large and permanent opening. The anatomic situation can be evaluated in advance on the basis of the CT scan. If fenestration is likely to be difficult, either the indication should be reconsidered or an extended frontal sinus operation should be considered.
3. The patient must be prepared to undergo regular follow-up examinations and topical treatment.

Visualization of the anatomy of the frontal sinus in a CT scan is a general precondition for endonasal surgery of the frontal sinus. A high-resolution coronal and wide axial scan in width window is required and if necessary, three-dimensional reconstruction can also be carried out.

There are a number of significant variants of the frontal sinus recess [478, 935] that may play an important pathophysiological role but are not always discernible in the diseased ethmoid cell system and are therefore only rarely regarded as an indication for or as determining the choice of surgical procedure.

The anterior ethmoidal artery is one of the most important anatomic landmarks in endonasal surgery of the frontal sinus. It is located in the frontal plane of the anterior wall of the ethmoidal bulla, directly below or slightly below the base of the skull in a mu-

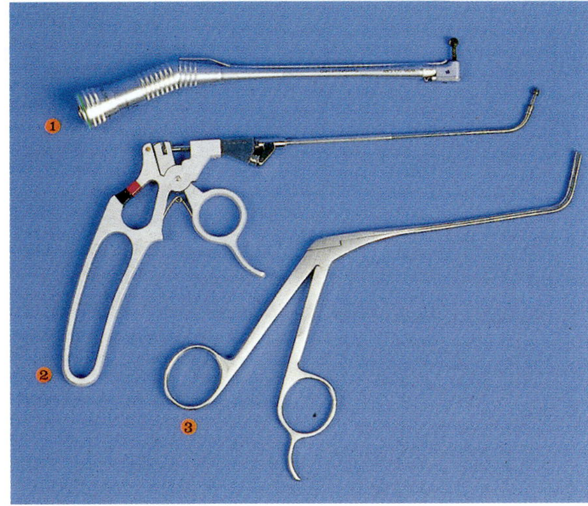

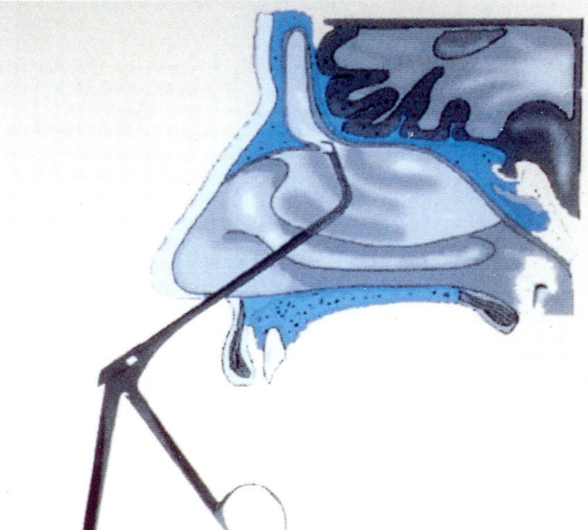

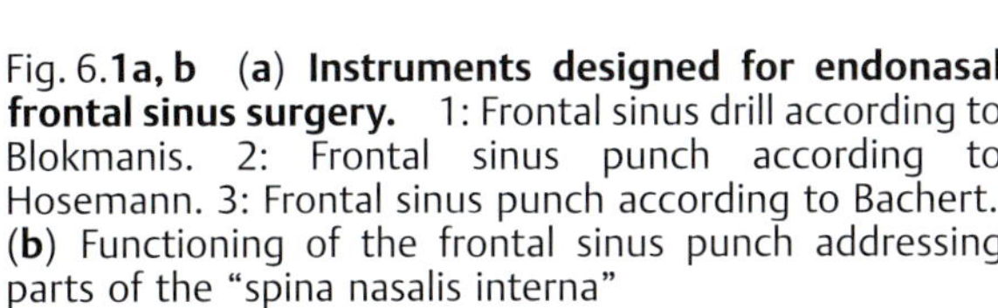

Fig. 6.**1a, b** (**a**) **Instruments designed for endonasal frontal sinus surgery.** 1: Frontal sinus drill according to Blokmanis. 2: Frontal sinus punch according to Hosemann. 3: Frontal sinus punch according to Bachert. (**b**) Functioning of the frontal sinus punch addressing parts of the "spina nasalis interna"

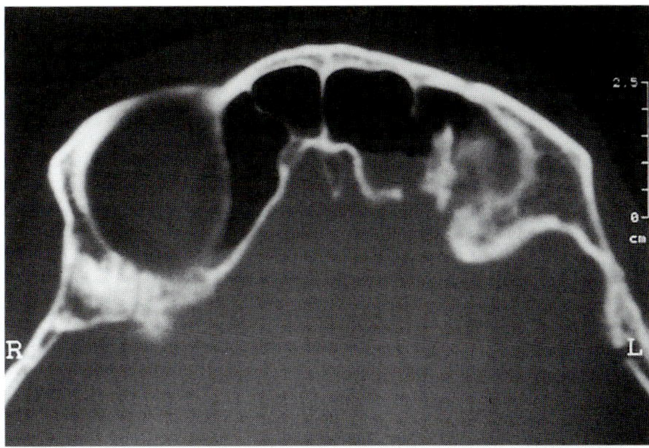

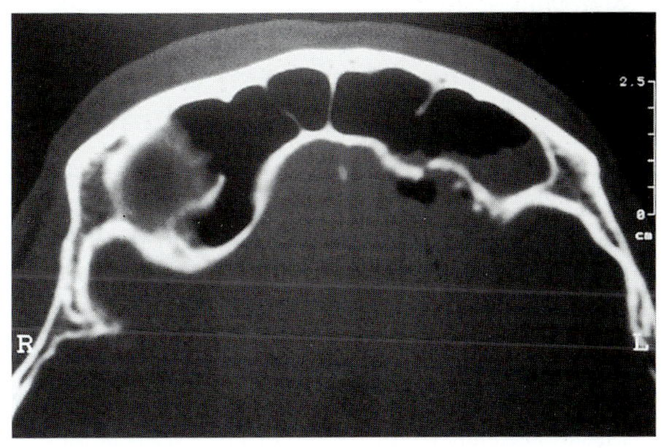

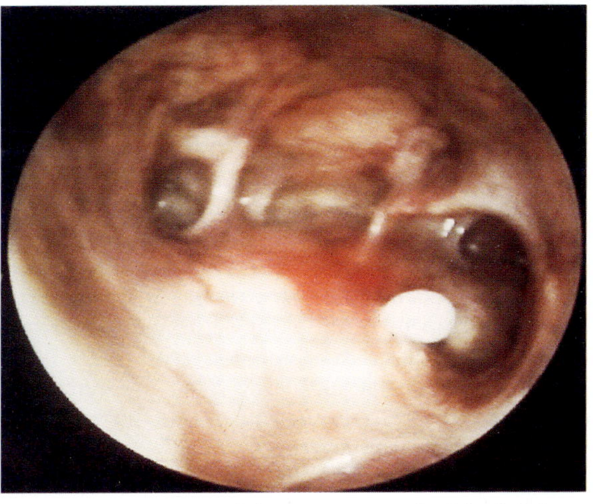

Fig. 6.**2a-c** Fracture of the posterior wall of the left frontal sinus with CSF-leak which could be repaired by an endonasal approach (negative fluorescein test six months postoperatively).(**a, b**) Axial CT preoperatively. (**c**) Endoscopic view six months postoperatively

cosal fold. In over 70% of cases it is possible to identify the artery with certainty [636], though this should obviously be done with care. The frontal recess is usually located anteriorly and medially [433, 996]. In the frontal sinus or frontal sinus recess, various forms of "frontal cell" can be found. Bent et al. [51] distinguish four types:

1. A cell above the agger nasi in the region of the frontonasal recess
2. A collection of cells in the region of the frontonasal recess above the agger nasi
3. A large cell projecting into the frontal sinus from the frontal recess in the form of a "bulla frontalis"
4. An isolated cell within the frontal sinus.

When the frontal sinus becomes diseased, the type of cell involved and whether these cells or the remaining frontal sinus compartments can be safely and adequately removed or drained endonasally must be decided on the basis of the preoperative CT scan and an exact intraoperative endoscopic examination [51, 729, 806]. In animal studies, the mucosa of the frontal sinus has been shown to be highly vulnerable and damage readily leads to the formation of prominent scar bands with impairment of mucociliary drainage [324]. Circular injuries to the mucosa led to complete occlusion of the frontal sinus access by scarring in 25 % of the patients [327]. These investigations must be taken into account when planning of operations of the frontal sinus access.

Endonasal Fenestration of the Frontal Sinus via the Natural Ostium

Operations on the frontal sinus recess are usually preceded by an anterior ethmoidectomy with removal of the agger nasi cells and visualization of the attachment of the middle turbinate medially, the lamina papyracea laterally, and the anterior skull base with the ethmoidal artery superiorly [750]. It may be necessary to reduce the middle turbinate [307], though other authors have recommended preservation of the ethmoidal bulla [516] or the agger nasi [636] or stated that middle turbinate resection does not result in a lower incidence of postoperative frontal recess disease [894]. Continuing the dissection strictly anteriorly, the base of the skull anterior to the anterior ethmoid artery is cautiously palpated with a curved curette. Cell septa are resected with preservation of the surrounding mucosa. Each step of the dissection must be conducted under endoscopic guidance. A 70° suction-irrigation endoscope is used by some surgeons for such procedures. The frontal infundibulum is frequently opened almost without resistance close to the attachment of the middle turbinate, 2–4 mm anterior to the anterior ethmoid artery. Finally, bony spicules of the superior nasal spine are removed, taking care to preserve the mucosa in the posterior part of the frontal sinus recess.

The aim is to create a frontal sinus neo-ostium with a diameter not less than 4 mm [747, 750, 838, 996]. Ostia with diameters up to 15 mm are technically possible [358, 781] but usually unnecessary. Special instruments such as curved curettes or rasps were used to effect the enlargement and as long ago as 1905 and 1933; Fletcher Ingals [222] and Watson-Williams [953] created openings measuring 5–7 mm using drills or rasps. Some authors attempt to keep the smaller neo-ostia patent by placing a catheter with a diameter of about 3.5–4 mm to serve as spacer that can be advanced into the frontal sinus through a curved suction tip or a guidewire and fixed to the septum caudally [362]. However, external incisions for insertion of silastic tubing [246] should be avoided. It is recommended that the spacers remain in situ for some weeks (3–8 weeks) [246, 306, 307, 362, 604, 706, 781] or 6 months [973], but it is better to avoid stenting wherever possible by not enlarging the frontal ostium circumferentially.

Where the anatomic conditions are unclear, it may be possible to perform the endonasal fenestration with the guidance of an endoscope advanced into the frontal sinus after performing trephination by Beck's procedure [173, 335, 996]. As early as 1907 Good [282] instructed his assistants to palpate the medial canthal ligament during manipulations in the frontal sinus access so as to be able to establish as soon as possible when the orbit had been reached. In 1899 Spiess [853] reported using an intraoperative plain radiograph of the lateral skull as an aid to orientation, a measure that is still recommended today [576, 604]. The use of these latter strategies remains reserved for unusual circumstances. Alternatively, irrigation of the frontal sinus may be performed using the Cloue Lemoyne technique as described by Klossek and others [462].

Despite recent developments in the field, the length, curvature, and caliber of the instruments impose more or less strict limitations on manipulations in the frontal sinus [636] and more extensive endoscopic frontal sinus surgery is not currently possible [993].

Table 6.**1** summarizes results on endonasal surgery of the frontal sinus. It is difficult to ask patients about the specific subjective outcome of an operation since in chronic rhinosinusitis frontal sinus surgery is usually only one of a number of procedures conducted to remove disease from several sinuses. The endoscopic follow-up examination is therefore of major importance. After frontal sinusotomy, closure of the neo-ostium due to scarring is to be expected in all cases. The diameter of the neo-ostium decreases on the average from 5.6 mm to 3.5 mm during the first few months after the operation. A further reduction after several months may be found in the case of further local inflammation, and cases in which the intraoperative diameter is less than 5 mm are especially vulnerable [347, 358, 604].

If the frontal sinus is opened intraoperatively, in about one-third of cases passage of a probe will not be possible after healing [341]. This percentage can be reduced to 19% by performing intensive intraoperative dissection at the frontal sinus ostium. Postoperatively, access to the frontal sinus is frequently achieved through a scarred stenosis of the nasofrontal recess distant from the neo-ostium. As a prophylactic measure, the vertical lamella of the middle turbinate should be preserved and not fractured, though reduction of an anterior wedge of the middle turbinate may be helpful [358].

After frontal sinus fenestration, postoperative CT scans show residual or new areas of opacification in 71% of cases. These foci can persist even if the ostium of the frontal sinus is patent, particularly in patients with aspirin intolerance. Conversely, some of the frontal sinuses that cannot be probed postoperatively are

Table 6.1 Outcome of endonasal frontal sinus operations via the natural access

Author(s)	No. of frontal sinuses	Surgical technique	Post-operative interval	Results	Additional remarks
Friedrich [247]	7	Endoscopic enlargement of natural ostium	13 mo	7/7 frontal sinuses normal	Silastic stenting of the nasofrontal recess through small external opening
Perko [706]	7	Endoscopic enlargement of natural ostium	11 mo	6/7 patients symptom-free 7/7 ostia patent	Isolated cases of frontal rhinosinusitis
Schaefer and Close [781]	36	Endoscopic enlargement of natural ostium	16 mo	58% symptom free 31% one recurrence of rhinosinusitis 3% unchanged 8% worse	Placement of silastic tube in ostia of less than 6 mm
Wigand and Hosemann [997]	162	Endoscopic enlargement of natural ostium, using diamond burr in some cases	3.5 y	40% ostia patent by endoscopy 28% ostia patent by probing 32% ostia closed by probing	
Metson [606]	7	Endoscopic enlargement of natural ostium	19–24 mo	6/7 ostia remained patent 1/7 ostia stenosed	
Moriyama et al. [636]	105	Endoscopic enlargement of natural ostium	6–42 mo	73.4% ostia widely patent 17.1% ostia narrowed 9.5% ostia occluded by polyps/granulation tissue	No bony occlusion of ostium observed
Otori et al. 1996 [684]	172	Endoscopic enlargement of natural ostium	> 1 y	Patent rate of 90.1%	Significan lower rates of patency in cases with preoperative severe lesion of frontal sinus and with small ostium
Draf et al. [179]	72 (471)	Endoscopic visualization of frontal sinus ostium (Draf type I)	5 y	Mucosa: 55.6% normal 11.1% polyps 33.3% "pathological"	
Hosemann et al. [358]	201	Endoscopic enlargement of natural ostium	13 mo	81% ostia patent by probing 71% frontal sinuses opacified postoperatively	Ostia < 5 mm have poorer prognosis

shown to be ventilated in the follow-up CT scans. In neither case is there a clear correlation with local symptoms. Even patients whose frontal sinuses are completely opacified and cannot be probed postoperatively are often free of complaints [307, 358, 384]. These latter cases must none the less be classed as potential failures and require careful follow-up.

After limited procedures in the region of the ostiomeatal complex, postoperative inflammation of the frontal sinus may be expected to occur as a side effect in about 1.5% [606] or 10% [229] of patients.

Table 6.2 summarizes current indications for endonasal fenestration of the frontal sinus via the natural ostium [358].

Extended Endoscopic Frontal Sinus Surgery, Median Drainage According to Draf

Draf has systematically extended the surgical approach to the frontal sinus and distinguishes three types of endonasal frontal sinus surgery [174, 179, 966] (Fig. 6.3, Table 6.3).

➤ *Type I: Simple drainage.* Simple drainage is established by conventional ethmoidectomy after removing cell septa in the region of the frontal recess, [478]. The superior part of the frontal ostium and its mucosa remain untouched (see p. 54). This ap-

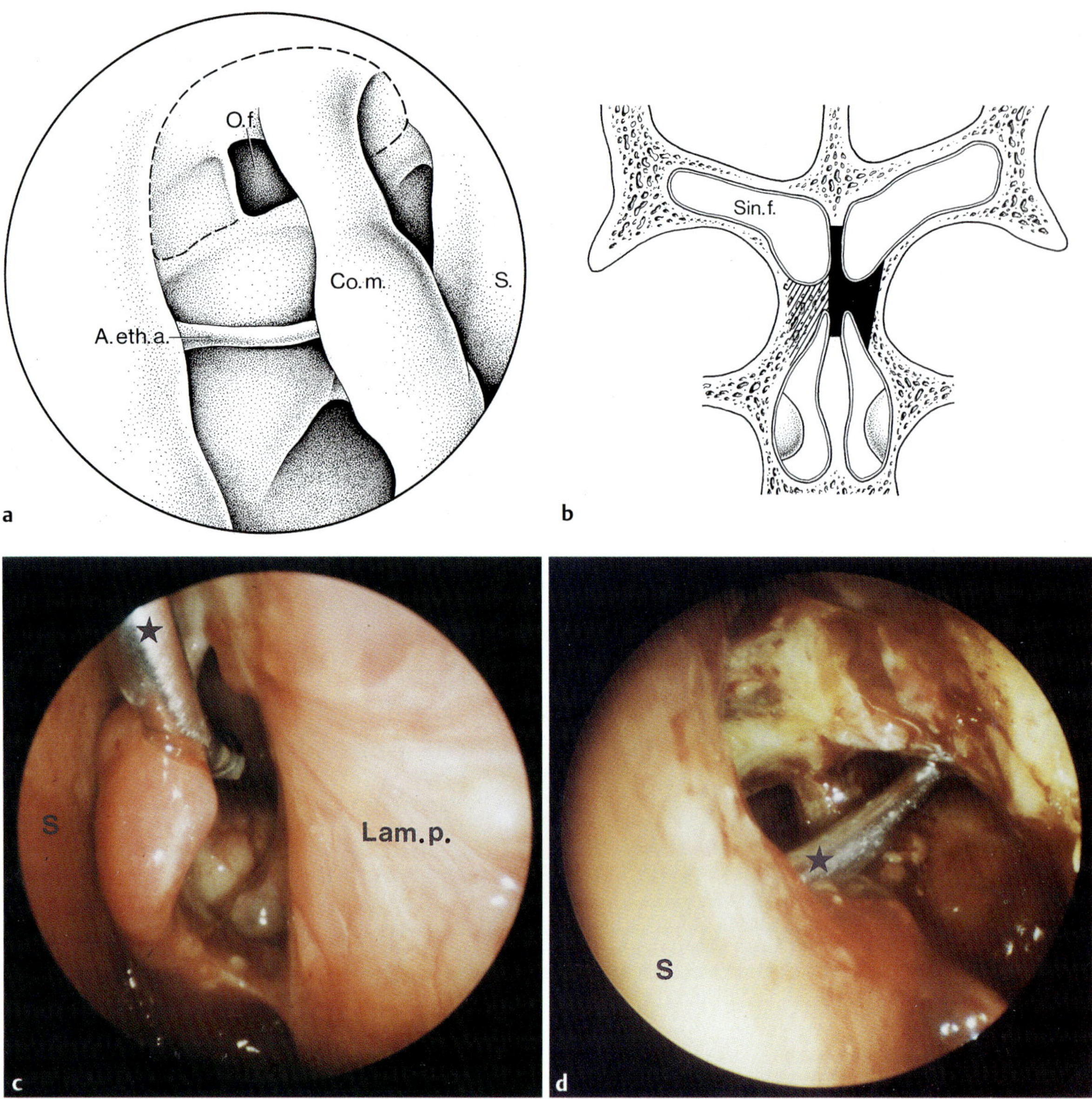

Fig. 6.**3a-d** **Simple and extended endonasal frontal sinus surgery**
(**a**) Endoscopic view of the right frontal sinus ostium after clearance of the anterior ethmoid with visualization of the base of skull and anterior ethmoidal artery (A.eth.a.). Simple drainage of the frontal sinus ostium (Draf I) is established by removing the inferior portion of the frontonasal recess. The frontal ostium (O.f) and its mucosa are preserved. Broken line: Enlarged frontal sinus ostium (Draf II). Type III cannot be represented in this diagram. Co.m., middle turbinate, S, nasal septum. (**b**) Frontal section through the skull showing extended endonasal frontal sinus surgery. Cross-hatched area, enlargement of the frontal sinus ostium as described by Draf (II). Area shaded black, additional enlargement according to Draf (III). Sin. f.: Frontal sinus. (**c**) Endoscopy three months after endonasal fenestration of the frontal sinus according to Draf (type II) in chronic frontal sinusitis: view of the left frontal sinus with a 70° endoscope. The window extended as far as the ipsilateral nasal septum. ★, curved maxillary sinus suction tip. Lam.p., lamina papyracea. (**d**) Endoscopy three days after endonasal fenestration of the frontal sinus as reported by Draf (type III) in chronic frontal sinusitis: view of the left frontal sinus with a 70° endoscope. A suction cannula (★) is passed into the left frontal sinus through the right nasal cavity. The septum of the frontal sinus is partially resected. S, nasal septum

Funktionelle Endoskopische Nasennebenhöhlenchirurgie

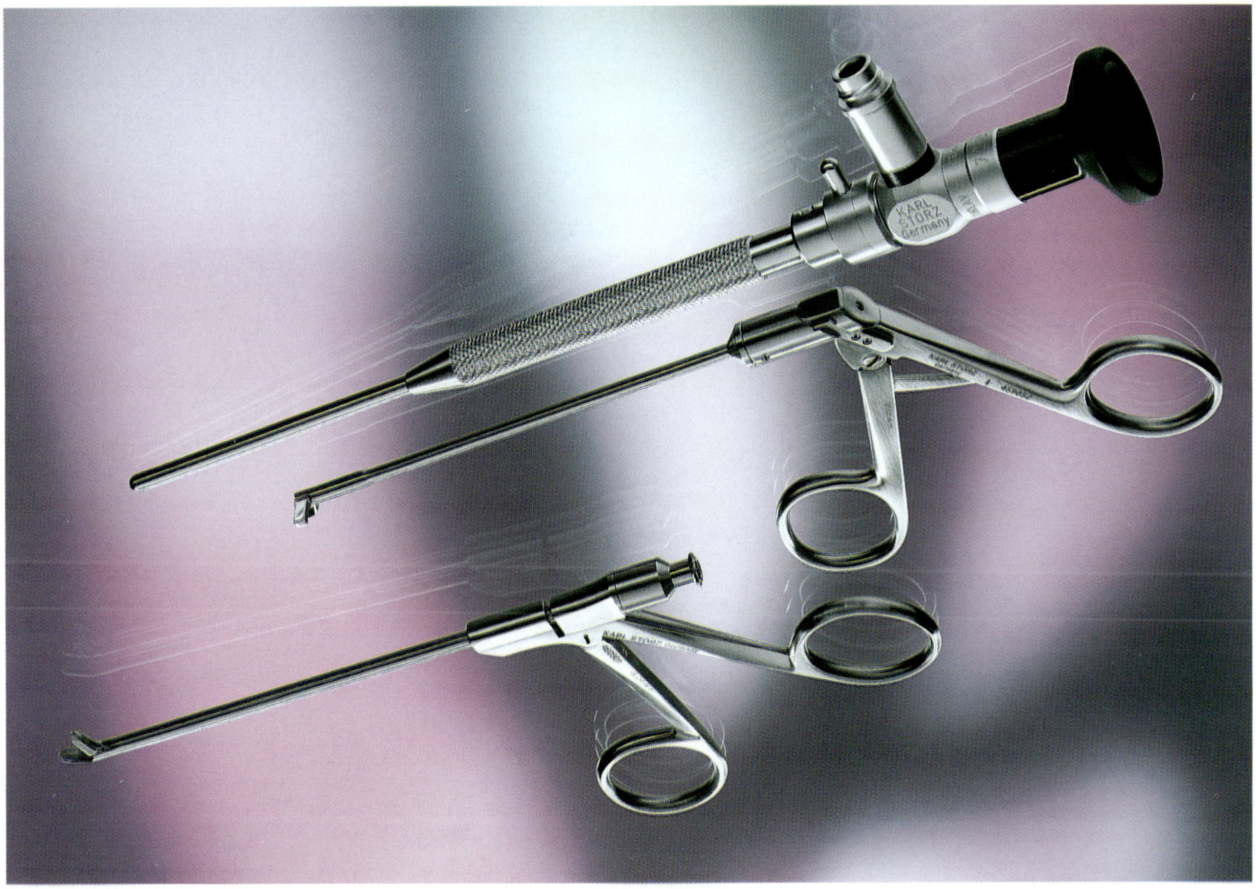

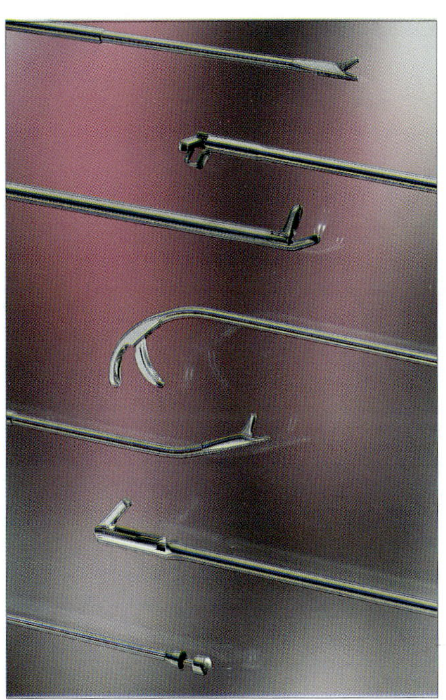

Als präzise und sichere Technik für chirurgische Eingriffe in den Nasennebenhöhlen hat die Funktionelle Endoskopische Nasennebenhöhlenchirurgie weltweite Anerkennung gefunden.
Die ersten speziell für diese Technik entwickelten Instrumente wurden von KARL STORZ gefertigt und KARL STORZ ist auch heute noch die erste Wahl, wenn es um Instrumente für die FEN geht. Denn in Verbindung mit dem glasklaren Bild einer HOPKINS®-Optik ermöglichen die in Zusammenarbeit mit namhaften Praktikern entwickelten, schlanken und ergonomisch ausgewogenen Instrumente ein unerreicht präzises und atraumatisches Vorgehen.

KARL STORZ GmbH & Co.
Mittelstraße 8, D-78532 Tuttlingen/Germany
Postfach 230, D-78503 Tuttlingen/Germany
Telefon: +49/74 61/708-0
Telefax: +49/74 61/708-105

KARL STORZ Endoskop Austria GmbH
Landstraßer-Hauptstraße 146/11/18
A-1030 Wien, Austria
Telefon: +43/1/715 60 470
Telefax: +43/1/715 60 479

E-mail: karlstorz-marketing@karlstorz.de
Internet: http://www.karlstorz.de
http://www.karlstorz.com

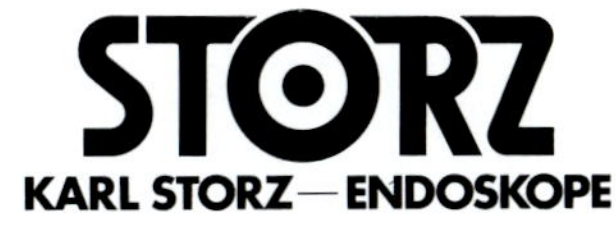

THE DIAMOND STANDARD

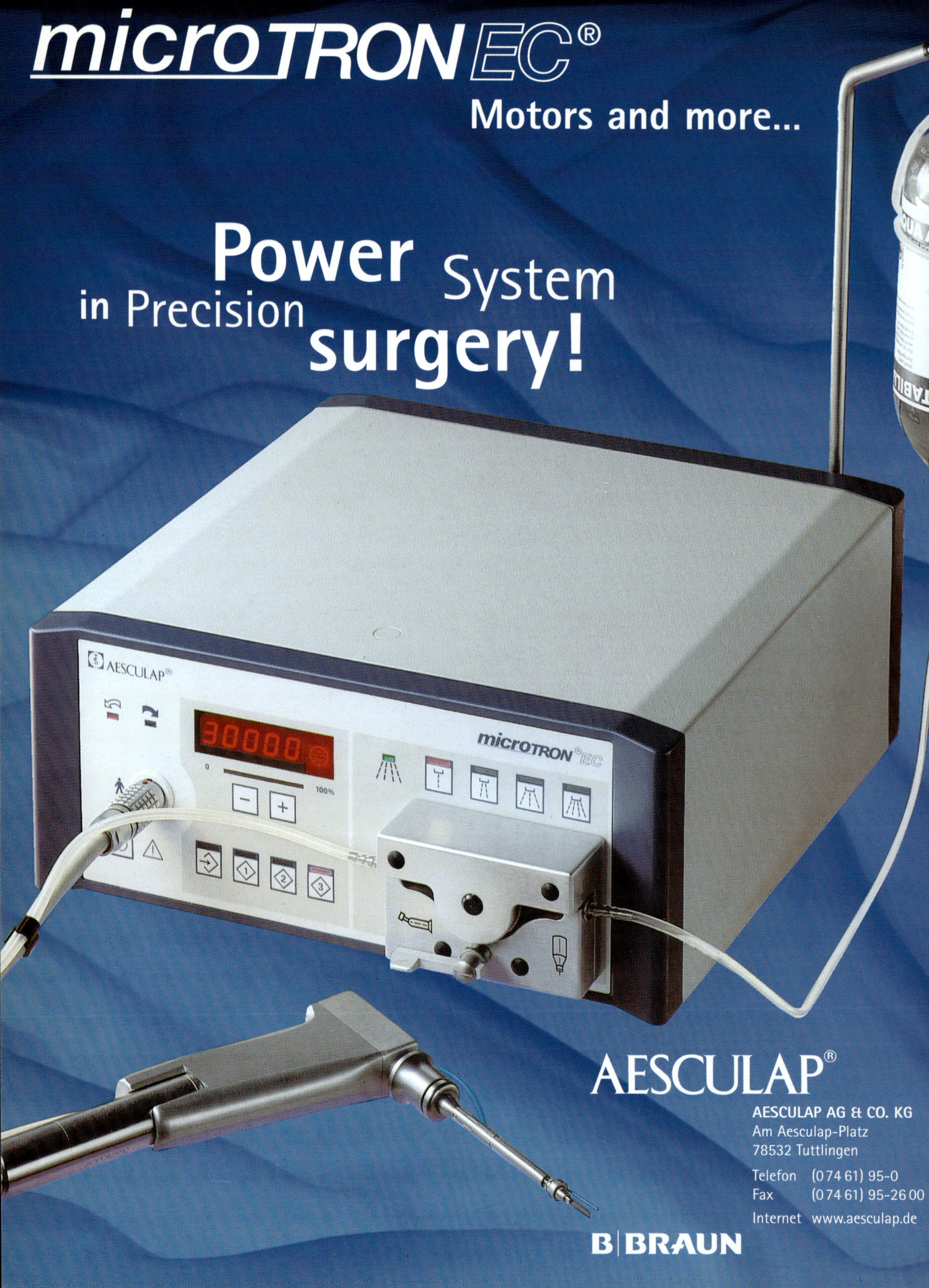

microTRON EC®
Motors and more...
Power System
in Precision surgery!
AESCULAP®
30000
microTRON® EC
100%
AESCULAP®
AESCULAP AG & CO. KG
Am Aesculap-Platz
78532 Tuttlingen
Telefon (0 74 61) 95-0
Fax (0 74 61) 95-26 00
Internet www.aesculap.de
B|BRAUN

Table 6.**2** Guidelines for establishing the indication for endonasal fenestration of the frontal sinus via the natural ostium in the surgical management of uncomlicated chronic mucositis

	Endonasal frontal sinusotomy indicated	**Confine surgery to frontal recess; CT control if possible**
Frontal sinus mucosa (CT)	Severe mucositis, polyps, fluid level	Minimal mucosal transformation
Spina nasalis interna (CT)	Hypoplastic	Hyperplastic
A.-p. diameter of the inferior frontal sinus (CT)	Large	Small
Anterior ethmoid	Broad	Narrow
Anticipated minimum diameter of the frontal sinus neo-ostium	5 mm or more	Below 5 mm
Local aftercare	Possible	Uncertain

proach is indicated when there is only slight involvement of the frontal sinus mucosa in chronic rhinosinusitis.

- *Type II: Extended drainage.* Extended drainage is achieved by resecting the floor of the frontal sinus medially from the natural ostium to the nasal septum. A neo-ostium is created that extends from the lamina papyracea to the nasal septum. This intervention is carried out in cases with significant mucositis of the frontal sinus, e.g. in cystic fibrosis, in ciliary dyskinesia, or in the presence of mucopyoceles or orbital complications and also in frontal sinus barotrauma.
- *Type III: Endonasal median drainage.* The extended opening is enlarged by resecting portions of the superior septum and inferior intersinus septum as far as the contralateral lamina papyracea. The neoostium drains both frontal sinuses. Endonasal median drainage as described by Draf is indicated in revision surgery of the frontal sinuses (especially where previous surgery was performed by an external approach), in orbital complications arising from the frontal sinus, and after previous operations and endocranial complications arising from the frontal sinus, without bone defects.

In the frontal sinus operations described by Draf, the agger nasi and portions of the frontal process of the maxilla are removed with a diamond burr under microscopic guidance and the lacrimal sac is exposed. The junction between the anterior wall of the frontal sinus and the floor of the frontal sinus is thinned laterally from the head of the middle turbinate stepwise in an anterior and superior direction. Early recognition of complete removal of the bone can be achieved by palpating the medial canthus from the outside with a finger. The frontal infundibulum is identified and the anterior ethmoid cells are resected. The diamond burr is introduced into clearly visible gaps in the infundibulum and drawn across the bone in an anterior direction. Care is taken to ensure that the frontal sinus ostium is bordered by bone on all sides and that the mucosa is preserved on at least one side. After conclusion of median drainage, a rubber finger stall can be introduced into the frontal sinus [174, 179]. Recently,

Table 6.**3** Endonasal frontal sinus drainage type I-III according to Draf [174, 179, 966] respectively Nasofrontal Approach (NFA) I-IV according to May and Schaitkin following Draf [584a]

		Extend of surgery
Type I	(NFA I)	Ethmoidectomy with removal of cells in the region of the frontal recess
Type II	a (NFA II)	Resection the floor of the frontal sinus between lamina papyracea and middle turbinate
	b (NFA III)	Resection the floor of the frontal sinus between lamina papyracea and nasal septum
Type III	(NFA IV)	Type II Drainage on both side and resection of portions of the superior nasal septum and inferior intersinus septum

the use of the diamond burr is minimized and the lacrimal sac is not exposed routinely in order to minimize the surgical trauma and to reduce subsequent scarring.

A number of authors use a diamond burr to enlarge the frontal sinus ostium, usually following a procedure similar to Draf's type II [292, 307, 576, 994]. Wound healing in the ostia enlarged with the drill is comparable to that in conventionally opened sinuses. At follow-up 40% were patent by endoscopy, 30% could only be probed, and a further 30% were patent neither by endoscopy nor by probing [997].

A special form of endonasal median drainage was presented by Close et al. [117]. The technique begins with bilateral endoscopic ethmoidectomy and frontal sinusotomy performed in the usual manner. A segment measuring 2 × 2 cm is then excised from the anterior-superior nasal septum. The resection is performed immediately inferior to the floor of the frontal sinus, anterior to the middle turbinate and the natural ostia of the frontal sinuses. Both frontal ostia can then be visualized endoscopically through one naris, while passing a drill through the contralateral side of the nose. The median frontal sinus floor is removed and the interfrontal septum extensively resected in a su-

Table 6.**4** Results of extended endonasal frontal sinus surgery

Author(s)	Technique	No. of operations	Follow-up period	Healing of frontal sinus ostium	Complications	Remarks
Close et al. [117]	Median drainage	11	5.8 mo	100%	1 CSF leak	In 5/11 patients additional small external incision
Draf et al. [179]	(a) Extended drainage (Type II) (b) Median drainage (Type III)	(a) 128 (b) 57	5 y	Normal/polyps/ pathological: (a) 61.7%/14.8%/ 23.5% (b) 67%/9.1%/23.9%	?	
Har-El and Lucente [307]	(a) Simple drainage (b) Extended drainage (c) Median drainage	(a) 16 (b) 5 (c) 1	10–50 mo	1/22 patients with ostium occlusion 2/22 patients with CT opacification but patent ostium	–	In 1/22 patients additional small external incision
Gross et al. [292]	Median drainage ("endonasal Lothrop procedure")	10	7 mo	100%	–	
Becker et al. [35a]	Median drainage	14	9 mo	100%	–	Special drill system
Rudert 1997 [766]	Type II and Type III drainage	40	1–3 y (?)	Restenosis in 3 cases		
Simmen 1997 [830]	Type II and Type III drainage	55	23 mo	62% symptomfree 29% improved		No data on endoscopic results
Weber et al. [966]	(a) Extended drainage (b) Median drainage	(a) 96 (b) 43	51 months 34 months	70% reventilation 76% reventilation		
Weber et al. [973]	(a) Extended drainage	21	12–16 mo	33% endoscopically patent, 71.4% aerated frontal sinus	-	Prospective study, statistically significant difference a : b
	(b) Extended drainage with silicone spacer for 6 months	15	12–16 mo	80% endoscopically patent, 93.3% aerated frontal sinus	-	

perior direction. Posteriorly, a bridge of bone is preserved to protect the remaining natural frontal sinus ostia with their mucosa. Becker et al. [35a] use a drill system with integrated suction for median drainage procedures without such a bony bridge.

Table 6.**4** gives an overview of results of extended endonasal frontal sinus surgery.

From a surgical view stenosis within the frontal recess most commonly occurs for three reasons [806]:

- Inadequate removal of agger nasi and frontal cells
- Overly aggressive dissection
- Excessive removal of the middle turbinate with lateralization

From a physiological view stenosis can take place in three partially related ways (general wound healing [111, 119]; wound healing after paranasal sinus surgery [349, 968–971]):

1. As a result of persisting obstruction of the opening with blood and fibrin in the immediate postoperative phase. During the proliferative phase of wound healing beginning on the second to third postoperative day, fibroblasts migrate into the fibrin mesh and granulation tissue is formed. Finally, collagen is deposited and the opening is occluded by scar tissue.
2. Marked swelling beginning in the third postoperative week [968–971] leads to contact zones between adjacent or opposite parts of the opening to the frontal sinus. As a result of either primary absence of epithelialization or secondary epithelial

damage due to pressure-induced maceration or inflammatory cell damage, contact between areas of granulation tissue leads to formation of tissue bridges. Here, too, the final stage is occlusion by scar tissue.

3. As a result of realignment of collagen fibers in the remodeling phase beginning in the third postoperative week. In this case the fibers form "scar bands" on concave surfaces as the distance can only be shortened by making use of the free lumen. This can lead to circumferential narrowing.

Weber et al. [973] performed a prospective survey to investigate the influence of stenting the neo-ostium on re-stenosis. They found out that long-term stenting of the frontal sinus significantly reduces the rate of restenosis of the frontal sinus neo-ostium (Table 6.**4**). They pointed out that the stent can only prevent restenosis if it not only prevents occlusion by fibrin meshes and edema during the initial postoperative phase but also affords resistance against the narrowing tendency during the phase of collagen remodeling, which lasts several months.

The optimal design for such a stent has not yet been clearly defined. It should not exert too much pressure on the mucosa. On the basis of experience with pressure-induced tracheal damage, this should not exceed 25 mmHg [889]. Furthermore, it should be self-anchoring in order to prevent dislocation and aspiration and to make additional fixation measures unnecessary. In selected cases this could be achieved using a transseptal U-intubation (type II drainage on both sides) or an H-shaped stent (type III drainage) with positioning on the nasal septum (Weber).

It should also be noted that stenting is not employed by a number of endoscopic surgeons (Stammberger, Kuhn, Lund).

Endonasal Decompression of the Optic Nerve

Endonasal decompression of the optic nerve after fractures in the region of the optic canal probably goes back to Takahashi [897], Tsutsumi [926], and Fujitani [251]. In 1974 Fujitani [252] reported on 16 cases treated with an endonasal approach without optical guidance. Like most authors, Fujitani later [253] began to use a microscope. As early as 1978 Belal [39, 40] mentioned the use of the microscope for the endonasal approach [39].

During sinus surgery, the optic nerve can be exposed by a variety of approaches. The endonasal approach has the obvious advantage of preserving soft tissues of the face and the bony skeletal structures. The optic nerve need not be approached tangentially, as in transfacial procedures, but can be visualized at an angle of about 60° through a microscope or endoscope. The main problem with decompression surgery in cases of indirect trauma to the optic nerve lies in establishing the indication. Chilla [103] and Stoll [887] and also Jorissen and Feenstra [397] and Joseph [398] give overviews on the various indications.

Endonasal decompression should be considered where there is

- radiographic evidence of fracture or narrowing of the optic canal,
- suspected edema, hematoma, vascular spasm in the region of the optic canal, blindness of the only seeing eye or bilateral blindness,
- no response to high-dose corticosteroids treatment after 24 hours' observation,
- post-traumatic deterioration of partial vision loss or scotoma,
- secondary funduscopic signs of increased intracranial pressure or papilloedema in an otherwise normal eye,
- operability, if a neurosurgical approach is not necessary for other reasons,
- availability of CT (proofing that the endonasal approach is anatomically possible) and an experienced surgeon,
- absence of serious injury to the globe,

and observing the following exclusion criteria: transsection of the optic nerve, total ischemia of the eye, injury proximal/distal to the optic canal, trauma more than, for example, 7 days previously, particularly in primary amaurosis.

Adequate visualization of the regional anatomy on an axial CT is a basic prerequisite for endoscopic decompression surgery. A poorly pneumatized sinus system, as with the conchal type of sphenoid sinus, can make an endonasal procedure impossible. If the sphenoid bone is intact, in doubtful cases intraneural hematoma or edema can be demonstrated by performing additional MRI. The surgeon must be thoroughly familiar with the sinuses' anatomy and their relationship to adjacent structures.

The optic canal is about 5–10 mm long. Proximally its wall is thin (0.2–1 mm). Here the bone can often be raised with an elevator without previous thinning. Distally the bone thickens to about 0.6 mm, forming the tubercle of the optic nerve (optic ring), an important landmark. Since the canal is narrow in the region of this ring, decompression with the drill must be carried out cautiously but completely at this point [298, 478, 479, 550].

The anatomy of the lateral junction between the ethmoid bone and sphenoid sinus varies, as do the location and extent of the protrusion of the optic canal into the sinus lumen. In 80% of cases the optic canal borders medially on the sphenoid sinus. In the remaining cases a posterior ethmoid cell envelops the optic canal medially (sphenoethmoidal cell, called Onodi cell). The relationship between the common tendinous ring and the posterior ethmoid bone is variable [479, 1014].

Another important landmark is the orbital apex, with its natural junction with the optic canal. An imaginary line drawn between the points of exit of the anterior and posterior ethmoidal arteries in the region of the superior lamina papyracea points in the direction of the optic nerve. In 16% of cases the ophthalmic artery is located inferomedially in the region of the optic canal. In these cases it is endangered if the sheath of the optic nerve is incised. Incision must be done with special care when cutting through the relatively thick ring of tissue at the tubercle of the optic nerve and the common tendinous ring.

It is frequently impossible to examine injured patients thoroughly as they are not fully conscious. In such cases the visual field and visual acuity cannot be tested. The indication for surgery is then established on the basis of an adequate radiographic evaluation (CT) and funduscopy, examination of the direct and consensual pupillary reflex (especially the "swinging flashlight test"), and recently by additional visual evoked potentials [264, 397, 900].

Radiological evidence of fractures of the optic canal is found in only one-quarter of indirect injuries to the optic nerve [397].

Endonasal decompression of the optic nerve is usually performed under general anesthesia, although there have been reports of its being conducted under local anesthesia [252]. The procedure starts with ethmoidectomy. Fenestration of the maxillary sinus in the middle meatus is extended posteriorly as far as the posterior wall of the maxillary sinus. Where microscopic guidance is employed, the operative field is exposed with self-retaining retractors. The entire anterior wall of the sphenoid sinus is removed. The junction between the orbital apex and the optic canal is visualized. Starting from the posterior orbital apex and using a diamond burr, the bone over the orbit and optic nerve is thinned or debrided under microscopic/endoscopic vision. Thorough irrigation and cooling of the operative field must be ensured. According to Aurbach [18, 19] a safe method is to advance the drill step-by-step from the posterior/superior/medial end portions of the maxillary sinus toward the anterior/superior/lateral portion of the sphenoid sinus. After thinning of the bone, the last bony lamella of the periorbita is elevated with a round knife as used in ear surgery. The exposed strip of the periorbita then serves as a guide rail along which the optic canal can be located posteriorly without risking injury to the adjacent carotid artery. The bone over the optic nerve is again thinned and raised and about 7 mm of the nerve is exposed. If necessary, the nerve sheath can be slit [550, 552, 896]. Finally, the optic nerve is covered with gelatin or pressed collagen sheets soaked in cortisone. Small CSF leaks can also be sealed with pressed collagen sheets or a small flap of autologous mucosa. The operative field is loosely packed for two days. Systemic corticosteroids and an antibiotic are given for one week, if necessary combined with neurotropic vitamins. Locally, the operative zone is gently cleansed and irrigated in the conventional manner [18, 19, 252, 552, 896].

Stammberger uses an endoscope for nerve decompression [538, 861]. After ethmoidectomy and broad fenestration of the sphenoid sinus he removes 7–10 mm of the lamina papyracea of the orbital apex. The bone of the optic canal is thinned with a special intranasal drill. The last layer of bone is elevated with a dissector to up to 180° of the medial circumference. The nerve sheath and the annulus of Zinn is opened carefully with a sickle knife [538], bearing in mind the position of the ophthalmic artery.

To date only a relatively few cases of endonasal optic nerve decompression surgery have been performed and the indication criteria often vary widely, making it difficult to compare results. Spontaneous return of vision after indirect trauma to the optic nerve can be expected in about 34% of cases. High-dose corticosteroids (e.g. methylprednisolone 30 mg/kg body weight, followed by 15 mg/kg body weight every six hours for one day) lead to improvement in about 60% of cases. The percentage of improvements in vision (visual acuity and/or visual field) after surgical decompression is also about 60% (0–100%) [123, 252, 253, 397, 398, 896]. The best results are reportedly achieved with a combination of surgery and corticosteroid therapy.

Postoperative recovery of vision often takes 3–4 weeks. The prognosis is poorer in primary amaurosis. Apart from this one parameter, there is no regular correlation between posttraumatic vision and the outcome of decompression. Evidence of fracture of the optic canal has no influence on the prognosis. Better results are obtained if the operation is carried out on the first day after the trauma or within the first week [397].

Opinions vary with regard to the necessity of incising the nerve sheath. Mann et al. [552] perform this procedure routinely and report a case of hematoma of the optic nerve sheath that was evacuated after incision of the nerve sheath. The preoperative CT had been normal.

Endonasal Surgery of Inflammatory Complications

With a few exceptions, *mucoceles of the ethmoid and sphenoid sinus* can be managed by endonasal surgery. The same applies to medial frontal sinus mucoceles provided that, despite any injuries or previous surgery, the bony skeletal framework is such that access is technically possible and the created access will not collapse (Fig. 6.**4**) [524].

The principle of the operation consists in establishing wide drainage into the nasal cavity (marsupialization). Complete excision of the mucosa is not necessary. The individual steps of the procedure are the conventional endonasal techniques carried out as dictated by the location and extent of the mucocele. Goodyear [284] recommended as long ago as 1944 that mucoceles of the anterior ethmoid and inferior frontal sinus should be drained by means of an anterior ethmoidectomy and the displaced, parchment-like bone in the medial canthus pressed into the correct shape with the thumb from without.

Today, bony erosion of the walls of the frontal sinus by a mucocele is no longer a contraindication for endonasal techniques. Even mucoceles extending intracranially or into the orbit can be managed by an endoscopic approach [50, 307, 438, 861]. The same applies to pyoceles associated with destruction of the anterior wall of the frontal sinus. Prefrontal abscesses are evacuated through a stab incision while the rest of the operation is conducted endonasally [194, 350]. The pathogenetic mechanism may be pressure on the nerve or a spread of inflammation. Mucopyoceles of the dorsal ethmoid or sphenoid sinus may cause vision loss. The mucopyoceles are marsupialized endonasally in the same way as the other mucoceles (Fig. 6.**5**) [634]. If the loss of vision is complete and has been present for more than 24 hours, the prognosis is much poorer [634].

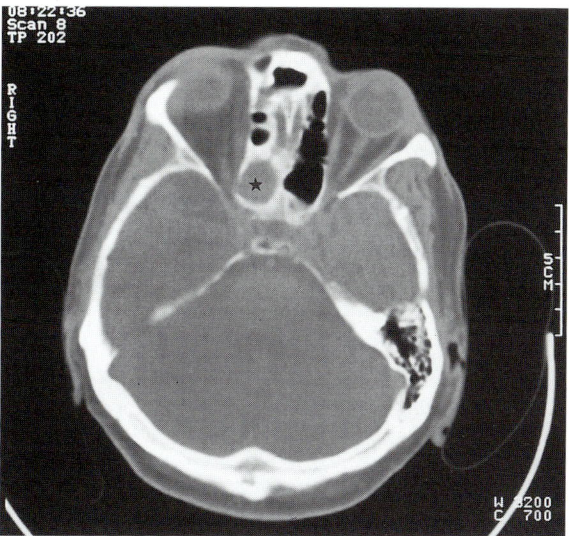

Fig. 6.**4** **Endonasal surgery in the region of the optic nerve.** Axial CT of a sphenoethmoid pyocele (★) with increasing loss of vision. Treatment started eight days after complete loss of vision. After marsupialization, the patient's visual acuity improved gradually and incompletely to 0.3 over a period of 14 days

A large mucocele in a concha bullosa is an ideal indication for endonasal therapy [25]. Rudert [764] re-

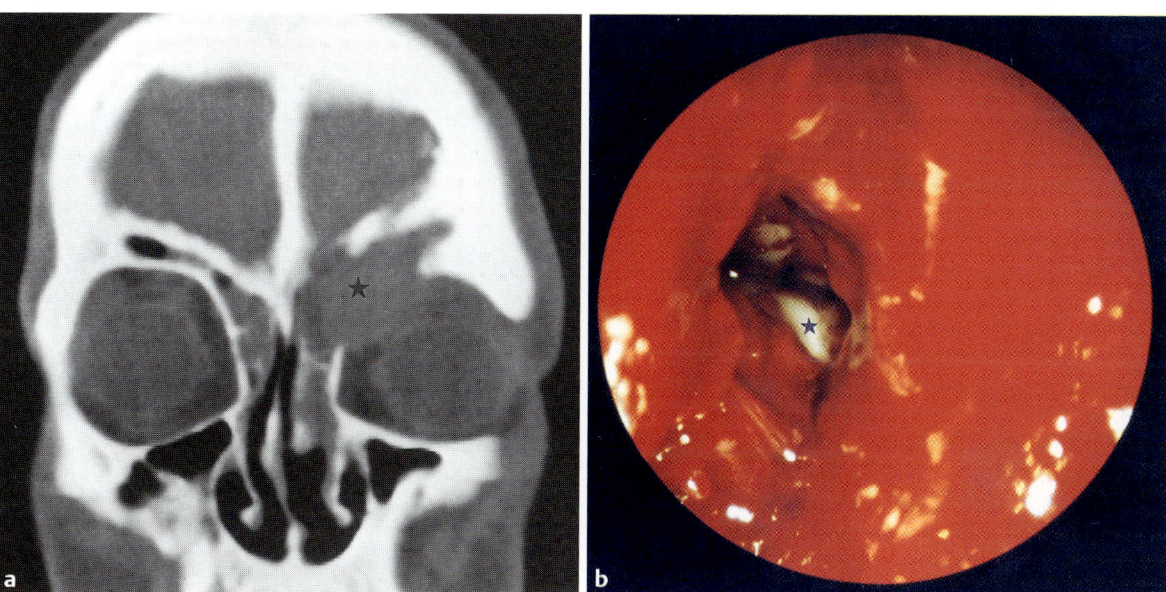

Fig. 6.**5a,b** **Endonasal surgery of frontoethmoidal mucopyoceles**
(**a**). Coronal CT of a 23-year-old man with a left frontoethmoidal mucopyocele (★). (**b**) View into the frontal sinus with a 70° endoscope following opening of the mucopyocele. Purulent mucus is evacuated (★)

Table 6.**5** Outcome of marsupialization of mucopyoceles in the paranasal sinuses

Author(s)	No. of patients	No. and location of mucoceles	Surgical technique	Follow-up	Results
Kennedy et al. [438]	18	11 frontal sinus 5 ethmoid complex 2 sphenoid sinus	Endoscopic	17 mo	External revision surgery in 2/11 frontal sinuses
Levine [503]	4	4 ethmoid complex	Endoscopic	17 mo	100% success
Draf [173]	26	26 frontal sinus	Microscopic–endoscopic	?	?
Hosemann et al. [350]	18	18 frontal sinus	Endoscopic	11 mo	Subjectively 100% cure/improvement Endoscop. success in 81% External revision surgery in 11%
Serrano et al. [811]	8	2 sphenoid sinus 2 maxillary sinus 4 frontal sinus and ethmoid complex	Endoscopic	10 mo to 4 y	100% success
Moriyama et al. [634]	25 patients with impaired vision	9 sphenoid sinus 5 ethmoid complex 11 mixed form	Endoscopic	?	100% endonasal marsupialization In 8/25 cases marked improvement in vision
Moriyama et al. [635]	47	41 ethmoid complex 8 sphenoid sinus	Endoscopic	1–10 y	100% success
Kennedy [443]	7	1 ethmoid complex 3 frontal sinus 3 ethmoid and frontal sinus	Endoscopic, ethmoidal mucosa completely removed, frontal sinus catheter for 3–6 weeks	18 mo	External revision surgery in 2/7 patients Endonasal revision surgery 1/7 patients
Har-El [306]	2	frontal sinus with intracranial involvement	endoscopic	12 and 42 mo	Both patients symptom-free
Benninger and Marks [50]	15	ethmoid/sphenoid sinus with intracranial/orbital involvement	Endoscopic, 2/15 additional transfacial procedure	20 mo	Recurrence in 2/15 successfully managed by endonasal revision surgery

ports on a huge mucocele in the region of the maxillary, ethmoid, and sphenoid sinuses and extending into the posterior cranial fossa. Marsupialization was achieved primarily through an endonasal procedure.

Small, lateral maxillary sinus mucoceles surrounded by scar tissue after previous transoral operations often present with technical problems. However, it is none the less advisable to attempt marsupialization by the endonasal approach. If it proves impossible to establish adequate drainage, transoral techniques can be employed in the same session. Large mucoceles in the maxillary sinus are treated by the conventional fenestration procedure via the middle meatus. In individual cases an additional external approach has occasionally been employed to manage secondary enophthalmus following loss of the bony floor of the orbita [35].

Thorough long-term follow-up care of the operative field is especially important. Occasionally, aftercare of mucoceles in the frontal sinus is carried out through a drainage tube, but this is rarely required [306]. Stenosis of the frontal sinus ostium can also be prevented by performing Draf's extended frontal sinus operation [175]. The results reported in the literature are summarized in Table 6.**5**. It is well known that it often takes 15–25 years for a mucocele to become clinically manifest [634, 635]. This must be kept in mind when reporting recurrence-free intervals.

In isolated cases, the endonasal procedure is performed as part of the combined treatment of severe *acute inflammatory complications of rhinosinusitis*. This includes endonasal treatment of the infection as part of the treatment of patients with rhinogenic thrombosis of the cavernous sinus. The operation is conducted after institution of intensive antibiotic treatment, for example, with cefotaxime and metronidazole. This treatment is continued for three weeks postoperatively. Unless contraindicated, 7500 IU heparin is also given every six hours [217, 1016].

In frontal osteomyelitis, an inflammatory focus can be eliminated or reduced by endonasal techniques. Removal of the diseased focus combined with intensive postoperative antibiotic therapy over 4–6 weeks can often replace or reduce the extent of external surgery [194, 308, 861].

Patients with inflammatory endocranial complications of frontal rhinosinusitis have been treated by endonasal sinus surgery after institution of conservative antimicrobial treatment and exclusion by CT of a bony defect in the posterior wall of the frontal sinus [174].

Gerber et al. [266] report on a child with an epidural abscess of the face of the sphenoid in rhinosinusitis. Surgical treatment consisted of endonasal sinus surgery combined with endoscopic drainage of the abscess via an image converter. The abscess was evacuated by suction through an opening in the face of the sphenoid. Healing was achieved after additional antibiotic treatment.

Endonasal Orbit Surgery

Acute orbital complications of bacterial rhinosinusitis are classified on the basis of their etiology and extent as inflammatory orbital edema, orbital periostitis, subperiosteal and intraorbital abscess, and orbital cellulitis with the risk of secondary thrombosis of the cavernous sinus. The diagnosis and principles of treatment have been thoroughly discussed by Stammberger [861].

These conditions are diagnosed on the basis of CT with contrast medium or MRI after examination by an ENT specialist and ophthalmologist. Subperiosteal abscesses are often missed on CT scans as they are sometimes difficult to distinguish radiologically from thickening of the periosteum due to inflammation [113, 205, 304]. The patients are often children. Surgical treatment is indicated if there is no response to antibiotics after 24 hours and the patient has a persistent or fluctuating fever, if there is evidence of visual compromise, if the local findings increase, or if there is radiographic evidence of an abscess or gas formation. In some cases of subperiosteal abscess it is considered justifiable to try conservative treatment for a limited period [861]. Endonasal techniques under endoscopic and/or microscopic guidance are the method of choice for removal of disease. Depending on the anatomic conditions, a 4-mm or 2.7-mm endoscope (e.g., 0°, 25°/30° or 70° endoscope with suction-irrigation handle) is employed.

Gamble [256] reported on an endonasal procedure for subperiosteal abscess as early as 1933. A relatively extensive ethmoidectomy is performed to gain access and remove the inflammatory foci that are the source of the disease. Mucosal bleeding may be controlled by packing with pledgets soaked in 1:1000 epinephrine or 0.05% oxymetazoline. The lamina papyracea is visualized and palpated under direct optical guidance. Inflamed fissures or canals can often be recognized by discoloration of the tissue, dehiscence, or change in consistency. Application of pressure to the globe (see p. 84) helps to locate dehiscences in the lamina papyracea. If dehiscences are suspected, the lamina papyracea is raised egg shell-fashion with an elevator and removed. A subperiosteal abscess can be gently and adequately drained by this procedure. In principle, the orbital periosteum is preserved. However, if there is evidence of more extensive inflammatory infiltration, it can be incised locally with a sickle knife under endoscopic guidance for diagnosis and treatment. If the inflammation originates in the frontal sinus, it is opened through an endonasal approach. In cases where the abscess cannot be satisfactorily drained endonasally, it may be combined with a limited external approach [86, 174, 205, 210, 259, 557].

Intraperiosteal intraorbital abscesses were treated endonasally by Seiffert as long ago as 1930 [807]. Now that optical aids have been introduced, the indication for surgical procedures should in principle be broad, taking into account the location and size of the abscess and concomitant factors. Localized intraperiosteal abscesses in the medial orbit can be managed well by endonasal surgery [861, 1003]. The ethmoid cells on the affected side are usually completely cleared by the endonasal route and the lamina papyracea is visualized. Under endoscopic guidance, a suitable elevator is cautiously inserted under the lamina papyracea, which is then removed piece by piece. The intact periorbita is incised from posterior to anterior at a suitable place, using a scalpel or a strongly curved sickle knife. The orbit can be explored under minimal suction with a blunt maxillary sinus suction cannula, and the abscess drained (Fig. 6.**6**). A 70° suction-irrigation endoscope as described by Wigand [990] has proved suitable for optical guidance for this procedure. After adequate drainage has been ensured, the remaining surgical steps are adapted to the individual case; for example, bearing in mind the difficulties encountered in the aftercare of young patients. If the natural ostium of the maxillary sinus is diseased or cannot be preserved with certainty intraoperatively, it is advisable to create a large window in the maxillary sinus. The vertical bony lamella of the middle turbinate can be reduced; however, fracture should be avoided. Surgical exploration of the frontal sinus will depend on the individual case [1003].

The children usually recover surprisingly quickly postoperatively [210]. If possible, packing is left in place for no longer than 24 hours. A postoperative ophthalmological examination soon after the operation is mandatory. The systemic antibiotic medication instituted before the operation is continued and fol-

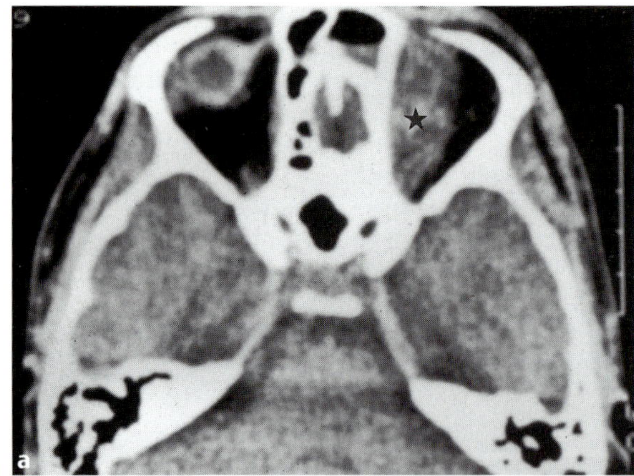

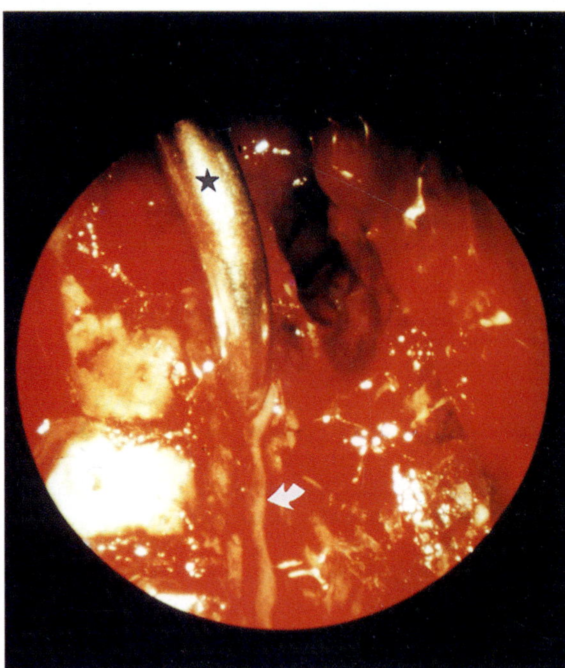

Fig. 6.**6a,b** **Endonasal surgery of an intraorbital abscess in a 13-year-old girl**
(**a**) Axial CT: right-sided intraorbital abscess (★). (**b**) View through the 70° endoscope of the exposed right periorbita and frontal sinus ostium following ethmoidectomy with fenestration of the frontal and maxillary sinuses. The blunt suction cannula (★) is draining the intraorbital abscess; purulent mucus is evacuated (arrow)

low-up is conducted by inspection, endoscopy, repeated smears, and monitoring of the conventional laboratory parameters. Depending on the patient's age, compliance, and the local findings, in children a follow-up examination under anesthesia may be required to clean the surgical cavity.

Orbital Decompression

In patients with progressive endocrine ophthalmopathy with or without optic neuropathy, endonasal decompression of the orbit can be undertaken when the possibilities of conservative treatment (steroids, radiation, and/or, where necessary, immunosuppressive therapy with cyclosporin A or plasmapheresis) have been exhausted. The first reports of this technique were published by Kennedy et al. [440] and Michel et al. [613]. The goal of treatment is to reduce the proptosis, treat keratitis, and maintain or improve visual acuity. Extended indications are refractory orbital congestion, pain, and severe cosmetic disfigurement [555]. Rarely, endonasal surgery is prevented by excessive bone formation on the floor of the orbit [440].

It is usual to operate on both sides simultaneously; in rare cases both orbits are operated on separately at an interval of one week [608]. The indication is usually established together with an ophthalmologist, internist, and radiotherapist. The basis for the indication is an ophthalmological and otolaryngological examination with adequate radiographic evaluation (coronal CT). The patient should be informed that existing diplopia may worsen, that ophthalmological revision surgery may be necessary, and that impairment of vision is theoretically possible. Postoperative eye training is important for all patients. A total ethmoidectomy with wide fenestration of the sphenoid sinuses is performed under general anesthesia with endoscopic or microscopic guidance. Maximum fenestration of the maxillary sinus is carried out in the middle meatus. An additional inferior meatotomy can be performed to ensure drainage of the maxillary sinus after the expected herniation of the orbital fat. If necessary the nasal septum is corrected. The middle turbinate is often substantially resected [608, 613]. Using an elevator, an angled spoon, or a nerve hook, it is possible to raise and remove the exposed lamina papyracea under direct vision. Decompression in the posterior orbital apex extending to the tubercle of the optic nerve is particularly important. Where necessary, it should be followed by decompression of the optic canal. The bony floor of the orbit is removed from the direction of the lamina papyracea as far as the infraorbital nerve. In the frontal recess, portions of the bony wall of the orbit are left in place to stabilize the frontal sinus ostium. To prevent the eye from sinking too far, Michel et al. [613] occasionally leave a bone remnant in place medially. As a rule, the exposed periorbita is slit from posterior to anterior with a strongly curved sickle knife, making several incisions of the same shape (Fig. 6.**7**) and taking care to spare the eye muscles. Fibrous bands on the periosteum must be divided under direct vision. In rare cases, the periorbita is excised [447]. The orbital fat then protrudes into the ethmoid and maxillary sinus and quickly mucosalizes. Several authors resect excess fat under optical guidance [555, 608], but this is unnecessary and potentially increases the chances of complications. Mann et al. [555] usually supplement the endonasal operation by transmaxillary inferior decompression or by lateral decompression via a bifrontal approach. Various other combinations of approaches have been

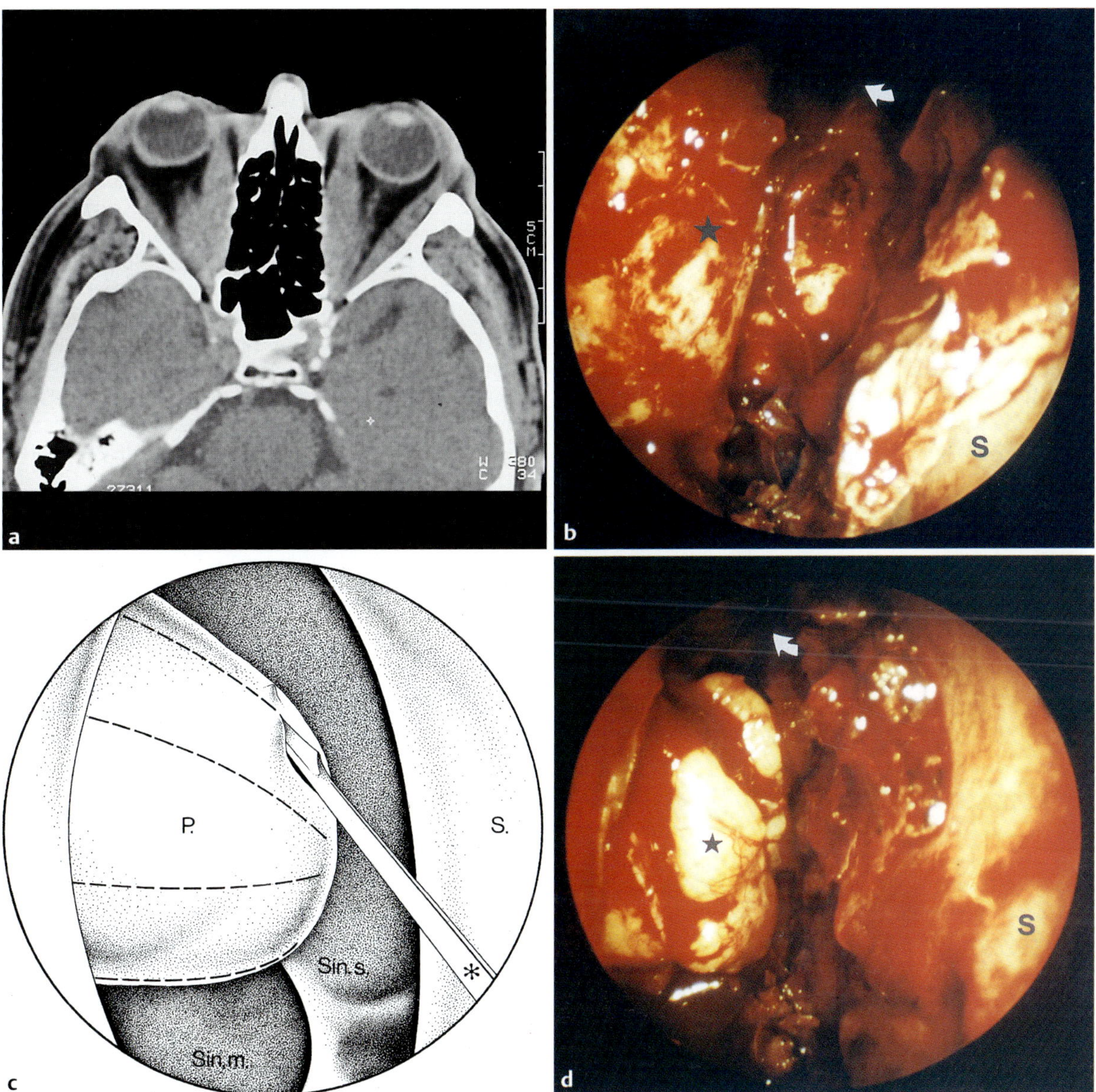

Fig. 6.**7a-d** **Endonasal decompression of the orbit in endocrine ophthalmopathy**. A 54-year-old man with deterioration of visual acuity in the right eye despite radiotherapy and corticosteroid administration. Bilateral endonasal medial decompression of the orbit in combination with lateral decompression performed by an external approach resulted in a gradual increase in visual acuity in the right eye from 0.03 to 0.5. The results of Hertel exophthalmometry improved by 5.5 mm on the right side and 3.5 mm on the left. Secondary surgery for strabismus was performed
(**a**) Preoperative CT. Fusiform distension of the rectus muscles of the orbit (**b**) View of the right nasal cavity after total ethmoidectomy with visualization of the skull base. Arrow: frontal sinus ostium; ★: exposed periorbita. (**c**) After removal of the lamina papyracea as far as the infraorbital nerve and cutting away the distal optic canal, the periorbita (P.) is slit several times from posterior to anterior using a sickle knife (★) beginning with the most cranial incision. S., nasal septum; Sin.m.: sinus maxillaris (maxillary sinus); Sin.s., sinus sphenoidalis (sphenoid sinus) (**d**) Operative site after the first incisions of the periorbita. Fat (★) is bulging into the ethmoid cavity. Arrow: frontal sinus ostium

described [440, 447]. Interestingly, a comparison of external and endoscopic approaches did not show any significant difference [532] in terms of resolution in axial proptosis.

If packing of the operative site is carried out at all, it is left in place for only 24 hours. The patients are given oral antibiotic cover and in some cases discharged as early as the first to third postoperative day [440, 555, 608, 613]. Aftercare of the operative field should be undertaken carefully with the aid of an endoscope.

Visual acuity improves postoperatively in over 75% of patients with infiltrative ophthalmopathy and simultaneous optic neuropathy, although there is no correlation between resolution of the exophthalmus and improvement in vision [440, 608, 613]. Proptosis is usually reduced by an average of 4 mm (1.5–4.5 mm) after endoscopic decompression alone and by almost 6 mm (3.5–7 mm) after combination of endoscopic decompression with other approaches. The final outcome cannot be established until about six months after the operation. There is no clear correlation between the extent of preoperative proptosis and the reduction achieved [440, 555, 608, 613]. Patients with keratitis can be freed from their symptoms without exception [440]. Two-thirds of patients with preoperative diplopia complain of an increase in symptoms after the operation that returns to the preoperative situation in most by three months. First-time occurrence of diplopia must be expected in one-quarter to one-third of patients postoperatively [440, 555, 608, 613] and may require correction with prisms on spectacles in the immediate postoperative period and occasionally muscle surgery if present after three months. The endoscopic approach described above leads to a smaller drop in the globe than after transantral resection of the floor of the orbit [608].

A relatively large percentage (39%) of patients suffer from episodes of rhinosinusitis postoperatively that can be minimized by a large middle meatal antrostomy and preservation of the frontal recess. However, this responds well to conservative treatment [555]. In isolated cases, mucopyoceles of the maxillary sinus or ethmoidal shaft are observed after transmaxillary decompression. Treatment of the former requires surgery of the maxillary sinus with fenestration in the inferior meatus. The middle third of the inferior turbinate can be resected simultaneously in order to extend the neo-ostium from the inferior meatus to the natural ostium of the middle meatus [332].

Median fractures of the orbit are discussed on p. 80.

Endonasal Surgery of the Lacrimal Drainage System

The first report of endonasal lacrimal duct surgery was published by Caldwell in 1893 [92]. He described a procedure whereby the inferior turbinate was partially resected and the nasolacrimal duct was followed from its inferior extremity to the lacrimal sac. The present-day endonasal surgical technique with fenestration of the lacrimal sac is based on the description presented by West [981]. The optically aided procedures were developed by H. Heermann [312]. The advantages of the endonasal procedure are that it does not require an external incision, bleeding in the operative field is minimal, and it can be accomplished in a short time. Inflammatory disease of the paranasal sinuses is considered to play a role in the pathogenesis of lacrimal duct stenoses. With the endonasal approach it is possible to deal with such changes in the adjacent sinus system in the same operation. Endonasal surgery is indicated where there is evidence of saccular and postsaccular stenoses of the lacrimal ducts with the corresponding symptoms, including re-stenosis after endonasal and transfacial operations. Active infections, including abscesses of the lacrimal ducts, are not a contraindication once conservative treatment has been instituted; in fact, the course of the disease is shortened [297, 961].

Before the operation, the patient should undergo a thorough ophthalmological examination, also rhinoscopy with endoscopy and diagnostic probing, and irrigation of the lacrimal ducts [600]. The radiographic evaluation may be performed by dacryocystorhinography or digital subtraction dacryocystography [951]. In medicolegal terms, a combination of CT and dacryocystography is useful following iatrogenic stenosis of the lacrimal ducts [569].

Endonasal surgery on the lacrimal ducts is carried out under local or general anesthesia (see pp. 17, 18) with the aid of an endoscope, a microscope or a headlight, where necessary in combination. To begin with, the intranasal mucosa is thoroughly decongested. In 10% of cases septal correction is necessary in order to be able to adequately expose the operative field [978]. A piece of mucosa measuring 15 × 8 mm is then excised anterior to the head of the middle turbinate and above the frontal process of the maxilla. The excision can also be performed by electrocautery [388]. It does not appear to be necessary to apply special mucosal flaps. The exposed bone is removed with a 4-mm chisel or a diamond burr so that the lacrimal sac and the nasolacrimal duct are exposed. The arm of a bayonet forceps can be passed into the nose for orientation. When the second arm of the forceps is lying on the medial canthus externally, the first arm indicates the position of the lacrimal sac on the inside [881]. Holding a cold light against the medial canthus from the outside can also help with orientation within the nose [588]. Threading suitably thin light fibers ("retina light pipes" or the Karl Storz endoilluminator) through the small lacrimal ducts into the lacrimal sac

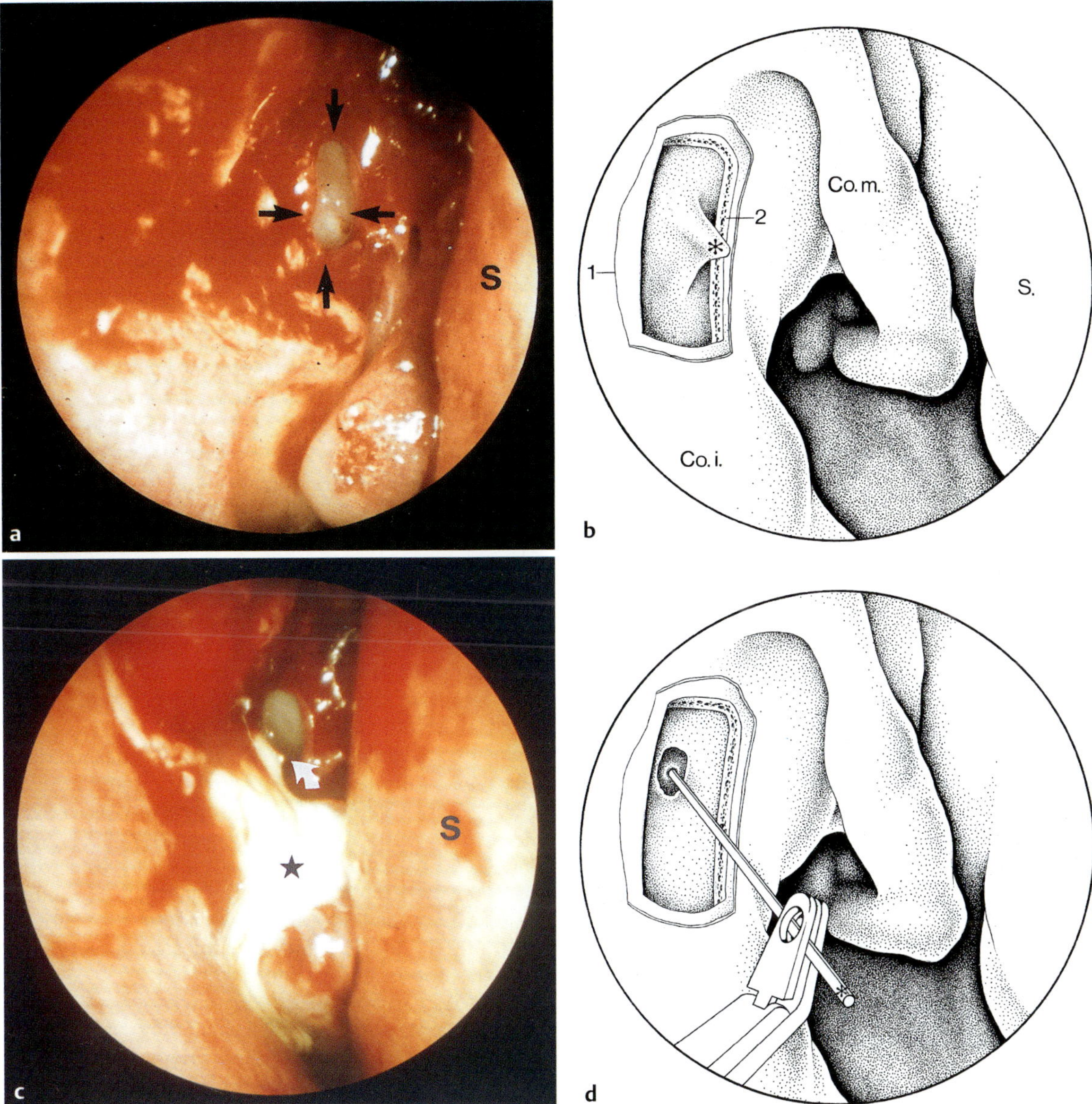

Fig. 6.**8a-d** **Endonasal lacrimal duct surgery**
(**a**) View of the right lateral nasal wall following excision of a square of mucosa and chiseling away of the corresponding bone superior to the sac and nasolacrimal duct. Arrows indicate borders of defects (enlargement advisable). (**b**) Fenestration of the right lateral nasal wall superior to the sac and nasolacrimal duct (1, resection of the mucosa; 2, bony window created with a chisel or diamond burr with exposure of the nasolacrimal duct). A probe (★) is advanced through the lacrimal ducts and marks the site of the incision of the lacrimal sac by stretching the wall of the duct. S., nasal septum; Co.i., inferior turbinate (concha inferior); Co.m., middle turbinate (concha media). (**c**) Pus drains from the lacrimal sac (★) after the incision. Arrow indicates the tip of the probe. (**d**) After cleaning and aspiration the lacrimal duct probes (★) are advanced through the superior and inferior lacrimal puncta, grasped one after the other with grasping forceps, and pulled out. They are finally joined together intranasally or knotted and trimmed

serves the same purpose [281, 567, 734, 737]. The bony window created should be relatively large and extend as far as the fundus; traumatization of the soft tissue must be minimized. Irregular edges of bone and mucosa are removed. In one-fifth to one-half of cases, anterior ethmoid cells overlie the superior portion of the efferent lacrimal ducts to a varying extent [915, 985], so that the anterior ethmoid complex is inevitably opened. The metal probe of the lacrimal duct intubation set (e.g., Guibor) is introduced through one lacrimal punctum. The probe stretches the medial mucosa of the lacrimal ducts endonasally (Fig. 6.**8**). An incision is made at this point in the lacrimal sac with a sickle knife. The medial portions of the sac and duct are then successively resected. It is necessary to explore the opened lacrimal sac carefully to ensure adequate drainage of possible diverticula and to avoid missing any debris. The tip of the metal probe is then grasped intranasally and pulled out (Fig. 6.**8d**). The second probe is passed through the second lacrimal punctum. The ends of the two tubes are knotted intranasally, tied together with suture, or joined with a small vascular clip.

Draf describes a modification of the procedure of Veis, Claus, and Güttich to be used in confined anatomic conditions [172, 961]. The technique involves visualizing the piriform crest and removing a 1.5 cm wide segment from the frontal process of the maxilla in the direction of the lacrimal sac. The lacrimal duct is opened from a more anterior direction.

Revisions of previous West or Toti procedures can also be performed endonasally under local or general anesthesia. The probe is advanced through the small lacrimal ducts and in such cases causes the scar tissue to bulge endonasally. An area measuring 10 mm across is cut round the scar with a sickle knife or small scalpel and excised. Angled grasping forceps are used to grasp the tissue in the vicinity of the tip of the probe and aid in exposure and excision. When the tip of the probe is exposed, the newly opened lacrimal sac can be inspected with a 70° endoscope and the opening can be enlarged. When there are stenoses in the area of the common duct, a funnel-shaped wedge of scar tissue is excised together with the stenotic segment of the duct and the scar contraction keeps the neo-ostium patent [316, 605]. The lacrimal ducts are intubated in the conventional fashion.

Nasal packing is frequently inserted unilaterally for only 24 hours. The silicone tubes remain in situ for six weeks, or, better, eight weeks. They are removed on an outpatient basis under endoscopic guidance. In the case of first operations, some authors do not intubate the lacrimal ducts [787, 961, 989]. In contrast, intubation for up to six months is recommended after revision surgery [605, 683].

Endonasal dacryocystorhinostomy can be carried out on an outpatient basis in uncomplicated cases. However, depending on the concomitant procedures, patients may also be discharged later, i.e., on the first to fourth postoperative day [554, 604, 609, 787, 961, 962, 977, 978]. The tissue obtained intraoperatively should always be examined histologically. Suspicious lesions should be biopsied to avoid overlooking tumors or specific inflammation.

A number of authors have reported on the use of *laser-assisted dacryocystorhinostomy*. This has the advantage of a relatively bloodless operative field, which makes it possible to carry out the procedure on an outpatient basis. Elaborate safety precautions are required to protect patients and staff against laser-induced damage and the time required for the operation is longer. An average of over 100 minutes is required for video-endoscopic laser surgery [609]. Increased scarring due to thermal damage must be avoided by selection of suitable settings and careful operative technique [1007].

In laser-assisted procedures the lacrimal sac is located endonasally by introducing thin fiberoptic light probes for transillumination. Using a carbon dioxide or potassium titanyl-phosphate laser [281, 737], an argon laser [70, 567] or a holmium:YAG laser [609, 734, 1007], neo-ostia of different sizes (5 mm in diameter to 15 × 20 mm) are created from the endonasal approach. Conjunctivorhinostomies are also performed [567]. Packing is often not required postoperatively; however, long-term lacrimal duct intubation is usually carried out.

The technique of *translacrimal laser dacryocystorhinostomy* was developed by ophthalmologists [107]. Slim, flexible fiberoptic light probes are passed through the small lacrimal ducts into the lacrimal sac from without and used to resect the medial wall of the sac by laser and create a fistula to the nose. The operation is monitored via an endoscope in the nose. According to initial reports, the success rates are between 50% and 75%. Dacryoliths are a contraindication for this procedure [107, 573, 712].

Generally no special aftercare is considered necessary following endonasal surgery of the lacrimal ducts [951]. Often only a single irrigation is required after the operation [961]. Conventional endonasal care of the operative field can be carried out and an intranasal steroid is given [70, 737].

Results of endonasal surgery of the nasolacrimal ducts are summarized in Table 6.**6**. The comparatively poorer performance of laser-supported procedures stands out. A number of laser operations have to be concluded by conventional methods [70]. No further attempts with laser should be made after a failure [609]. The overall success rate is about 85%. Patients with posttraumatic stenosis or revision surgery after Toti operations, and patients who lose their lacrimal duct tubes early on have reduced chances of success [978]. Patients with ectatic lacrimal ducts, dacryoliths, or empyema have a very good prognosis [559, 787, 961]. The only major complication with this procedure is injury to the periorbita, which occurs in about 6% of cases, though usually without any sequelae [961].

Some patients note air blowing through the medial canthus when they blow their noses. However, this need hardly be considered a complication [986].

There is no satisfactory agreement between postoperative endoscopic findings and residual symptoms. Even after extensive removal of bone, only relatively small neo-ostia result [508], but openings with diameters of 1–2 mm are functionally adequate. Granulation tissue can form in the vicinity of the ostium, especially after intubation of the lacrimal ducts, and can obstruct tear flow. It can be removed endoscopically on an outpatient basis [69, 605, 743, 978, 1007].

Endonasal dacryocystocele of newborns leads to the formation of a generally yellowish cyst in the inferior meatus, and frequently also to a swelling in the region of the ipsilateral medial canthus. The prolapsed hy-

Table 6.**6** Results of endonasal surgery of the nasolacrimal ducts

Author(s)	No. of lacrimal ducts operated on	Type of stenosis (operation)	Results	Additional remarks
Taylor et al. [905]	18	First operation	80% success	
Metson [604]	5	5 revisions	100% success	
Metson [605]	13	13 revisions	75% success	
Orcutt et al. [683]	8	5 revisions, 3 iatrogenic injuries	86% success	
Weber et al. [961, 962]	123	Pre-, intra-, and post-saccular stenoses	82% success	
Mann et al. [554]	23	20 first operations 2 revisions	96% success	
Walther et al. [951]	103	?	87% success	
Weidenbecher et al. [978]	56	45 first operations 11 revisions	86% success	
Wielgosz et al. [989]	(a) 594 (b) 45	(a) saccular/postsaccular (b) common duct	(a) 98% success (b) 84% success	
Gutiérrez-Ortega et al. [297]	20	Only surgery on dilated lacrimal sac	100% success	In 50% postoperative endonasal inflammation at the neo-ostium
Gonnering et al. [281]	15	First operations	100% success (follow-up in some cases with intubation)	CO_2 laser in 3 cases, potassium-titanyl-phosphate laser in 12 cases
Reifler [737]	19	First operations	68% success	Potassium-titanyl-phosphate laser
Whittet et al. [986]	19	18 first operations, 1 revision	95% success	CO_2 laser in some cases
Woog et al. [1007]	40	First operations	82% success	Holmium: YAG laser
Boush et al. [70]	46	First operations	70% success	Argon laser
Metson et al. [609]	46	27 first operations 13 revisions 6 conjunctivorhinostomies	85% success	Holmium: YAG laser N.B.: 4/4 revisions with laser were unsuccessful
Gleich et al. [273]	5	First operations	80% success	Holmium laser

drops of the lacrimal ducts can be located in the inferior meatus under local anesthesia using a 2.7-mm endoscope or a microscope and eliminated by means of an incision or marsupialization. Often several narrow points of the lacrimal ducts are present. Accurate evaluation and close cooperation with the ophthalmologist are important. Péloquin et al. [704] reported on the treatment of four dacryocystoceles. We have also successfully treated four cases endoscopically as outpatients. Postoperative intubation of the lacrimal ducts as described by Hulka et al. [367] was not necessary.

A comprehensive overview that includes almost all surgical procedures conducted to reconstruct the lacrimal drainage system is available on CD-ROM (Keerl and Weber). The main emphasis is on endonasal dacryocystorhinostomy. The CD-ROM contains 15 video films lasting 46 minutes [Keerl R, Weber R (1999) The interdisciplinary surgery of the lacrimal drainage system. Giebel Verlag, Eiterfeld].

Endonasal Tumor Surgery

In isolated cases, intranasal tumors were resected or snared endonasally even before the introduction of optical aids [193, 644], but the limitation of such approaches was clearly recognized.

The use of an optically guided endonasal approach to tumors, be they benign or malignant is controversial. In order to undertake such surgery it is mandatory to have considerable experience in the management of sinonasal neoplasia with expert imaging, histopathology, and the full range of oncological therapies available. The surgeon must be familiar with the natural history of the many histologies that can

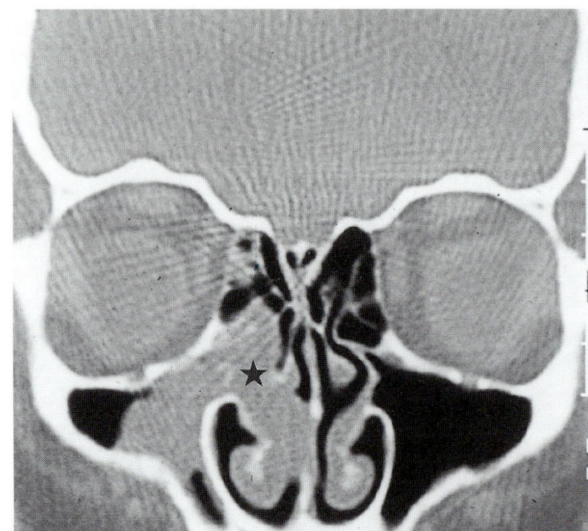

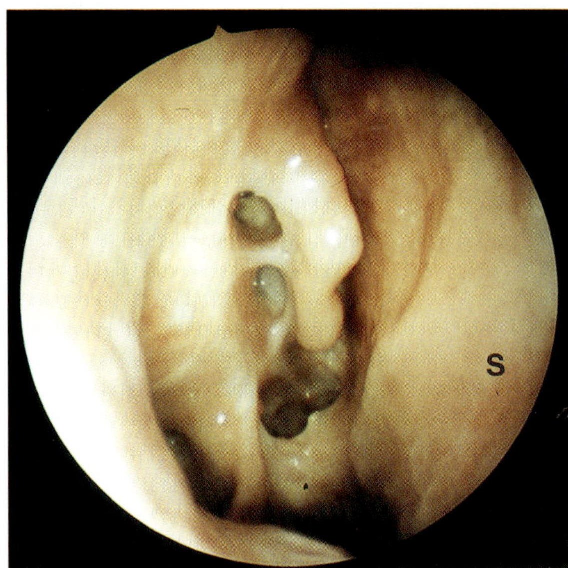

Fig. 6.**9a,b** **Endoscopic follow-up examination after endonasal surgery for inverted papilloma.**
(**a**) Preoperative coronal CT of a 46-year-old man with an inverted papilloma of the right middle nasal meatus (★).
(**b**) Follow-up endoscopy eight months after an endonasal operation in which the lamina papyracea was removed: the operative site shows no signs of inflammation

occur in this area and be experienced not only in endoscopic sinus surgery but also in the more radical external approaches that may be required if the tumor has been under-staged for any reason. Clearly, when an endonasal approach is undertaken, the removal is piecemeal and en-bloc resection is not attempted. It is therefore fundamental that preoperative imaging includes fine detail axial and coronal CT scanning combined in the case of all malignant and of some benign tumors with magnetic resonance imaging, [106, 469, 1020]. Frozen section facilities should be available in theater and a range of suitable instrumentation including endoscopic drills and suitable knives and rasps. Exact illumination of the operative field, including remote corners, must be ensured by employing a microscope and/or endoscope with a sufficiently large viewing angle (25/30°, 70°; suction-irrigation shaft) [177]. The patient must be informed about the procedure and consent to the possibility of more extensive surgery or additional measures with an external or transoral approach, should these be needed. Long-term, in some cases life-long, monitoring of the operative site with a flexible or rigid endoscope is particularly important (Fig. 6.**9**).

The use of endonasal surgery obviates the need for external incisions or tissue mobilization but from the oncological point of view still offers the same possibility of "on-the-spot" tissue resection as classical surgery. Morbidity is often surprisingly low and acceptance is correspondingly high. None the less, endonasal tumor surgery forms the sensitive border zone between the indications for endonasal and classical surgery, particularly in the case of malignant tumors. The choice of surgical approach must be reassessed in each individual case. In view of the availability of cosmetically acceptable classical procedures, inappropriate extension of the indications for endonasal surgery must not be undertaken [91, 650].

Endonasal Surgery of Benign Tumors

Before the operation, a thorough endoscopic examination must be performed after maximal decongestion of the mucosa. This provides a basis for initial evaluation of the extent and natural history of the tumor. The actual depth of infiltration is indicated by CT and MRI. Tumors often grow exophytically on a narrow base and their extent is overestimated owing to concomitant polypoid inflammation. The type of tumor is confirmed by biopsy before the operation. Removal of large amounts of tissue for biopsy is avoided so as not to interfere with an exact endoscopic evaluation of the borders of the tumor owing to blurring as a result of scars and inflammation. Endonasal surgery for tumors consists of the following steps (Fig. 6.**10**):

- Exposure of the operative field
- Visualization of the tumor borders
- Resection of exophytic portions of the tumor
- Excision of the tumor pedicle with safety margin
- Removal of tissue specimens from the marginal area

The operative field is first optimally exposed. This may necessitate septoplasty and concomitant procedures, e.g., on the inferior turbinate. Placement of a self-retaining retractor leaves the surgeon using a microscope free to use both hands [177]. It is then possible to free the area around the tumor by endoscopically guided removal of areas of secondary inflammation including neighboring portions of the sinuses, and thus to establish its extent. Tumors in the middle meatus usually require total ethmoidectomy. The turbinates are substantially reduced or removed if they bear any relationship to the tumor. In the case of pedunculated tumors, exophytic portions may also be resected earlier on, so as to be able to visualize the base of the tumor with certainty. Once the borders of the tumor are visible, the indication for endonasal surgery is again reassessed. Resection is completed by total removal of the tumor together with a margin of healthy tissue. If necessary, portions of the nasal septum, the medial wall of the maxillary sinus with the inferior turbinate, the floor of the sphenoid sinus, the palatine bone or the bony anterior skull base, and the lacrimal bone can be removed with a punch or diamond drill. If the nasolacrimal duct has to be opened or resected, the neo-ostium should be intubated as in endonasal lacrimal duct surgery. The lamina papyracea can be removed egg shell-fashion as in surgery of subperiosteal abscesses. Finally, biopsies of marginal tissue are taken. The exposed bone can be polished with a drill.

Endonasal tumor resection is only acceptable if the specimens of marginal tissue that have been carefully and self-critically removed are tumor-free and if it has been possible to remove a similarly broad margin of healthy tissue around the base of the tumor as in conventional operations.

The complications are no different from those encountered with surgery for chronic rhinosinusitis.

The domain of endonasal tumor surgery includes tumors of the nasal septum, the inferior turbinate and medial portions of the ethmoid complex, the middle meatus, and the sphenoid sinus. Depending on the type of tumor, neoplasms of the lateral and superior borders of the ethmoid complex and the maxilloethmoid junction can also be managed endonasally. Tumors extending further toward the maxillary sinus can be managed by a supplementary transoral procedure [333]. Depending on the histology of the tumor and the anatomic conditions, involvement of the frontal infundibulum may require an extended endonasal frontal sinus procedure [174] or a limited external approach [173, 996]. Smaller resections of the dura can also be conducted endonasally. Covering of the defect is carried out in the same manner as for management of CSF leaks [174].

There are reports in the literature of microscopic endonasal surgery for smaller, median frontal sinus osteomas whose base is situated on the posterior wall of the frontal sinus or in the infundibulum [174] (Fig. 6.**11**) and for angiofibromas. The last-named tumor may only be resected in combination with adequate embolization. Other authors create an additional limited external opening for management of osteomas in the frontal sinus access [87, 804]. Purely endoscopic endonasal surgery has been reported for a *sinus hamartoma* [910], a *giant cell granuloma*, and a *schwannoma* of the middle turbinate [59, 463], and for a *chondromyxoid fibroma* [374]. Excision of a schwannoma from the retromaxillary space under endoscopic guidance has also been reported [461].

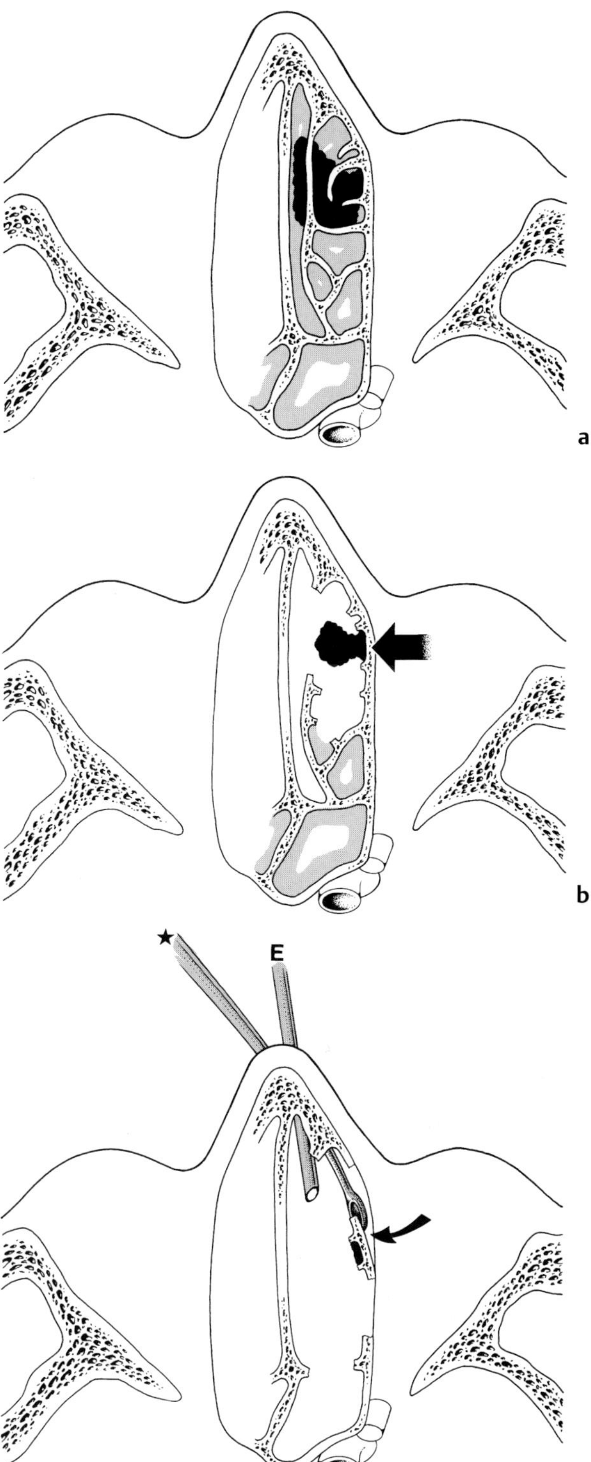

Fig. 6.**10a-c** **Steps of endonasal ethmoid surgery for benign tumors (a)** Axial section through an ethmoid cell system with a tumor (inverted papilloma, black) and concomitant secondary rhinosinusitis (gray). (**b**) Visualization of tumor base (arrow) following partial ethmoidectomy with resection of exophytic tumor mass. (**c**) Excision of the tumor base under constant endoscopic control, concomitant excision of the lamina papyracea (arrow) as safety zone. The periorbita is preserved. Completion of the ethmoidectomy. E, endoscope; ★, slim curette

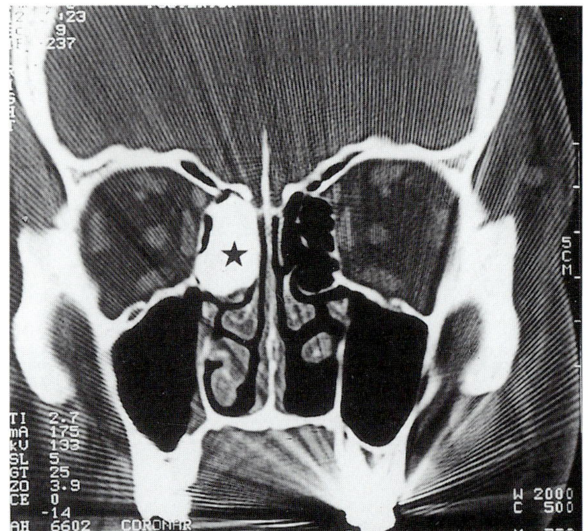

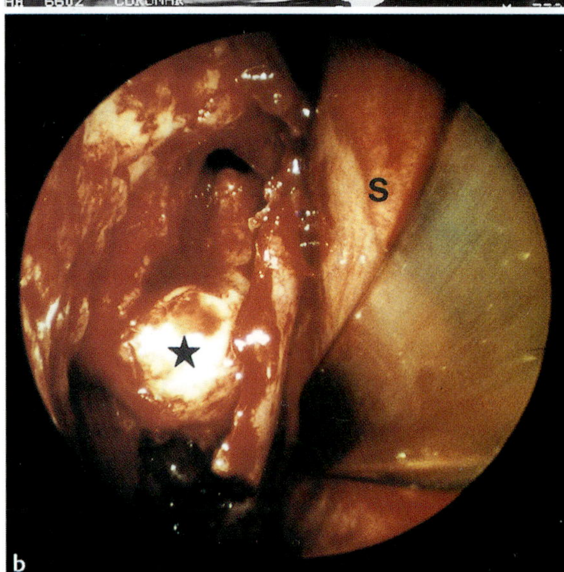

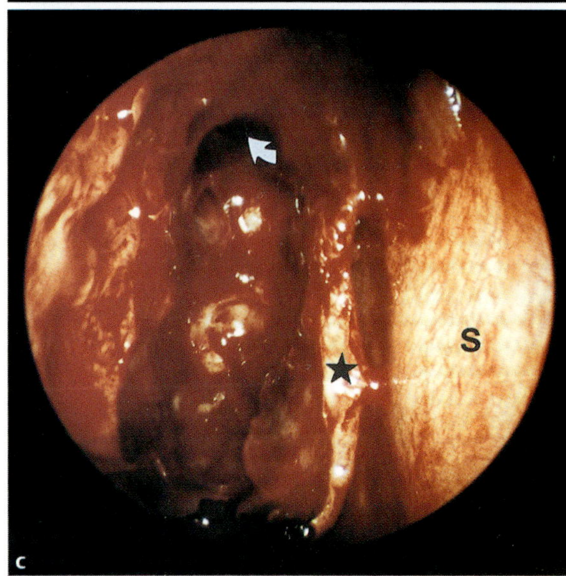

Fig. 6.**11a-c** **Endonasal surgery of benign tumors**
(**a**) Coronal CT of an osteoma (★) in the region of the right anterior ethmoid in a 29-year-old woman. (**b**) Exposure of the tumor (★) during an anterior ethmoidectomy. (**c**) View into the ethmoid complex following mobilization and extraction of the tumor. The vertical lamella of the middle turbinate (★) is preserved; the frontal sinus ostium (arrow) is patent

The most commonly encountered tumor that may be suitable for an endonasal resection is the *inverted papilloma*.

The rates of recurrence previously reported for endonasal ethmoid surgery performed without optical aids are unacceptable (Table 6.**7**). All authors report that inverted papillomas often show exophytic growth and may have a relatively narrow tumor pedicle that is concealed by sometimes severe concurrent secondary rhinosinusitis [408, 487–489]. Involvement of the nasopharynx is frequently only simulated [408]. Thus the indications and principles of treatment are essentially those already described [383] (Fig. 6.**12**). In isolated cases, the use of a potassium titanyl phosphate laser has been reported [502]. Caution must be exercised with tumors involving supraorbital cells or peripheral portions of the maxillary sinus, perilacrimal projections, and fingers of tumor extending into the frontal sinus ostium and olfactory groove [408]. Kamel [410] describes transnasal endoscopic medial maxillectomy for tumors of the medial wall of the maxillary sinus. Endonasal surgery is contraindicated in all cases where the tumor borders are not clearly visible, where the extent of the tumor or the prevailing anatomic conditions render it impossible to observe the above rules, or where there is invasion of extranasal structures with malignant transformation. Recurrences usually occur within 24 months [946]. While a number of authors advise against endonasal operations for recurrences [408, 487], others expressly recommend endonasal revision surgery [879, 946]. This also applies to recurrences after lateral rhinotomy [80].

Endonasal Surgery of Malignant Tumors

To a very limited extent, the criteria of endonasal tumor surgery also apply for malignant tumors. However, in these cases the decision to use an endonasal approach is associated with a special responsibility. Only tumors that can be excised with a broad safety margin in all directions are suitable. Malignant tumors with infiltration of, for example, the floor of the nose, the maxillary sinus, the base of the skull, the orbit, the retromaxillary space, the pterygopalatine fossa, and the nasopharynx are generally contraindicated.

Table 6.**7** Results of endonasal surgery for inverted papilloma

Author(s)	Patients	Size/location of tumors	Surgical technique	Follow-up period recurrences	Additional remarks
Cummings and Godman [135]	22 patients	?	No optical guidance Polypectomy, ethmoidectomy	2 y 73% recurrences	
Lawson et al. [487]	4 patients	?	No optical guidance Endonasal ethmoidectomy	24 mo	
Weissler et al. [979]	112 patients	?	No optical guidance	Ca 1 year, 71% recurrences	
Lawson et al. [489]	15 patients	Septum, inferior turbinate, middle meatus	No optical guidance? In some cases additional transoral surgery	6 y; 20%, recurrences	2 additional patients with endonasal revision surgery after recurrence following classical surgery
Stammberger [854]	15 patients	Middle meatus, ethmoid complex	Endoscopic	Follow-up?, 20% recurrences	
Hoffman et al. [333]	1 patient	Posterior septum	Microscopic	60 mo, no recurrences	3 further cases with additional transoral/transfacial surgery
Benninger et al. [47]	1 patient	?	Endoscopic	36 mo, no recurrences	66% recurrences after surgery without endoscope (n=6)
Kamel [408]	2 patients	Maxillary sinus, nasal cavity, nasopharynx	Endoscopic	23 mo, no recurrences	1 further case with additional transoral surgery
Waitz and Wigand [946]	27 patients	Ethmoid complex, skull base, sphenoid sinus, frontal sinus ostium	Endoscopic	46 mo, 17% recurrences	8 further cases with additional transoral surgery
Stankiewicz and Girgis [879]	10 patients	Nasal cavity, ethmoid complex, sphenoid sinus, medial wall of maxillory sinus	Endoscopic	36 mo, 33% recurrences	5 further cases with additional transoral surgery
McCary et al. [586]	7 patients	Lateral nasal wall, frontal recess, maxillary sinus	Endoscopic	19 mo without recurrences	
Buchwald et al. [80]	5 patients	Lateral nasal wall, ethmoid complex maxillary sinus	Endoscopic	24 mo without recurrences	Additional 6 recurrences after lateral rhinotomy, successful endoscopic operation
Kamel [410]	17 patients	(a) (n=8) lateral nasal wall; (b) (n=9) medial maxillary sinus.	Endoscopic (9 endoscopic “medial maxillectomies”)	(a) 43 mo, no recurrences (b) 28 mo, no recurrences	
Draf et al. [179]	14 patients	Ethmoid complex, maxillary sinus	Combined microscopic and endoscopic	1–5 years 1 recurrence in maxillary sinus	

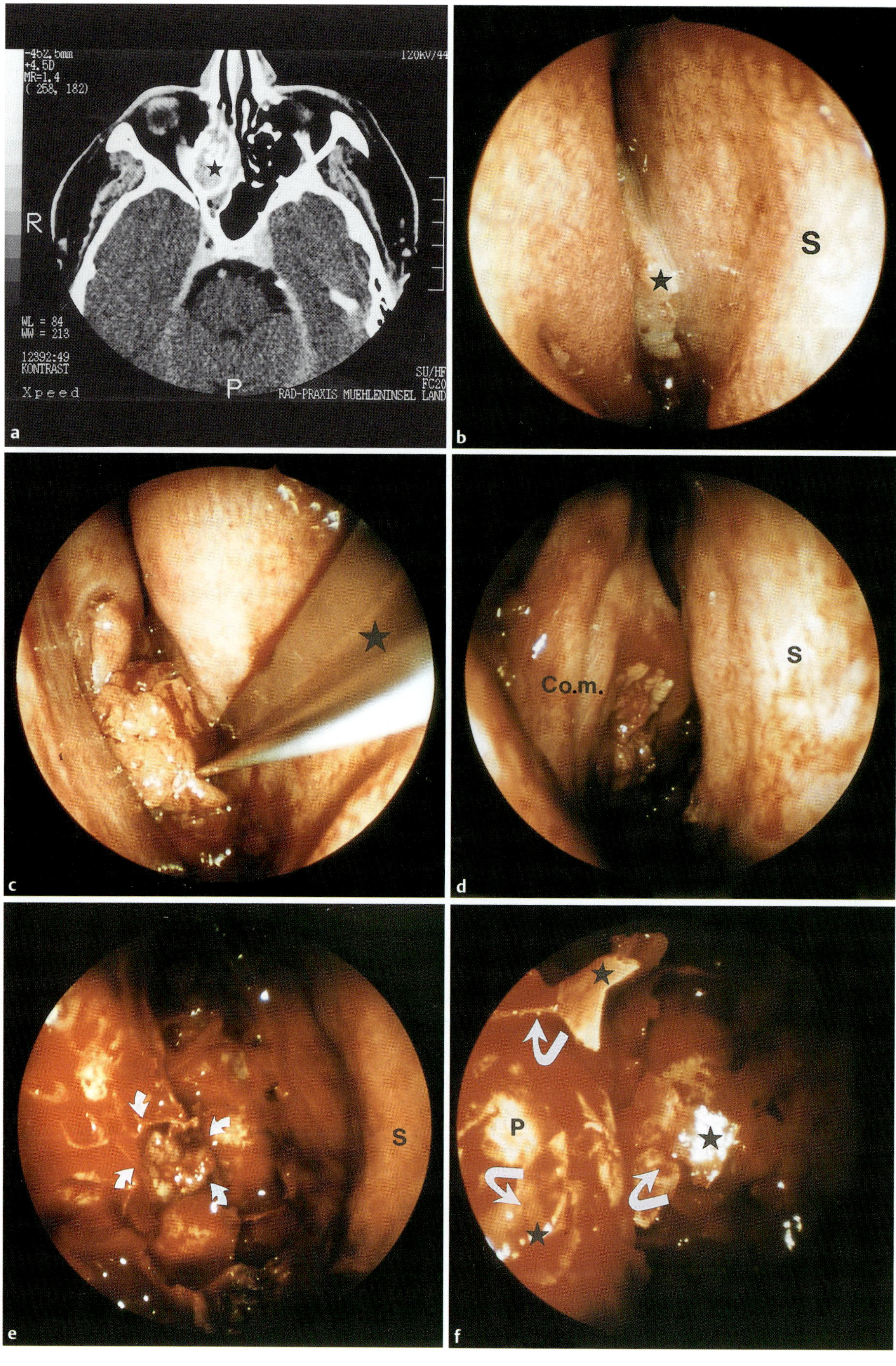
-452.5mm
+4.5D
MR=1.4
(258, 182)
120KV/44
R
WL = 84
WW = 213
12392:49
KONTRAST
Xpeed
P
SU/HF
FC20
RAD-PRAXIS MUEHLENINSEL LAND
a
S
b
c
Co.m.
S
d
S
e
P
f

◁ Fig. 6.**12a-f** **Endonasal surgery of an inverted papilloma of the right ethmoid complex in a 44-year-old man**
(**a**) Axial CT with visualization of the tumor mass (★). (**b**) Endoscopic view of the right nasal cavity before septoplasty. ★, tumor. (**c**) Endoscopic view following septoplasty (★, speculum). Tumor mass above the inferior turbinate. (**d**) After removal of exophytic portions of the tumor, the tumor can be followed into the superior meatus. The middle turbinate was displaced laterocaudally by the papilloma. Co.m., middle turbinate (concha media) S., nasal septum (**e**) After excision of further exophytic portions of the tumor and generous resection of the ethmoid it was possible to visualize the pedicle of the tumor (arrows) in the region of the superior lamina papyracea. (**f**) The tumor pedicle is removed together with the lamina papyracea. For demonstration purposes the lamina (★) is lifted "egg-shell" fashion and hinged back (arrows). The pieces are then removed. The tumor pedicle is excised under endoscopic control. The periorbita (P) is preserved

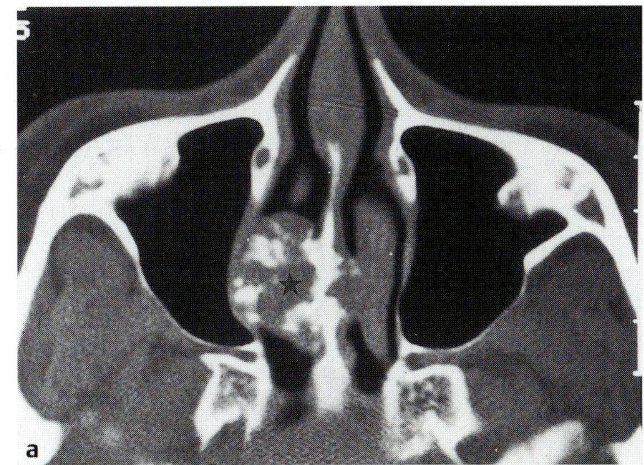

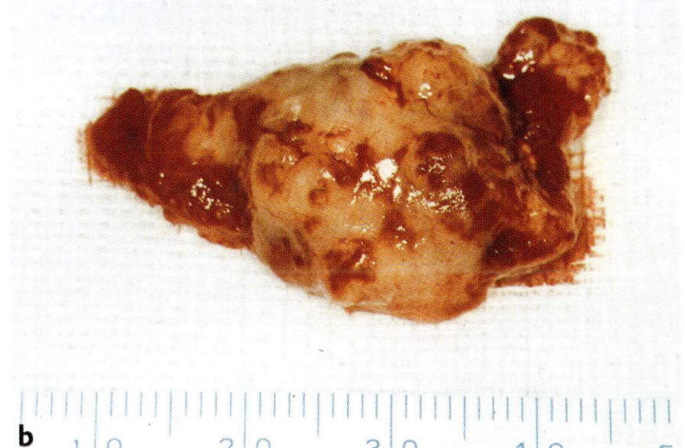

Fig. 6.**13a,b** **Endonasal surgery of a chondrosarcoma of the vomer in a 51-year-old man** ▷
(**a**) Axial CT showing the tumor (★). (**b**) Surgical specimen. Further revision resections were performed endonasally under endoscopic control

In 1986 Arnhold-Schneider and Minnigerode [17] presented two cases of ethmoid carcinoma in elderly patients that were managed by endonasal ethmoidectomy. The follow-up periods were 10 years and about two years, respectively. Stammberger [854] described a successful endonasal endoscopic operation for a malignant inverted papilloma. In a relatively small series, Hosemann and Wigand [352] reported the successful endonasal surgery of two carcinomas, two sarcomas, one malignant histiocytoma, and one esthesioneuroblastoma, with follow-up periods of 11–24 months (Fig. 6.**13**). Draf [177] describes endonasal microscope-assisted resection of five malignant tumors (one transitional cell carcinoma, one plasmacytoma, one esthesioneuroblastoma, one adenocystic carcinoma, and one metastasis of a breast carcinoma) with a follow-up period of 2–6 years. Recurrences occurred one and four years postoperatively in the case of the plasmacytoma and one year postoperatively at a different site in the case of the adenoid cystic carcinoma and were removed endonasally.

However, these anecdotal cases with a short follow-up must be compared with the gold standard of craniofacial resection, which has doubled the prognosis for some tumors such as adenocarcinoma and olfactory neuroblastoma while demonstrating the prognostic importance of adequate dural and orbital clearance [533]. The actuarial survival of most sinonasal malignancy cannot be judged in terms of five-year actuarial survival and long term data is mandatory before endoscopic approaches can be recommended.

Biopsies and Palliative Operations

Areas of unclear tissue hyperplasia in the region of the nose and paranasal sinuses are biopsied under endoscopic control. In isolated cases, this is also done for tumors of the medial orbit or the retromaxillary space [86]. The choice of surgical approach, e.g., partial ethmoidectomy, depends on the particular situation. In the latter cases, partial removal of the orbital floor, the lamina papyracea, or the posterior wall of the maxillary sinus is also performed. Similar techniques may also be used by ENT specialists for biopsy of tumors of the pituitary gland with minimal damage to the surrounding tissue [789]. Endoscopy also offers advantages in therapeutic surgery of the pituitary [257, 318, 1010].

In very advanced neoplastic disease, palliative endonasal removal of a tumor can lead to an improvement in the patient's quality of life [177]. Endonasal fenestration surgery conducted prior to radiation for maxillary carcinoma prevents retention of secretions and secondary inflammation.

Endonasal Surgery of the Skull Base

Endonasal management of *cerebrospinal fluid fistulas*was first described by Hirsch [331]. Modern optical aids often permit excellent endonasal visualization of the dural defect, precise and tissue-sparing dissection of the margin of the defect, and accurate placement of the graft material. Depending on the location of the dural opening, the patient's sense of smell is intact after the operation [348].

Stammberger [861] presented a detailed description of the specific diagnostic evaluation of frontal CSF fistulas in 1993. This was updated in 1997 by Stammberger and Wolf, including a special emphasis on the intrathecal administration of sodium fluorescein [868, 1002a]. Established CSF leaks in the anterior skull base are an absolute indication for surgical repair. A "wait and see" policy is not to be recommended [504, 590, 692, 877, 942].

Endonasal repair is suitable for small and middle-sized defects in the anterior skull base, i.e., leaks in the region of the sphenoid sinus, foveae ethmoidales and cribriform plate. More superiorly located defects of the posterior frontal sinus wall are not accessible endonasally. Leaks at the horizontal anterior skull base and sphenoid sinus can be visualized very well with a microscope. Defects in the lateral or inferior recesses of the sphenoid sinus can sometimes only be satisfactorily visualized with endoscopes with the appropriate viewing angles [11, 691, 692].

After endoscopic (fluorescein test) or radiographic (CT, cisternography) location of the defect, sinus operations of varying dimensions are conducted to gain access. The foveae ethmoidales are visualized by means of a conventional ethmoidectomy, and the sphenoid sinus by wide fenestration. Where necessary, the area of the defect is debrided and the fistula is visualized precisely with an endoscope or microscope (Fig. 6.**14**). The mucosa around the leak is pushed back 5 mm or removed. The defect is then closed. The recommended procedures for this vary widely. If the defect has a diameter less than 10 mm, a covering of soft tissue is sufficient. Mattox and Kennedy [572] are of the opinion that larger defects must be provided with a bony scaffold. Bone or cartilage is removed from the septum or nasal turbinates. In some cases, combined grafts consisting of both mucosa and bone are employed [164]. Wigand [994] obtains a free autologous flap of mucosa from the inferior turbinate, in some cases also from the middle turbinate. This is placed over the exposed defect in an overlapping fashion and fixed with fibrin glue. Free mucosal grafts of this kind are better for repairing small defects than are pedicled grafts [528], which can develop folds, become arched, or retract in an irregular fashion in the course of the healing process [164]. Pedicled grafts are, however, to be preferred after radiation [572]. Other authors use a single layer of allogenic connective tissue, muscle, fascia, or perichondrium and insinuate the pieces of tissue between the bone and the dura at the edges of the defect. The use of specially prepared allogeneic connective tissue is reportedly safe as regards the transmission of infection [157a, 967]. Fibrin glue is used as adhesive [32, 572, 942]. More reliable repair is expected if a second layer of tissue is stuck over the filled defect from below [861, 1022]. The muscle and fascia can be obtained from an incision in the region of the ear, though occasionally fascia lata is required and fat and fascia from the rectus abdominis muscle may be obtained from the periumbilical area [164, 504, 691, 877]. Often several materials are combined: pedicled turbinate flaps with free fascia and muscle [692] or fascia above the defect and muscle below it [877].

Lesions of the dura in the sphenoid sinus can be covered with a single layer like other lesions [348, 691, 792]. Other surgeons line the sinus generously with fascia, muscle, and fat after removing the mucosa [9, 572, 692, 733]. If the sinus is lined with fascia and filled with fat, it can also be sealed with a bony lamella on the side of the nose [11]. If the window created in the anterior wall of the sphenoid sinus is not made too large, the graft or inserted gelatin is well supported and packing in the main nasal cavity may not be required. In isolated cases, small defects in, for example, the sphenoid sinus are repaired with gelatin and fibrin glue alone [73, 877].

Defects of the anterior skull base due to fractures are often located posterior to the superior nasal spine in the inferior region of the frontal sinus ostium. In such cases, unobstructed drainage of the frontal sinus must be maintained after insertion of the graft. To achieve this, a large window is created in the frontal sinus or an extended frontal sinus operation is carried out. The graft is kept correspondingly thin and stuck on or pushed into the defect.

The grafts are secured with a layer of gelatin or pressed collagen sheeting placed against loose nasal packing [861, 877]. The packing is left in situ for 2–10 days [32, 164, 572, 960, 996]. The patients are instructed to remain in bed and to avoid straining and nose-blowing. The head end is raised [504, 789, 861]. Penicillin (3 × 10 000 000 U i. v. for two days followed by 3 × 1 000 000 U orally) is recommended as antibiotic prophylaxis. The antibiotics are stopped one day after removal of the packing [960]. Occasionally no antibiotics are given [877, 942, 967].

Some authors recommend postoperative insertion of lumbar drains for 3–4 days [572]. Others advise against use of lumbar drains or consider them indicated only in individual cases [861, 877, 942]. The results of surgery for repair of dural defects are summarized in Table 6.**8**. Weber and Draf [960] recommend investigating the outcome of the operation with fluorescein six weeks postoperatively [861]. They have subsequently changed this recommendation and performed the fluorescein-test after postoperative edema has completely disappeared.

Smaller *meningoceles and encephaloceles* of the anterior skull base can be managed in the same way as CSF fistulae [164]. Care should be taken that the choice and combination of grafts are suitable.

Mattox and Kennedy [572] report on the surgery of one meningocele and one encephalocele. The meningocele, which had a narrow base, was coagulated externally with a bipolar electrode. This caused the outer sac to shrink and withdraw into the relatively small bony defect in the base of the skull. The remaining bone defect was covered with a free mucosal graft. In the case of the encephalocele, the overlying mucosa was removed, the sac was reduced and the 1 × 1.5 cm bony defect in the skull base was closed with a piece of bone from the middle turbinate. The bone graft was covered with a pedicled mucosal flap from the turbinate.

In other cases, dural defects have been sealed after removal of smaller encephaloceles with a piece of septum between two layers of fascia [775] or with lyodura and fat [305]. In interdisciplinary operations in which a neurosurgeon closes an intracranial defect, remnants of the encephalocele can be removed endonasally without complications [999].

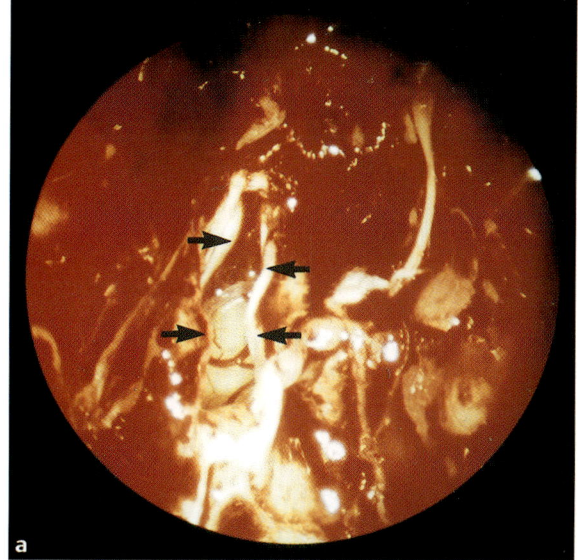

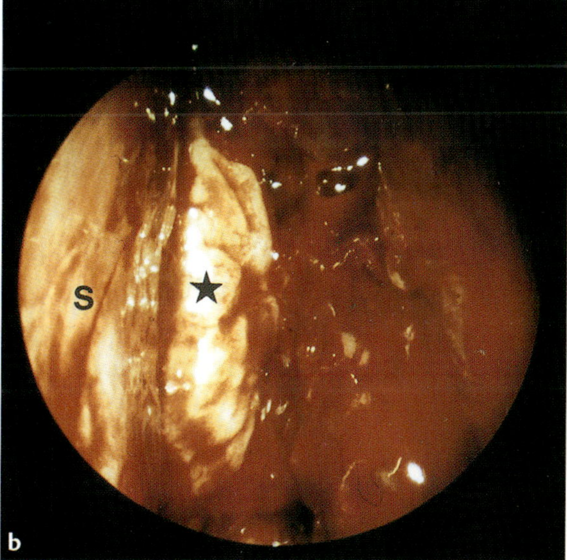

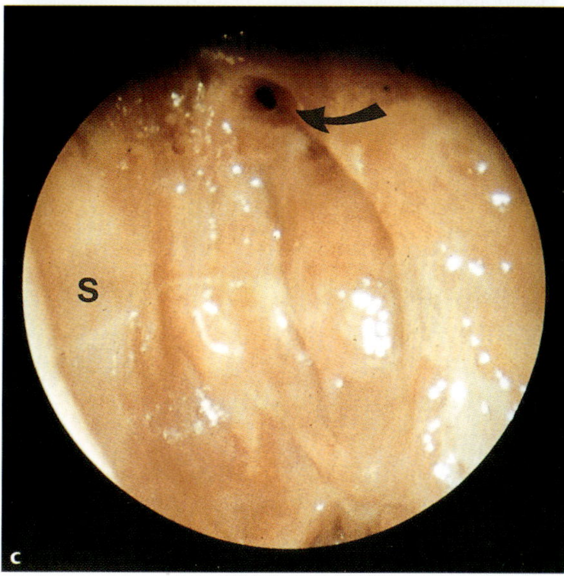

Fig. 6 **14a-c Endonasal closure of a defect in a patient with a left-sided iatrogenic CSF leak** ▷
(**a**) Defect in the anterior skull base (arrows) with CSF leak caused by avulsion of the superior attachment of the middle turbinate in a 38-year-old man with chronic diffuse rhinosinusitis. (**b**) The leak is covered with a free autologous turbinate graft (★). (**c**) Incorporation of the graft after three months. The frontal sinus ostium (arrow) is not obstructed

Table 6.**8** Endonasal repair of defects in the anterior skull base: review of the literature

Author(s)	Patients (no.)	Defect repair (method)	Follow-up	Results	Complications	Additional remarks
Wigand [993]	6	Autologous mucosa (free)	12 mo	100% success	None	
Papay et al. [692]	4	3 × fascia and muscle; 1 × additional mucosa (pedicled)	6–12 mo	100% success	1 × meningism postoperatively	
Mattox and Kennedy [572]	(a) 5 CSF fistula (b) 2: encephalocele	Autologous mucosa (free or pedicled)	?	(a) 80% success (b) 100% success	(a) 1 recurrence after nose-blowing (b) none	Recurrence with pedicled mucosal flap
Scher and Gross [789]	2	Autologous mucosa (free) (sphenoid sinus: filling consisting of temporal muscle)	3–4 mo	100% success	None	
Hosemann et al. [348]	18	Autologous mucosa (free)	17 mo	94% success after first operation	None	1 × second operation with healing
Stankiewicz [877]	8	5 × fascia/muscle (temporal muscle) 1 × fibrin glue	17 mo	100% success on intervention 50% success with conservative management	None	2 × conservative management
Weber et al. [973]	15	Preserved dura, fibrin glue	20–120 mo	100% success at first operation	None	
Amedee et al. [11]	22	12 × mucosa (free) 6 × abdominal fascia, fat, and pedicled mucosa 4 × fascia, fat, and bone	36 mo	95% success	2 × meningitis	10 × lumbar drainage
Dodson et al. [164]	29	Dermis and fat; fascia and fat; mucosa (free) +/− bone	3–443 mo	76% success after first operation	1 × cerebral abscess (2 months postoperatively)	4 patients closure by second craniotomy
Zeitouni et al. [1022]	4	Fascia lata	15 mo	75% success	1 × thigh infection	
Schick et al. [794]	72	Allogeneic connective tissue, fibrin glue, mucosal flap, underlay and onlay technique	1–16 y, on average 6 y	97% success after first operation, 100% success including endonasal revision		
Weber et al. [967]	42	Allogeneic connective tissue, fibrin glue, mucosal flap, underlay and onlay technique	6 mo – 15 y, on average 5 y	100% success	17% olfactory disturbances	Fluorescein test conducted in 20 patients 6 weeks postoperatively negative in all cases

Table 6.8 (continued)

Author(s)	Patients (no.)	Defect repair (method)	Follow-up	Results	Complications	Additional remarks
Schick et al. [793]	12	Allogeneic connective tissue, fibrin glue, mucosal flap, underlay and onlay technique	4 mo–12 y, on average 61 mo	92% success after first operation, 100% success including endonasal revision		12 out of 23 patients with late manifestation of prior cranial trauma, recurrence at cribriform plate
Stammberger et al. [868]	35	Allogenic connective tissue, mucosa, turbinate, fibrin glue	17–65 mo	91.7% success after first operation on the basis of individual operations	None	Success rate is based on total series of 72 patients 35 of whom underwent endonasal surgery, 24 external surgery, and 13 a combination
Schick et al. [792]	14	Allogeneic connective tissue, autogenic fascia lata, fibrin glue, mucosal flap, underlay, onlay, obliteration	on average 5 years	93% success after first op., 100% success incl. endonasal revision	None	

Endoscopic Surgery of Choanal Atresia

Transnasal, microscope-assisted surgery for choanal atresia is already one of the standard procedures of nasal surgery [313]. The reader is referred to the recognized text books on operative surgery [153] and reviews [714]. Operative methods and instrumentation have only recently begun to include endoscopic sinus surgery. Additional consideration of the more recent literature would therefore appear justified.

Transnasal choanal atresia surgery is suitable for well-defined atretic plates that are thin or that consist of connective tissue and in the absence of pronounced regional deformities (severe septal deviation, craniofacial malformation, substantial hyperplasia of the turbinates). An axial CT is required as a basis for planning the operation. The angle and thickness of the atretic plate, and the dimension and course of the lateral nasal wall, nasopharynx and nasal septum are analyzed.

The transnasal, microscope-assisted procedure can be carried out with a 250-mm or 300-mm endoscope [313, 714]. In the past, carbon dioxide and argon lasers have been used to remove atretic plates that were membranous or less than 1 mm thick [311, 565, 646]. A chisel or drill is better for removing thick bone. The operation can be performed transorally under the control of a rigid 110° or 120° endoscope or a flexible endoscope ("retropalatal endoscopic surgical technique") [43, 202]. The success rate for unilateral atresia is about 75% [149, 371, 565].

Endoscopes have also been employed in transnasal surgery. They provide good vision of the operative site, even under constricted anatomic conditions. However, in neonates the small nares make it difficult to manipulate the endoscope and drill simultaneously satisfactorily.

Following thorough decongestion, a cruciform or rectangular incision in the mucosa is made with a sickle knife above the atretic plate under the control of a 2.7-mm or 4-mm endoscope (0.25/30°). To improve visualization, the inferior turbinate is fractured laterally or upward. Otological microinstruments are used to raise the mucosa and a small inferomedial perforation is made in the exposed atretic plate with a chisel or diamond drill. Then the pharyngeal membrane is incised, forming further mucosal flaps. A pledget placed in the nasopharynx or an additional endoscope with a 110° or 120° angle of view in the oropharynx serves as an aid to orientation. The perforation can be extended medially with a punch by removing the posterior vomer and laterally using a drill. A back-biting punch is particularly suitable for insertion through the contralateral nasal cavity to punch out the vomer under direct vision. Finally, the mucosal flaps are placed over the exposed edges of bone. A silicone tube is placed for 2–12 weeks [202, 409, 876]. Intubation is not necessary in older patients with unilateral atresia [134]. The current literature on endoscopic surgery includes altogether 15 cases of unilateral and four cases of bilateral atresia in children or patients aged between five days and 18 years. Surgical revision was necessary in four cases, more frequently in small children or bilateral atresia.

Other Indications

The advantages of endonasal surgery also apply to certain areas of *fracture management*. External incisions are avoided or minimized even when a combination of approaches is employed and the supporting bony skeleton and mucosa are spared. Uncomplicated, closed fractures of the ethmoid without suspicion of concomitant fracture of the anterior skull base or trauma to the optic nerve are not an indication for endonasal debridement of the ethmoid complex. Even when severely traumatized, the ethmoid cell system has a strong tendency to spontaneous reventilation [354]. Two exceptions should be noted:

Blowout fractures of the medial wall of the orbit are relatively frequently associated with fracture of the orbital floor. In a small percentage of cases entrapment of the medial rectus muscle or a clinically relevant herniation of the orbit into the ethmoid complex with enophthalmus and persisting diplopia may ensue. In such cases, surgical treatment is indicated after examination by an otolaryngologist and ophthalmologist and adequate imaging (CT).

Ozawa et al. [688] presented an endonasal microscopic and endoscopic operation technique in 1984. The anterior ethmoid is carefully opened by a modified technique. If possible, the uncinate process is preserved and only the bulla ethmoidalis is resected to permit visualization of the lamina papyracea. For Michel [611], the technique of choice is ethmoidectomy with broad fenestration of the frontal sinus and reduction of the middle turbinate. The ethmoid complex is debrided, sparing periorbita and fat (Fig. 6.**15**). The herniated orbital contents are exposed, reduced back into the orbit and fixed laterally with silicone film. Alternatively, a piece of allogenic connective tissue or a piece of PDS film may be inserted between the remains of the lamina papyracea and the periorbita and fixed with fibrin glue. The reconstructed area may be closed with autologous mucosal flaps if desired. A piece of 0.5-mm thick silicone film is then folded and pushed into the ethmoid shaft with the convex side facing superiorly. A piece of antibiotic-impregnated gauze is inserted as spacer between the two leaves of the film. Alternatively, sponge packing (Merocel) can be swelled in doxycycline solution. Reduction and fixation can also be achieved by insertion of an ethmoid balloon catheter as described by Milewski. The gauze must be changed every week. After 4–6 weeks it is removed completely. Michel [611] leaves the packing for only eight days. The operation can be conducted under microscopic, endoscopic, or video-endoscopic control [611, 1012]. All seven patients in Michel's report were free of diplopia after healing. Whether similarly good results can be obtained where enophthalmus is the presenting symptom remains to be demonstrated in view of the different pathophysiology in such cases [302].

In cases of *fracture of the frontoethmoidal junction* with obstruction of the frontonasal recess, endonasal reventilation of the frontal sinus may be indicated. Even after reduction of the external skeleton, between one-third and one-quarter of cases of fractured frontal sinus ostia react with chronic frontal rhinosinusitis [354, 577]. In these cases, endonasal frontal sinus fenestration is indicated as part of the overall fracture management after adequate radiographic diagnosis (CT) and may be performed either immediately or after an interval with CT monitoring. In doubtful cases, a combination of the endonasal approach with transfrontal endoscopy of the frontal sinus permits simultaneous exclusion of fractures of the posterior wall of the frontal sinus [336].

Midface fractures can lead to a persistent disturbance of maxillary sinus drainage. In up to 50% of cases of severe trauma there is radiological evidence of chronic maxillary rhinosinusitis after reduction and refixation. There is often thickening of the mucosa in the region of the medial wall of the maxillary sinus and solitary or multiple polyps and mucoceles [354, 470]. Permanent mucosal reactions are also observed in the presence of functioning sinus ostia [788]. Thus, as a rule there is no correlation between the symptoms and endoscopic and CT findings. Treatment is therefore selected individually on the basis of all findings and complaints.

Treatment-resistant, *paranasal rhinosinusitis of dental origin* can be managed by nasal surgery following dental treatment of the primary focus (Fig. 6.**16**). Depending on the severity and extent of the sinus involvement, the endonasal surgery is performed, after institution of antibiotic therapy, either immediately after the dental treatment or at a later date after a follow-up CT scan. Draf and Weber [178] perform endonasal maxillary sinus surgery following removal of the dental focus in all cases. Davidson and Stearns [140] report on a dental implant that was extracted from the floor of the maxillary sinus through the middle meatus under transoral endoscopic control.

Patients in intensive care often show radiological opacification of the sinuses. This applies to 100% of patients with nasotracheal intubation and 43% of patients with a nasogastric tube, usually after 5–7 days [68]. The pattern of mucositis differs from that in

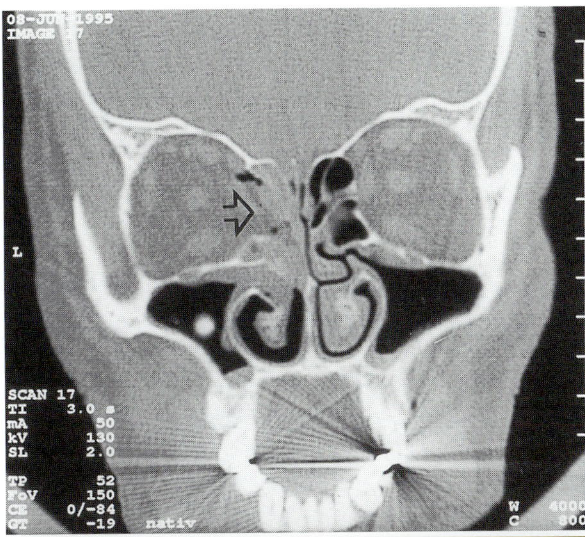

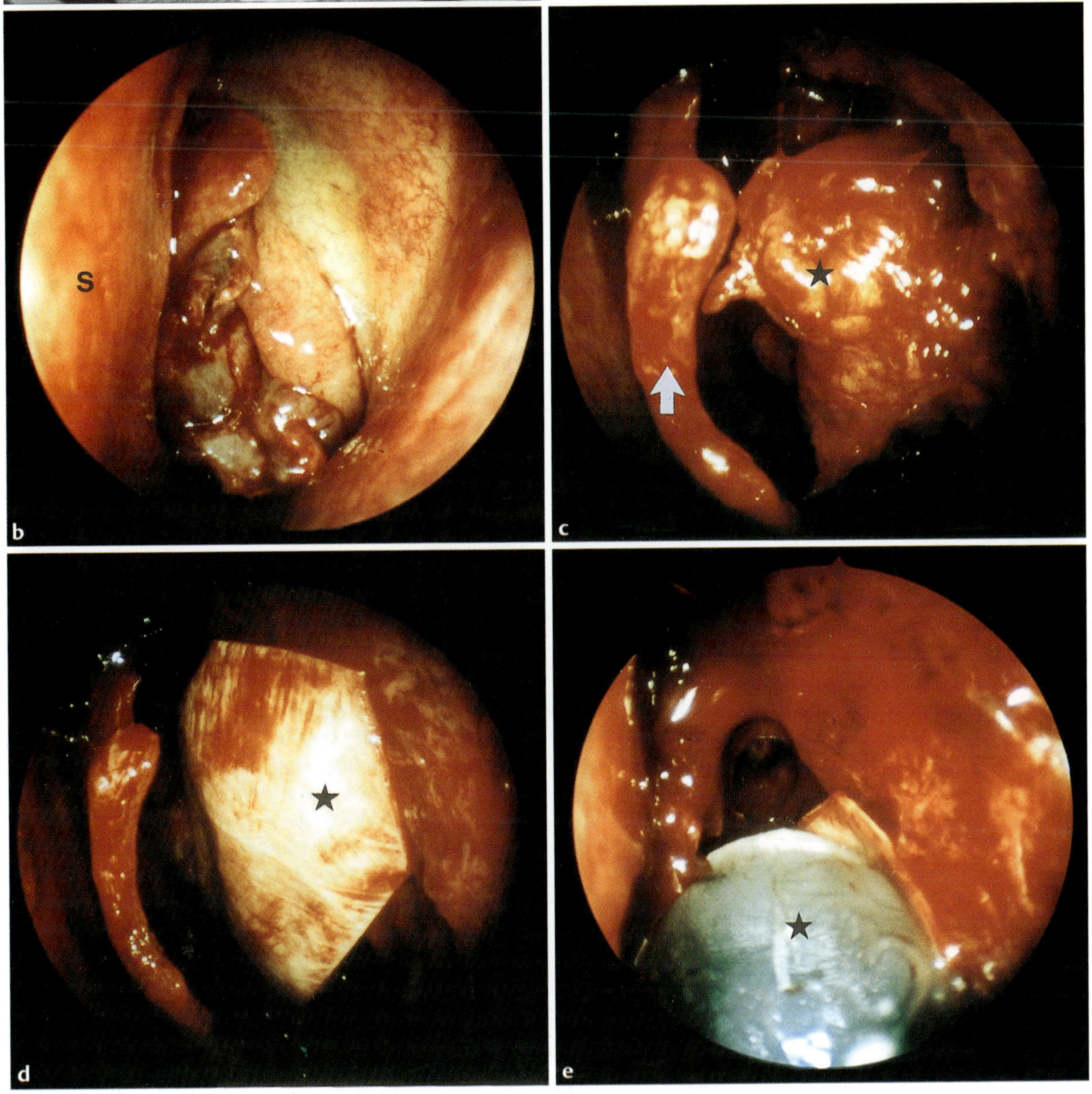

Fig. 6.**15a-e Endonasal management of left-sided medial fracture of the orbital wall in a 38-year-old man**
(**a**) Coronal CT showing herniation of orbital fat and muscle tissue into the ethmoid (arrow). (**b**) Endoscopy prior to surgery. (**c**) The herniated orbital tissue (★) is exposed during ethmoidectomy sparing other tissues. Arrow indicates preserved vertical lamella of the middle turbinate. (**d**) The herniated tissue is covered with a piece of allogenic connective tissue (★) and later reduced back in the direction of the orbit. (**e**) The outcome of the reduction is secured by inserting a small balloon catheter (★) for three weeks

S

b

c

d

e

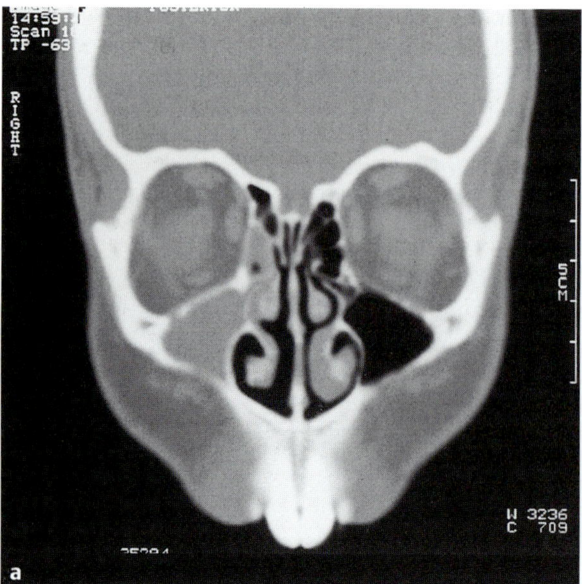

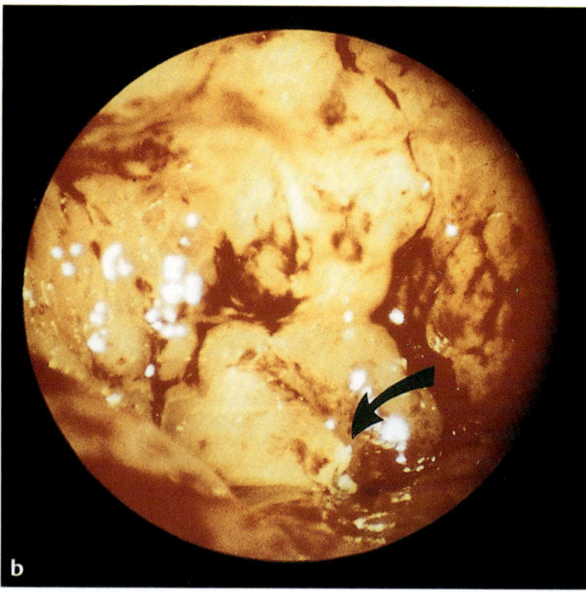

Fig. 6.**16a,b** **Endonasal surgery of the ethmoid and maxillary sinuses in paranasal rhinosinusitis of dental origin**
(**a**) Coronal CT showing total opacification of the right maxillary sinus with secondary involvement of the middle nasal turbinate. The dental focus was visualized by means of an orthopantomogram. (**b**) Performance of an anterior ethmoidectomy with fenestration of the ipsilateral maxillary sinus. The dental lesion and fistula (arrow) on the floor of the maxillary sinus can be visualized through the middle meatus using a 70° endoscope. This operation is immediately followed by appropriate dental surgery

chronic rhinosinusitis: the ethmoid is involved in only 50% of cases, while the sphenoid and maxillary sinuses are each affected in 87% of cases and the frontal sinus in 12.5% [215]. These findings gain significance in connection with the discussion on “fever of unknown origin” [294, 339, 509]. Despite the radiological signs described, clinically the fever can be attributed to the rhinosinusitis in only about 5% of cases. Conservative treatment is usually successful. Surgery is indicated only in rare cases after failure of conservative therapy and elimination of the triggering factors (nasogastric, endotracheal tube). The operation can be performed under endoscopic control at the patient’s bed in the intensive care unit.

Surgery of the vidian nerve is described in classical text books of operative surgery [153]. A number of more recent papers have appeared since the introduction of optical aids. However, the clinical significance of this operation is diminishing owing to its uncertain indication, poorly understood pathophysiology, and unpleasant side effects. Vasomotor rhinitis or excessive, watery rhinorrhea as presenting symptom are the indications given. Extended indications are refractory allergic rhinitis and recurrent nasal polyposis.

The local anatomy varies widely [29]. None the less, a number of standardized procedures are given in the literature. Portmann et al. [720] find the pterygoid canal 5–6 mm posterior to the sphenopalatine foramen using a microscope. The superior maxillary foramen is located 7–10 mm further laterally. The endonasal approach is helped by the fact that the sphenopalatine foramen is at an angle of 15–20° to the sagittal plane. The nerve is coagulated with a special bayonet-shaped electrode [220].

The operation is also conducted under endoscopic control by a similar approach [204, 411]. El-Guindy [201] presents a transseptal endoscopic technique; 88% of patients thus treated are reportedly satisfied with the postoperative result. Head and facial pain persisting for some weeks is frequently observed [220]. In smaller series, roughly 30% of patients suffer from postoperative xerophthalmia that requires treatment [201, 411].

Pneumosinus dilatans develops as a result of abnormal expansion of the frontal sinus. The walls of the sinus are of normal thickness, but bulge either outward or intracranially. The patient suffers from cosmetic disfigurement, diplopia, headache, or localized pressure. *Pneumocele* is a similar syndrome with similar symptoms and focal or generalized thinning of the sinus wall [932]. The development of both phenomena can be arrested by endonasal operative drainage and ventilation of the involved sinuses [1004]. Bachor et al. [24] report on a patient with pneumosinus dilatans of the sphenoid sinus. While mountain climbing, the patient developed frontal headache and a reversible loss of vision due to compression of the exposed optic nerve. The patient was freed of his symptoms by endonasal fenestration of the sphenoid sinus. A similar case was successfully treated endonasally by Som et al. [843].

Sinus barotrauma is a comparable condition. In severe barotrauma of, for example, the frontal sinus, surgical improvement of ventilation can lead to immediate resolution of symptoms [178]. Straatman and Buiter [891] report on several cases of baroheadache originating from the maxillary sinus. Diagnostic aspiration of the maxillary sinus led to immediate cure of acute symptoms. Definitive treatment consists of endonasal infundibulotomy with maxillary sinus fenestration [104]. When the location of the symptoms is unclear, surgical ventilation of several sinuses during exploration of the anterior ethmoid may become necessary. This technique is a blessing for pilots, most of whom are able to resume flying after the operation [62, 695]. The condition must be distinguished from the "*middle turbinate headache syndrome*" [279], which has been attributed to contact between an usually enlarged middle turbinate and the lateral nasal wall or septum and leads to headache located in the periorbital, supraorbital, or temporozygomatic regions. During a pain attack, application of cocaine to the specific sites of contact, e.g., in the region of the middle turbinate, leads to resolution of the symptoms. This test is the precondition for specific operative treatment, e.g., septoplasty or partial resection of the middle turbinate.

In rare cases, chronic subclinical maxillary rhinosinusitis can lead to atrophy of the bony walls of the maxillary sinus with retractions in the form of *hypoplasia or atelectasis of the maxillary sinus*. The exact pathological mechanism is not known, but suggested causes are stenosis or the formation of valves at the maxillary ostium. Characteristic CT findings are lateralization of the middle meatus and/or lateralization of the middle turbinate and a hypoplastic uncinate process. The collapse of the walls of the maxillary sinus may result in enophthalmus with depression of the middle third of the face [14]. Treatment consists in reventilation of the maxillary sinus by endonasal surgery. The anterior ethmoid is explored and the middle meatus is fenestrated. The middle turbinate is reduced if necessary. It may prove difficult to identify the hypoplastic uncinate process. Attention should be paid to the close proximity of the orbit [58, 976].

A number of authors also use endoscopy routinely for *septal surgery*. Endoscopic inspection of conventional mucosal tunnels offers limited benefit over conventional techniques, although circumscribed posterior deviations of the septum can be managed by making separate incisions in the mucosa within the nose under the control of a straight endoscope. The mucosa is incised immediately anterior to the spur and a circumscribed bilateral tunnel is created. The spur is removed with forceps or a chisel. The mucosal flaps are then approximated. Reimplantation of septal material is often unnecessary. The operation can be conducted under local anesthesia and is excellent for teaching purposes. As in all nasal surgery, occasional septoturbinal synechiae may develop [71, 268, 460, 860]. Nasopharyngeal cysts can, of course, also be removed endoscopically, either together with other procedures or as a separate procedure [899].

7 Complications, Side Effects, and Sequelae

Type and Incidence of Complications

The specific risks of endonasal sinus surgery have long been recognized [319, 540, 585, 756]. Stammberger [861] published a detailed report of iatrogenic complications in 1993. Medicolegal aspects of optically guided procedures have been described by Hosemann et al. [351] and Hosemann and Kühnel [356]. The comments below are limited where possible to the recent literature relating to routine sinus surgery.

In the United States, endoscopic sinus procedures are the commonest cause of medicolegal disputes in the sphere of ENT medicine [748]. In this connection, it is sensible to separate minor complications from major ones. Of the major complications, a further distinction should be drawn between those that can be corrected and those which cannot [955]. A modified classification by May et al. [582] gives the following summary. Among the major complications, disastrous events are underlined: death or neurological deficit, impairment or loss of vision and permanent diplopia.

Classification of complications of endonasal sinus surgery (modified after May et al. [582])

Minor complications

- Bronchospasm
- Periorbital emphysema
- Bleeding into the lids
- Epistaxis requiring nasal packing
- Dental or lip pain or numbness
- Adhesions requiring treatment
- Postoperative atrophic rhinitis

Major complications

- Epiphora requiring surgery
- Loss of intact sense of smell
- Hemorrhage requiring transfusion
- Cerebrospinal fluid leak
- Orbital hematoma (post septal)
- Postoperative meningitis
- Diplopia persisting for weeks/permanent diplopia
- Impairment or loss of vision
- Brain hemorrhage, cerebral abscess
- Injury to the carotid artery

The rate of complications depends on the extent of the operation, and also on the nature and severity of the disease, on previous procedures, the specific anatomy of the patient, and finally on various factors relating to the surgeon.

Larger collations of statistics reveal serious complications in less than 0.5% of patients, with a wide variation in reports. Minor complications must be expected in around 3% of patients [412, 442, 913]. Tables 7.**1**–7.**3** summarize the findings from the literature. To improve comparability, the results are grouped according to the categories shown in the summary above. The listing of more than one complication per patient may lead to some error in calculation of the percentages.

A review of the literature shows, surprisingly, that the overall rate of complications in endonasal sinus surgery has not been changed greatly by the introduction of *optical aids*. The risk is also low for procedures using the headlight, rates being comparable to those for optically guided or transfacial operations. It is worth noting, however, that a survey by Kennedy et al. [442] recorded disastrous sequelae, in particular, more often in surgery without optical aids. The profile of complications may therefore vary with the individual technique [583, 952], but statistically significant differences cannot be identified even comparing endoscopic, microscopic, and video-guided operating techniques [154, 218, 240, 442, 590, 733, 861, 942, 954].

Other surgeons have had the opposite experience and expect a higher rate of complications where optical aids are not used [960]. It has therefore been proposed that, for medicolegal reasons, surgeons should be under an obligation to use some form of optical aid [955] and, in spite of some opposition [840, 859], it is now standard procedure in most units to keep optical aids available at all times during endonasal procedures.

The individual operator has a *learning curve*, which can be seen from a decreasing rate of complications with increasing experience in handling the optical aids [370, 406, 428, 869–871, 955]. In analyses performed by Stankiewicz, the rate fell from 29–31% for the first 90 patients to 2.2% in the later course [869–871]. It is debatable whether serious complications tend to occur more often in younger colleagues [730, 955]. Serious complications in medicolegal cases might also be caused by older surgeons [346]. In a survey by Cumberworth et al. [133], serious complications were reported for doctors who had, on average, already performed 345 operations. In the overall statistics for larger departments, no learning curve can be observed after the establishment of endonasal surgical techniques, reflecting the constant change in the active operators [942]. In an analysis of the first

Table 7.1 Incidence of complications of endonasal ethmoid sinus surgery without optical aids. Authors' reports adapted to the classification of May et al. [582]

Author	No. of patients (P), sides (S)	Procedure Optical aids	Major complications Percentage of patients (P), sides (S)	Minor complications Percentage of patients (P), sides (S)
Eichel [195]	123 (P) 236 (S)	Ethmoidect.[a] without optical aids	1 diplopia for weeks 1 transfusion 1 CSF fistula 1 meningitis = 3.2% (P)/1.7% (S)	
Tylor et al. [905]	284 (P) 526 (S)	Ethmoidect.[a] without optical aids	3 CSF fistulae 1 retroorbital hemorrage = 1.4% (P)/0.8% (S)	2 postoperative hemorrage 2 × headaches 3 adhesions 1 palatine neuritis = 2.8% (P)/1.5% (S)
Stevens and Blair [884]	87 (P) 230 (S) (includes 60 (S) revisions)	Pansinus[a] without optical aids	3 retroorbital hemorrage 3 hemorrage requiring transfusion = 6.9% (P)/2.6% (S)	6 periorbital hemorrhages 2 postoperative hemorrhages = 9.2% (P)/3.5% (S)
Sogg [839]	146 (P) 276 (S)	Various procedures without optical aids	0%	1–2% of patients periorbital edema, ecchymosis
Friedman and Katsantonis [240]	1163 (S)	Pansinus without optical aids	4 CSF fistulae 3 hemorrhages = 0.6% (S)	17 cases of asthma 2 atrophic rhinitis 4 epistaxis 3 orbital edema = 2.2% (S)
Sogg and Eichel [841]	3000 (S)	Ethmoidect.[a] without optical aids	5 CSF fistulae 2 hemorrhages with transfusion = 0.2% (S)	270 lid hematoma 12 postoperative hemorrage = 9.4% (S)

[a] Abbreviations: Ethmoidect.: extensive (complete) ethmoidectomy; *Micr./end.* : combined microscopic and endoscopic surgery; Pansinus: pansinus operation.

300 operations of five now- experienced operators, it was shown that the risk of dural lesion was highest during the initial phase (approximately 30 procedures). In an analogy with traffic lights, this was described as the red phase. This was followed by a phase of increased numbers of orbital lesions (amber phase) until, after approximately 200 procedures, a stable low rate of complications was reached (green phase) [428, 430]. In a review of the literature, the rate of complications for departments with extensive surgical teaching activities was shown as 8–34% and that for departments with a low teaching capacity as 2–5% [730]. The figures given in publications from the larger training hospitals must therefore be assessed in the light of this [959].

Attendance of clinical training courses unfortunately has no positive effect in principle on the rate of complications. After such training, surgeons operate more extensively or with an increased feeling of self-confidence. Conflicting reports are given for training on cadaver specimens, which may offer a rather more reliable learning aid with regard to avoidance of complications [133, 442].

There is agreement in the literature concerning the increase in *surgical risk after a previous operation* leading to the loss of landmarks [154, 865]. This applies particularly to the risk of iatrogenic injuries to the base of the skull where the middle turbinate is missing and also to orbital complications where there is regional scarring [129, 942].

The majority of authors observe that in right-handed operators CSF fistulas and damage to the optic nerve and orbit occur more often on the *right side* [154, 546, 733, 873, 877, 960]. This connection is questioned in other reports [351, 364, 942].

The use of *local anesthesia* in sinus operations provides the possibility of important warning indications that complications are threatened or may even have occurred: manipulations to the base of the skull or lamina papyracea trigger pain stimuli, while alterations in the area of the optic nerve can produce pain or visual disturbances. A local anesthetic contributes indirectly to safety by reducing blood loss. The use of local anesthesia trains the operator to undertake circumspect or cautious dissection. In summary, local anesthesia is reported to contribute to the safety of

Table 7.**2** Incidence of complications in endonasal ethmoid sinus surgery with the microscope. Authors' reports adapted to the classification of May et al. [582]

Author	No. of patients (P), sides (S)	Procedure Optical aids	Major complications Percentage of patients (P), sides (S)	Minor complications Percentage of patients (P), sides (S)
Bagatella and Mazzoni [32]	155 (P) 290 (S)	Ethmoidect.[a] Microscope	6 CSF fistulae = 3.9% (P)/2.1% (S)	13 adhesions 8.4% (P)/4.5% (S)
Silverstein and McDaniel [829]	31 (P)	Pansinus[a] Microscope	2 hemorrhages 1 meningitis 1 possible CSF fistula = 13% (P)	1 reversible diplopia 1 hemorrhage = 6% (P)
Amedee et al. [10]	325 (P)	Pansinus[a] Microscope	(0%)	(0%)
McFadden et al. [590]	25 (P) 64 (S)	Partly with microscope Partly with endoscope	2 CSF fistulae 1 hematoma = 12% (P)/5% (S)	1 bronchospasm = 4% (P)/1.6% (S)
Ilberg et al. [370]	221 (P)	Various procedures Micr./end.[a]	3 CSF fistulae = 1.4% (P)	3 lid hematomas 2 hemorrhage = 1.8% (P)
Teatini et al. [906]	(a) 78 (P) (b) 22 (P)	(a) Micr.[a] (b) Micr./end.[a]	(a) – (0%) (b) – (0%)	(a) 15 lid hematoma = 19% (S) (b) lid hematomas = 14% (S)
Draf and Weber [175] (15 operators)	170 (P) 340 (S)	Pansinus[a] Micr./end.[a]	12 hemorrhages 15 dural injuries 2 carotid artery injuries = 17% (P)/9% (S)	2 x periorbital injury 1 x dental or lip numbness = 2.2% (P)
Weber and Draf [960]	1178 (S)	Pansinus[a] Micr./end[a]	30 injuries to dura (2.55%) (S) 2 injuries to carotid artery (0.17%) (S)	40 periorbital injuries (3.4%) (S)

[a] For abbreviations, see Table 7.**1**

the procedures [548, 860]. The fact that more extensive procedures tend to be carried out under general anesthesia no doubt plays a role in these observations.

Comparative investigations, however, frequently show no difference between general and local anesthesia with regard to the frequency of complications [269, 838, 942]. In rare individual cases, particular complications are observed after local anesthesia: Hill et al. [328] reported total spinal anesthesia after injection of around 3 mL lidocaine 2% with epinephrine into the anterior ethmoid during an anterior ethmoidectomy. The anesthetic must have entered the subarachnoid space either directly as a result of inadvertent puncture of the subarachnoid space or indirectly via the olfactory plexus. Three minutes later there was sudden dilatation of the pupils proceeding to apnea and coma. The situation was controlled by intubation and ventilation and persisted for 35 minutes. Where cocaine and epinephrine (1:1000) are given simultaneously, persistent swelling of the nasal mucosa is seen in rare cases, with a tendency to ischemic necrosis [4]. Because of this interaction, the simultaneous administration of these two substances must be regarded with extreme caution in nasal surgery. The maximum total dose of cocaine is 200–300 mg.

Individual Complications

Asthma attacks occur more often in patients treated under local anesthesia [583]. The incidence is around 1% [240, 247, 433]. Those affected are mainly patients with severe asthma in whom bronchospasm is recorded in up to 40% [207]. In rare cases, interruption of the procedure may be necessary [238]. Hoffmann [337] reported two fatal cases of status asthmaticus during procedures under local anesthesia.

The typical mechanism of *injury to the nasolacrimal duct* is excessive widening of the maxillary sinus window in the middle meatus in the anterior direction, particularly with the back-biting punch [65, 271, 810] (Fig. 7.**1a**). Overenthusiastic resection in the region of the root of the uncinate process or an agger nasi cell can also lead to damage. Caudally, the duct is protected by the slightly thicker ethmoid process of the inferior turbinate. Superiorly, however, it is surrounded only by the thin lacrimal bone. On the ethmoid side, the bony dividing wall may be absent here, aplasia of the lacrimal bone having been reported [221]. The mean distance between the natural maxillary ostium and the nasolacrimal duct is 9 mm (5–18 mm) [93]. In difficult cases it is advisable to expose the lacrimal ducts intraoperatively [175, 733].

Table 7.**3** Incidence of complications of endonasal ethmoid sinus surgery with the endoscope. Authors' reports adapted to the classification of May et al. [582]

Author	No. of patients (P), sides (S)	Procedure Optical aids	Major complications Percentage of patients (P), sides (S)	Minor complications Percentage of patients (P), sides (S)
Friedrich [247]	65 (P) 113 (S)	Ethmoidect.[a] Endoscope	1 Orbital hematoma = 1.5% (P), 0.9% (S)	1 hemorrhage 1 asthma attack = 3.1% (P), 1.8% (S)
Kennedy and Zinreich [437]	95 (S)	Various procedures Endoscope	2 × postoperative epiphora = 2% (S)	0%
Toffel et al. [919]	170 (P) 335 (S)	Various procedures Endoscope	1 hemorrhage = 0.6% (P); 0.3% (S)	1 × adhesions 5 hemorrhages = 3.5% (P); 1.8% (S)
Wigand [996]	220 (P) 419 (S)	Pansinus[a] Endoscope	2 CSF fistulae 1 orbital hematoma = 1.3% (P); 0.7% (S)	4 asthma attacks 4 neuralgias 1 adhesion (mucocele) = 4% (P); 2.1% (S)
Stammberger and Posawetz [865]	4500 (P)	Various procedures Endoscope	3 CSF fistulae 2 orbital hematomas = < 0.1% (P)	?
Stammberger and Posawetz [865]	500 (P)	Various procedures Endoscope	1 hemorrhage = 0.2% (P)	3 lid emphysemas 2 lid hematomas 11 hemorrhages 10 × operations discontinued due to hemorrhage 5 soft tissue infiltrates 1 pack left = 6% (P)
Kennedy [433]	120 (P) 224 (S)	Endoscope 108 Pansinus 74 Ethmoidect. 42 Partial ethmoidectomy	= 0%	1 bronchospasm = 0.8% (P); 0.4% (S)
Vleming et al. [942]	667 (P) 1235 (S)	Various procedures Endoscope	2 orbital hematomas 2 CSF fistulae 2 hemorrhages, 1 × epiphora = 1% (P), 0.6% (S)	16 injuries to lamina papyrocea 11 hemorrhages 15 adhesions = 6.3% (P), 3.4% (S)
Lund and MacKay [528]	650 (P)	Various procedures Endoscope	1 CSF fistula 1 orbital hematoma = 0.3% (P)	?
Ramadan and Allen [730]	337 (P)	Various procedures Endoscope	3 CSF fistulae 1 × epiphora = 1.1% (P)	21 adhesions 13 injuries to periorbital area = 10% (P)
Dessi et al. [154]	386 (P)	Various procedures Endoscope + monitor	3 orbital hematomas 2 CSF fistulae = 1.3% (P)	?

[a] For abbreviations, see Table 7.**1**

Complete transsection of the nasolacrimal duct may be clinically asymptomatic, provided that a fistula is formed into the nasal cavity. In other cases the duct is crushed or fractured [65]. In around 1% of all paranasal sinus operations, epiphora is seen immediately after the operation or up to two or three weeks later [810]. At most half of iatrogenic fistulas close in the course of postoperative scar formation, with the result that symptoms develop slowly. It is therefore possible to wait before performing corrective endonasal dacryocystorhinostomy [65, 569]. The diagnostic evaluation is as for spontaneous stenosis of the lacrimal duct.

Damage to the periorbita usually occurs during resection of the uncinate process, during removal of the bulla ethmoidalis, during fenestration of the maxillary sinus, or in general during manipulations following previous operations or fractures with existing dehiscence of the lamina papyracea [861, 873] (Fig. 7.**1b**). The incidence is around 2% (Tables 7.**1**-7.**3**). Fat bulges out through the lacerated periorbita and is readily identifiable by its yellow color and glistening appearance. The *pressure test described by Draf and Stankiewicz* is a useful aid to diagnosis [178, 873] (Fig. 7.**1**c): repeated careful application of pressure to the outside of the patient's eyeball with two fingers produces corresponding movements of the bulging fat that are easily identifiable with the endoscope or microscope. Limited injuries to the lamina papyracea are regarded as minor complications, provided that there is no secondary damage to the orbital cone. Only in half of patients is a limited defect clinically manifest in the form of lid emphysema or hematoma in the medial canthus [865]. Accompanying movements of the eye on endonasal manipulations with the forceps are serious signs of a threatening major complication. Removal of tissue to carry out the *float test* (fat and cerebral tissue float in water while mucosa sinks) is not encouraged [138].

Perforating injuries to the lamina papyracea can cause intraorbital hematoma or lead directly to more extensive damage to the ocular muscles, the nerves to the muscles, or the optic nerve. Muscles at risk are the medial rectus, inferior rectus, and superior oblique. Spontaneous healing of mechanically damaged muscles is rarely seen. In general, secondary strabismus surgery is required [185]. A feared complication is damage to the anterior ethmoidal artery, which after laceration retracts into the orbit, resulting in dangerous proptosis.

Possible sources of *increased bleeding in the operative field* are the sphenopalatine artery, the ethmoidal vessels and their branches, or, if there has been injury to the base of the skull, also from the meningeal vessels and branches of the anterior cerebral artery. Damage to the internal carotid artery is disastrous (see below). Bleeding from the medial posterior nasal artery at the lower edge of the window after fenestration of the sphenoid sinus can be troublesome [226]. There is profuse bleeding from the trunk of the sphenopalatine artery if the "spur" of the artery is inadvertently removed in cases with extensive pneumatization of the sphenoid sinus and ethmoid [733]. Rudert [765] describes an endonasal approach to coagulating the sphenopalatine artery in cases of severe epistaxis in order to avoid a Caldwell-Luc-like procedure. Bleeding from the vertical lamella following anterior shortening of the middle turbinate is similarly constant but less profuse. An anterior ethmoidal artery running in a mucosal fold at a distance from the anterior base of the skull is particularly at risk of injury.

Around 2% of endoscopically guided procedures without irrigation devices have reportedly been discontinued because of diffuse bleeding [865].

A strict distinction must be drawn between localized *CSF leaks or skull base injuries* and serious instrumental perforation of the skull base. Exposed dura may be recognized by its light, whitish color and fibrous structure, its springy resistance on palpation, and by its pulsation. The incidence of CSF leaks is around 1% (Tables 7.**1**-7.**3**).

Iatrogenic perforation of the base of the skull occurs mainly in the area of the anterior medial ethmoid roof in the region of the lateral lamella of the cribriform plate. The thinnest point in the anterior skull base is in the vicinity of the exit point of the anterior ethmoidal artery. A deep olfactory fossa (type III according to Keros) represents a particular hazard. In resection of the middle or more rarely superior turbinates near the base of the skull, the CSF spaces of the olfactory nerve bundles may be breached, resulting in microleakage of CSF fluid [733, 861, 877, 994]. Often, but not always, the defect becomes identifiable immediately owing to marked CSF rhinorrhea [42]. This may be provoked by brief compression of the neck veins [154]. Tamponade of the defect with cerebral tissue can, however, prevent CSF leakage. Medicolegal cases show than even severe injuries to the base of the skull of up to 8 cm^2 may not be noticed intraoperatively [351, 922]. Long periods often elapse before final clarification. The prognosis worsens considerably where defects are larger [364]. Stammberger [861, 868] has given full details of diagnosis and treatment.

Persistent postoperative headaches may be the result of an unnoticed pneumocephalus [682]. Clevens et al. [116] reported a case of tension pneumocephalus following injury to the cribriform plate. The patient was suffering from clouding of consciousness with headache but no meningism or rhinorrhea.

Unfortunately, in everyday clinical experience it is still frequently the case that a disastrous complication with penetration of the base of the skull (Fig. 7.**1d**) is recognized intraoperatively only by hemodynamic instability or postoperatively by a delay in regaining consciousness, clouding of consciousness, or focal neurological deficits [231, 351, 739, 922].

Fig. 7.**1a-f** **Complications of endonasal sinus surgery and their management** ▷
(**a**) Situation after fenestration of the left maxillary sinus in the middle meatus with injury to the lacrimal ducts (70° endoscope). The lacrimal duct fistula is asymptomatic (arrow: film of secretion in divided nasolacrimal duct).(**b**) Situation after injury to the left orbit (arrow) during ethmoidectomy with fenestration of the maxillary sinus in the middle meatus (postoperative CT, coronal plane). (**c**) Diagram of globe compression test according to Draf [960] and Stankiewicz [873] (figure from [873]). Axial section. The globe is carefully palpated with the finger. If there is periorbital injury, the movements transmitted to the orbital fat are indicated by similar movements of the herniated tissue visible in the operative field (white arrow) (E, endoscope). (**d**) Situation following injury to the base of the skull with penetration of the frontal lobe (MRI sagittal section; arrow indicates puncture canal). (**e**) Anatomic specimen of the sphenoid sinus in coronal section: situation after endonasal pansinus operation with perforation of the left internal carotid artery (arrow) during sphenoidotomy. S.i., sphenoidal septum. (**f**) Diagram of lateral canthotomy (1) and inferior cantholysis (2). Using an incision similar to (2) (under the outer skin of the lid), division of the lateral upper palpebral ligament should also be undertaken (superior cantholysis)

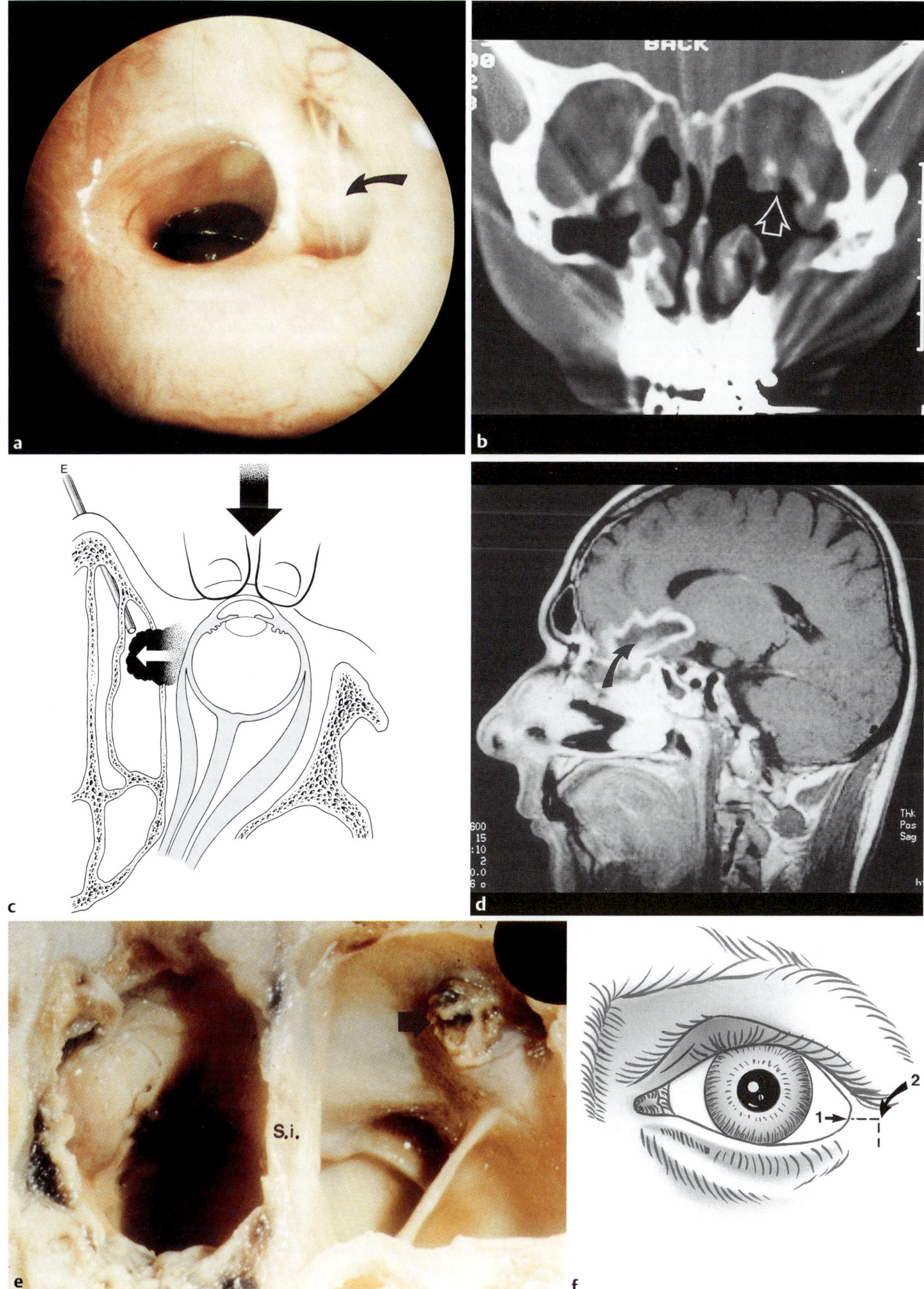
a
b
c
d
e
f
E
S.i.
1
2
Thk
Pos
Sag

Direct *damage to the optic nerve* is less common than indirect damage via an intraorbital hematoma. Damage may also be caused by epinephrine after injections into the mucosa or application of moistened cotton pledgets for hemostasis [315, 673, 780]. Typical locations for mechanical damage are the sphenoid sinus or a posterior ethmoid cell [861]. Extensive pneumatization of the sphenoid sinus and posterior ethmoid increases the risks [363]. All events of this kind are very rare individual cases. Nevertheless, bilateral blindness as a calamitous result of surgery has been reported [549]. In one case the optic chiasm was damaged during surgery for an osteoma of the sphenoid sinuses, and in a second case bilateral orbital hematoma occurred [546]. A third case involved bilateral transsection of the nerve during a routine ethmoidectomy [90]. It is not always major complications that need be the cause of visual impairment, as Kosko [466] reports. He noticed an anisoconia immediately after surgery due to injury to the postsynaptic parasympathetic fibers of the oculomotor nerve, without seeing damage to the adjacent structures of the sinuses. Fortunately, this returned almost to normal within two months. Mason [566] gives an interesting overview over the differential diagnosis of asymmetrical pupils and a recommends a strategy for their examination during surgery.

A worrying, though comparatively harmless, event is contamination of the conjunctiva with epinephrine solution, which may manifest as generally unilateral pupillary dilatation during or even before the operation [833]. If for some other reason orbital emphysema develops, damage to the optic nerve need not generally be feared in spite of the often considerable proptosis [873].

Injuries to the internal carotid artery occur in the area of the lateral sphenoid sinus or posteriorly projecting ethmoid cells (Fig. 7.**1e**). Direct damage occurs only in rare individual cases [861]. The prognosis in the event of injury to the artery is generally very serious [546]. Bogdasarian et al. [61] report more favorable therapeutic outcomes in a neurosurgical patient population. Weber and Draf [959] were able to definitively manage one of two cases after removal of the local mucosa by covering the defect with allogenic connective tissue, fibrin adhesive, and cellulose gauze via transfacial approach. The possibility of a false aneurysm must always be borne in mind, often occurring after weeks or even months [510]. Hollis et al. [338] reported a hemorrhage of this kind after one week. This was controlled by balloon occlusion of the artery and there was no secondary damage. Isenberg and Scott [375] reported an injury with an estimated blood loss of 4000 mL. Emergency treatment included administration of Ringer's lactate solution, plasma protein and platelet concentrates. Tight anterior and posterior packing was placed in the nose. After circulatory stabilization, radiological investigations were performed. These showed that there was already a pseudoaneurysm of the internal carotid artery. The artery was occluded with three balloons. The patient survived and remained free from side effects over a 5-year follow-up period. Chen [100] describes a series of six patients with pseudoaneurysms successfully treated with detachable balloon techniques and coils.

Side Effects, Sequelae

In 15% (6–22%) of cases, problematic *scarring* must be expected after paranasal sinus surgery in spite of adequate local aftercare [138, 436, 458, 730, 773, 865]. The most common unwanted sequel is scar formation between the middle turbinate and the lateral nasal wall (Figs. 4.**1 b**, 8 **1 b**) [782]. Depending on the extent and position of the wound created intraoperatively, adhesions may also be observed postoperatively between the septum and the middle and inferior turbinates. Where correction of a significant septal deviation was not performed, the percentage was higher [46]. Generous resection at the head of the middle turbinate may be undesirable from the rhinological point of view, but does prevent lateralization with scarring [919]. At any rate, preservation of mucosa and avoidance of fractures to the vertical lamella of the middle turbinate are a better policy. This requires particular attention when using self-retaining specula to spread the middle meatus. If septa and bony trabeculae are left in the anterior ethmoid, these can contribute to stabilization of the remaining middle turbinate [452]. Opposing wound areas should always be avoided.

Only around 20% of severe adhesions cause complaints requiring treatment [865, 869]. Endoscopic surgical division of the scar tissue is generally successful. For adhesions between the septum and turbinates, it is sometimes necessary to insert a silicone stent that is fixed with sutures and left in place for two weeks [32].

The presence of postoperative tissue swelling results in an increased tendency to sinusitis. It must be expected following partial ethmoidectomy and in some cases persists for several months. Localized mucosal swelling is aggravated by any correction of the septum [459].

Atrophic rhinitis is not observed after reduction the middle turbinate by half or two-thirds. On the contrary, in these patients there is a lower percentage of ostium stenoses in the middle meatus and the patients feel better postoperatively. The sense of smell is not impaired [477].

Indeed, atrophic rhinitis does not occur even after extensive operations on the sinuses [258]. However, a feeling of dryness of the inner nose is experienced by 46% of these patients and is regarded as a serious problem by 5% [218]. The feeling of dryness may decrease gradually after surgery [906]. Where this is not the case, patients will have to resort in the long term to salt water douches and other conservative forms of treatment.

A number of patients report an *impaired sense of smell* for the first time after extensive sinus surgery.

These disorders cannot always be measured objectively [959]. Unambiguous iatrogenic anosmia must be expected in 1.5% of cases [152, 353]. Most of these are patients with preexisting hyposmia [353]. Endoscopic investigation is necessary in all cases to exclude persistent or new mucosal pathology or inflammation in the olfactory fossa as a cause of the anosmia.

Prevention and Management of Complications

Prevention

Surgical complications are increased by the following factors:

- For right-handed surgeons, visibility and manipulation of instruments in the right nasal cavity is comparatively difficult.
- Inexperienced operators employ optical aids too late or to an insufficient extent.
- Important landmarks such as the middle turbinate are removed at an early stage or are already absent. The latter is often the case in revision procedures.
- Intraoperative orientation is made more difficult by the extent of the disease or by troublesome diffuse bleeding [485].

By way of prevention, the surgeon must, of course, master the usual operating techniques and local anatomy. The former also includes conventional procedures by the external approach for dealing with emergencies. Strategies to be followed in the event of a complication must be known and the necessary organizational preparations made in advance. The CT scans should be adequately studied preoperatively, and should be within view during surgery. The surgeon should be familiar with the patient's drug history and other factors that could lead to an increased bleeding tendency, and the appropriate laboratory tests must have been carried out. Patients taking antiplatelet drugs should discontinue these, if possible eight days before the operation [546].

Immediately preoperatively, the nasal cavity should be thoroughly decongested. In positioning the patient, care must be taken to ensure that the eyes are neither covered nor closed with tape. Intraoperatively, important landmarks should not be removed too early, and others should be exposed at an early stage by careful dissection. If the view is restricted, septoplasty, septum mobilization by partial removal of the vertical lamina, or procedures to the inferior turbinate may be helpful [351]. Surgeons should not be too quick to remove tissues of unknown origin for the float test (see p. 88). Biopsies for tissue identification as a topographical aid are mostly superfluous and dangerous [224, 231].

Resection of the uncinate process with a pointed sickle knife should be performed very cautiously. The use of other instruments such as a double-ended elevator, a nasal knife, or a back-biting punch may be preferable [65]. To avoid injury to the lacrimal duct, in case of doubt, the lacrimal sac may be exposed during operations on the anterior ethmoid [733]. In the area of the medial anterior ethmoidal artery in the transition to the lateral wall of the olfactory fossa, dissection must be undertaken with great caution. This does not mean, however, that there is any reason to leave any clear foci of disease in this area [877]. The basal lamella of the middle turbinate should be penetrated if necessary inferiorly and posteriorly [583]. Packs soaked in epinephrine must not be left in place for long in the area of the optic nerve as vasoconstriction of the accompanying vessels can lead to visual impairment [171]. Safe fenestration of the sphenoid sinus has already been mentioned. In the sphenoid sinus, septa often lead toward the bony canal of the internal carotid artery. The removal of these septa, which is not without risk, is generally unnecessary.

Where anatomical relationships are unclear, constant checking of landmarks and optimization of the overview and hemostasis are necessary. With increased caution and under constant optical guidance, an attempt is then made to clarify the situation. Haste is dangerous. The inexperienced surgeon will ensure competent assistance in good time. Where injury to the orbit is suspected, the globe pressure test described by Draf and Stankiewicz [178, 873] is helpful (see above). Provided that dissection is carried out carefully, a graduated measuring device and intraoperative radiographs should not be necessary [853, 871]. The same applies to measurements of orbital resistance to detect defects in the lamina papyracea and also to the monitoring of optic nerve integrity with visually evoked potentials [322, 446].

The type and number of packs should always be noted on completion of the procedure. Failure to remove packs can obviously lead to complications [547].

Management of Complications

Average Blood Loss

The amount of blood loss depends on the patient's primary and concomitant diseases and on the extent of the procedure and the technique. Blood loss is often lower where local anesthesia is used [269, 773]. Adjunctive measures such as those involving the inferior turbinate can considerably increase blood loss.

Many authors take operations of varying extent together and calculate a blood loss of around 120 mL for a bilateral ethmoidectomy [57, 62, 335, 564, 883]. However, a pansinus operation for diffuse disease together with the concomitant procedures to the septum and turbinates can lead to a blood loss of 500 mL

[993]. Extensive forms of polyposis and recurrences predominate here. The average volume reported is around 200 mL [433, 503, 877]. These average figures conceal the fact that in 2% of extensive routine procedures losses of up to 1200 mL are reported [730, 869, 877]. Red cell concentrates are given in less than 1% of cases (0.2–3.7%) [865, 919, 942, 959]. The blood loss decreases with the increasing experience of the surgeon [335]. Procedures for inverted papillomas are similar to a pansinus operation with regard to blood loss [879].

Circumscribed procedures in the middle meatus under local anesthetic cause a blood loss of around 25 mL, including revisions [269, 492, 677, 865]. If these operations are carried out under general anesthesia, the loss rises to around 70 mL [269, 433, 438]. In children, rather more limited procedures are performed, in principle under general anesthetic. Here the blood loss can be expected to be around 40 mL [183, 289, 492, 751].

Management of Intraoperative Bleeding

Diffuse bleeding is managed by insertion of cotton pledgets soaked in a vasoconstrictor solution (epinephrine stock solution 1:1000 or naphazoline 1:1000). The pledgets must first be squeezed out slightly to ensure that no excess solution escapes into the rest of the operative field [996]. Isolated bleeders are controlled with bipolar hemostasis forceps [994]. Other possibilities are monopolar needles or suction tips, clips, and, for bleeding from the bone, even a diamond burr (see p. 51). Kennedy and Zinreich [437] mix microfibrillary collagen with water and soak cotton pledgets in this solution. The solution or pledgets are placed over the wound.

A feared event is retraction of a damaged anterior ethmoidal artery into the orbit, resulting in a vision-threatening orbital hematoma. If the artery cannot be safely located and coagulated intranasally, and if the proptosis increases in spite of the appropriate decompression measures (see below), hemostasis must be achieved as an emergency measure by an intranasal or external approach [869]. Rarely, bleeding cannot be controlled locally. In these cases an adequate packing must be installed and the operation discontinued. Further evaluation can be carried out by selective angiography. Where the bleeding source is in the external carotid circulation, embolization may be considered as a therapeutic option [363]. In rare cases, transantral ligature of the maxillary artery may be necessary [702, 808] or an endonasal approach as reported by Rudert [765].

Bleeding from the cavernous sinus is treated by multiple long-term packs over 10–14 days combined with a covering of muscle or fascia [733].

Carotid artery injury may result in immediate or delayed profuse bleeding, the formation of a carotid-cavernosus fistula, or false aneurysm. Small nicks to the carotid artery may be managed by applying collagen sponges or similar materials [861]. In the event of spontaneous profuse bleeding, the nose should be packed as an emergency measure and the common carotid artery temporarily compressed from the outside. As soon as bleeding is under control and the patient's circulation is stable, emergency carotid angiography [100] should be arranged. Then, if the injury is more extensive, both angiographic balloon occlusion of the carotid artery and surgical sealing of the sphenoid sinus using muscle, fascia, or fat should be undertaken [441]. The grafts are held in place by means of tight packing. Sealing and packing alone do not prevent the development of a pseudoaneurysm with further episodes of bleeding. If the collateral supply of the cerebral circulation is radiologically unsatisfactory, establishment of an extra-intracranial arterial bypass may be discussed with the neurosurgeon prior to the neuroradiological intervention.

Skull Base Defects—CSF Fistulas

If detected intraoperatively and treated as described on p. 76, localized CSF leaks that are not associated with intracranial damage have an excellent prognosis.

Stammberger [861] has described the wide spectrum of lesions following deep intracranial perforation. Apart from injury to the dura, cerebral damage of varying severity, intracranial hemorrhages, and also secondary meningoencephalitis and disorders of CSF circulation can be expected. After an injury of this kind, immediate rhinological closure of the defect and wound should be attempted while the neurosurgeon is contacted. A follow-up CT scan is of the utmost urgency. Further action is then planned in consultation with the neurosurgeon. Failure to detect extensive injuries to the base of the skull intraoperatively considerably worsens the patient's prognosis [351].

Detection of CSF rhinorrhea after sinus surgery is an indication for immediate reexploration of the operative field. The revision should be primarily endonasal (see p. 76). Conservative treatment with bed rest and antibiotic cover [364, 380] is indicated only in specially selected circumstances. At all events, an urgent CT scan of the paranasal sinuses should be arranged. Radiological follow-up is also indicated for otherwise normal patients who complain of marked headache postoperatively and in whom a noncontrast CT scan is then performed to exclude defects of the anterior skull base, subarachnoid hemorrhage, intraparenchymatous hematoma, or pneumocephalus [363]. If a defect of the anterior base of the skull is detected and treated intraoperatively, a follow-up CT scan should be obtained postoperatively.

Injury to the Lamina Papyracea

Localized injuries to the lamina papyracea require no treatment. The patient is instructed not to blow the nose postoperatively [942] for at least two weeks. Ointments containing petrolatum should not be used for the final packing of the nose (see below). If too much fat penetrates into the ethmoid and thus obstructs visibility, the displaced tissue should be pushed back carefully. Cautious coagulation of the top layer of the tissue with a bipolar coagulation forceps is effective but not without problems [996]. After reduction, the defect is sealed with fibrin glue, or with fascia or allogenic connective tissue in the case of larger areas [733, 861]. Large defects are managed in the same way as blow-out fractures of the medial orbital wall (see p. 80). Patients are given antibiotics postoperatively, e.g., amoxicillin (2 g/day), and for periorbital hematoma steroids are also given (methylprednisolone 60 mg/day) [154]. Under no circumstances should herniated fat be resected. Cases where the mechanism of injury only becomes evident upon routine histological examination of fat or muscle tissue must be managed as well as possible by secondary procedures in the event of functional impairment such as displacement of the globe or diplopia [198, 351].

For all patients with marked proptosis, significant subcutaneous emphysema, or suspected visual impairment or diplopia, an immediate postoperative CT scan, usually in the axial plane, is urgently indicated [363].

Orbital Hematoma

Postseptal bleeding into the orbit can lead to direct pressure on the optic nerve, indirect nerve damage from compression of the ophthalmic artery and vein, and compression of the retinal vessels as a result of increased intraocular pressure. Further mechanisms of damage include traction on the nerve due to the exophthalmos and acute narrow-angle glaucoma. Nerve damage due to compression, traction, or ischemia of the intraorbital section of the optic nerve is the most likely. The optic nerve and retina can tolerate ischemia by means of compensating mechanisms for only 60–180 minutes [754, 778].

The majority of hematomas occur only during or after recovery from the general anesthetic, often in association with sneezing or coughing [129].

A hematoma with unimpaired vision is treated with ice compresses; the head of the bed is raised and the nasal packing is removed [658]. Immediate CT or ultrasound investigation will visualize the hematoma and any concomitant injuries. The ophthalmologist is consulted as a matter of urgency and vision is monitored constantly. Further action depends on findings and the clinical course.

A serious hematoma leads to severe proptosis and a rock-hard globe. The conscious patient is vagotonic and thus shows bradycardia with nausea and retching. Treatment is urgent. A stepped procedure is shown below.

Treatment of perioperative hematoma-related exophthalmos with the threat of optic nerve damage

Organization: inform ophthalmologist
Positioning, tamponade

- Remove nasal packing
- Raise upper body, apply cold compresses
- Ocular massage [114] (controversial issue)

Surgical treatment

- Transnasal decompression with removal of the lamina papyracea and incision of the orbital periosteum
- Lateral canthotomy and inferior cantholysis, superior cantholysis if necessary
- Hemostasis, e.g., of the anterior/posterior ethmoidal artery, possibly via an external approach

Drug treatment [851, 914]

- Acetazolamide 500 mg i. v.; repeat after 2–4 hours
- Mannitol 1 g/kg, 20-minute infusion; further administration of up to maximum 2 g/kg in 2 hours
- Dexamethasone 1 mg/kg [452, 703, 914]

Methods of treatment should be selected in the light of clinical findings and depending on whether the patient is still in the operating room [703]. If still in the operating room, any manipulation on the contralateral side is immediately stopped [90]. If necessary, decompression of the orbit is undertaken by incision of the periorbita. Rarely, direct observation of the hemorrhage or hematoma is then possible. An ophthalmologist is called in, though this should not delay the procedure. The next step is lateral canthotomy with cantholysis, if the transnasal orbital revision is not immediately possible or was unsuccessful. If necessary, an external approach may be considered [481]. Concomitant drug treatment is initiated.

For a hematoma occurring postoperatively, drug treatment and the removal of nasal packing combined with lateral canthotomy and cantholysis may help to gain time. At all events, not least for medicolegal reasons, an ophthalmologist must be called in as a matter of urgency. He should check the intraocular pressure, direct and consensual reactivity to light, and visual acuity, and evaluate the retina and pupil using an ophthalmoscope.

By means of *lateral canthotomy with cantholysis*, May succeeded in reducing the intraocular pressure by 17 mmHg [581]. The procedure can be carried out under local anesthesia. Hemostasis is achieved with a straight clamp, which is introduced horizontally into the lateral canthus and closed. The lateral canthus is then opened horizontally up to the lateral orbital margin using scissors (lateral canthotomy). The lateral superior and inferior palpebral ligaments are then divided (inferior and superior cantholysis) longitudinally along the bone (Fig. 7.**1f**). The globe of the eye can then move 4–5 mm anteriorly after this procedure [914]. Intraorbital and intraocular pressure decreases, but the tensile load on nerves and vessels increases [165]. Lateral canthotomy alone achieves no appreciable effect [769, 1021]. If these measures do not result in adequate decompression, in extreme cases an infraorbital incision is used to divide the orbital septum followed by a blunt orbital dissection in consultation with the ophthalmologist. After diagnosis, a subperiosteal hematoma can be relieved by an additional incision. In the last resort, transcorneal puncture of the anterior chamber is performed by the ophthalmologist [658, 754]. Stevens and Blair [884] report injection of the orbit with hyaluronidase as a treatment option. Stankiewicz [872] recommends orbital massage. This is said to achieve distribution of the hematoma. The eyeball is massaged carefully through the lids. Massage is contraindicated in the case of preexisting conditions such as lens implantation.

Unlike reduced vision, reduced mobility of the eyeball due to hematoma has a comparatively good prognosis even when it has persisted for a longer period. However, where there is also oculomotor nerve paralysis, the condition may take up to two years to resolve in some cases [280].

The prognosis for pronounced intraorbital hematoma is serious: in over one-third of cases blindness results. Even after surgical interventions, the precise source of bleeding generally cannot be stated [892]. Refixation of the palpebral ligament after lateral cantholysis is performed a few days later [658, 703].

Injury to the Ocular Muscles

Apart from orbital hematoma, postoperative diplopia may also be due to muscle edema, direct muscle damage, or neural damage. Direct injury most often involves the medial rectus muscle, less often the inferior rectus and inferior oblique muscles. Muscular damage is not necessarily accompanied by marked orbital hematoma [129, 185, 658]. In principle, the diagnostic procedures are as for orbital hematoma.

Muscle edema resolves spontaneously. In some cases posttherapeutic CT or MRI follow-up is recommended [129]. Laceration or tearing of the muscle should be repaired surgically by the ophthalmologist at an early date (within three weeks). Concomitant systemic treatment with corticosteroids may be instigated. Injuries to the medial rectus muscle often require secondary procedures, though these do not usually lead to complete recovery [705]. Division of scars alone on completion of wound healing is unsuccessful [224]. Entrapment of the muscle in the medial orbital wall defect is identified by the forced duction test. Immediate surgical revision is indicated [658]. Where a neurogenic disorder is suspected, a "wait and see" approach is justified. Improvement is often seen over a period of 6–12 months. After this time, a corrective neuro-ophthalmological intervention is needed [129, 658].

Damage to the Optic Nerve

Apart from orbital hematoma, damage to the optic nerve may be due to direct transsection of the nerve, a compression or crush injury, hematoma of the optic nerve sheath or central retinal artery occlusion [114, 703, 861]. The clinical signs may be stationary or progressive loss of vision, reduction of visual field or even blindness. Indirect injuries may not become evident until after a certain period [129].

In principle, an immediate ophthalmological examination should be performed, followed by urgent CT scanning of the paranasal sinuses, orbit, and optic nerve canal. Treatment with corticosteroids (dexamethasone 1 mg/kg i.v.; then 0.5 mg/kg i.v. after 6 hours) may be instituted as a precautionary measure [658, 703]. The patient is provided with antibiotic cover [861].

There is no specific treatment for transsection of the nerve. If occlusion of the central retinal artery is suspected, ophthalmological treatment is given. For a crush injury or sheath hematoma, treatment with corticosteroids is continued. If there is no improvement, surgical decompression of the optic nerve canal and posterior orbit should be considered after 24 hours at the latest. If vision improves, the cortisone dose should be continued for a maximum of five days and then tapered out. If the condition then worsens again, surgical decompression is indicated [658, 703].

CSF leaks are managed as described on p. **76**.

Myospherulosis, Petrolatum Granulomas

If nasal packs soaked in petrolatum are inserted after sinus surgery and there is also a surgically created defect of the lamina papyracea with bleeding, hydrocarbons may be carried in the blood from the packing material into the patient's eyelids, where they can cause petrolatum granulomas (sclerosing lipogranulomas). The period between the operation and development of the granuloma is usually 3–4 weeks but in individual cases may be up to two years [263, 428, 902, 964]. The solid yellowish pseudotumors do not respond to conservative treatment and must be removed by plastic surgery. Complete resection is made more difficult by diffuse spread of the granuloma. Extensive repair of the eyelid may become necessary [89, 330]. Since they almost always contain petrolatum as the base, ointments should not be used intranasally after sinus surgery, particularly where there are defects of the periorbita or bleeding into the lids. Gels may be applied instead or the packs may simply be moistened.

Lanolin and petrolatum as constituents of impregnated gauze strips in the paranasal sinuses may also be responsible for the development of *spherulocytosis (myospherulosis)* [278, 629].

Medicolegal Consequences

The costs of legal disputes concerning the sequelae and side effects of endonasal ethmoid surgery doubled in the United States during the period 1980–1985 [801]. In Germany, too, there has been an increase in the provision of expert opinion in connection with sinus surgery at some centers [351].

A number of papers have appeared concerning the medicolegal aspects of endonasal sinus surgery [351, 356, 733]. Many aspects have already been mentioned. Issues regarding *information of patients* are dealt with on p. **16**. The *medical documentation* must conform to high standards: operation reports and patients' notes must show clearly the indication and type of procedure carried out, the optical aids used, any change in the degree of difficulty or new diagnoses, and the use of special instruments and aids. The terminology should be as generally comprehensible as possible [802, 955]. The timing and prompt recording of medical decisions at the time of and after a surgical complication are of particular importance.

Education and Training

Mastery and availability of optical aids are now the standard for endonasal sinus surgery [955]. The consequences for *medical training* will be discussed against this background.

Thorough anatomic dissection exercises on the basis of demonstrated specialist knowledge and general skills are probably the only way of avoiding complications [442]. Appropriate techniques for the removal of the sinonasal block at autopsy have been described [28, 40, 342, 484]. Rivron and Maran [753] have developed the FESS trainer, a special cadaver-based benchtop practice system for surgical training. An animal (sheep) model for training in endoscopic nasal and sinus surgery has been developed by Gardiner et al. [260]. After this preparatory training, the trainee is gradually introduced to operations in patients, and should follow a series of procedures performed by experienced surgeons. Attendance at surgical courses is of additional benefit. The first procedures performed independently are carried out under constant supervision. Simultaneous observation is possible via an appropriate attachment to the operating microscope, an observer tube, or video monitor. It has been shown that a strictly organized and personally managed training program is beneficial in keeping the rate of complications low [560, 730, 883].

Hillen [329] has devised an interactive computer program as a teaching aid for general understanding of the anatomy of the paranasal sinuses and anterior skull base (Elsevier, Amsterdam) [425]. Keerl and Weber [427] have produced a program on CD-ROM which can be used by trainees to familiarize themselves with the anatomy, radiology, surgical technique, and special risks of paranasal sinus surgery according to their personal requirements. While comparing two groups of surgeons with and without multimedia training, they show that CSF leaks went down in the second group and periorbital lesions diminished significantly [426].

Ecke et al. [192] developed an nasal endoscopy simulator (NES) that combines computer graphics and virtual reality (VR) in order to enhance surgical education.

Duration of Inpatient Care, Outpatient Surgery?

The length of stay in hospital after endonasal surgery to the paranasal sinuses is determined essentially by the extent and technique of the operation, the type and extent of adjunctive procedures, and the primary and concomitant illnesses of the patient.

A pansinus operation with its adjunctive surgical measures to the turbinates and septum requires inpatient treatment for 5–8 days postoperatively [185, 341]. After limited procedures, patients often stay in hospital for only 2–3 days [162, 829, 856, 865].

Outpatient surgery or "day-case surgery" is regarded in the international literature as possible for the majority (50–90%) of limited procedures [32, 138, 269, 291, 301, 335, 437, 564, 838, 865]. Mucopyoceles are also treated in this way [438]. The same applies for children, in whom the procedure is in any case generally limited and who do not tolerate intensive topical aftercare in hospital. Performance of extensive ethmoid procedures in children is the exception [183, 289]. After the operation, patients are given verbal or written instructions. On the day following the operation, a routine telephone inquiry may be made by a member of the hospital staff [434].

Martin and May [564] only perform outpatient procedures in patients who live or have accommodation relatively near to the hospital [301]. All patients who have undergone extensive procedures stay in hospital, as do those with complications, a blood loss of more than 350 mL, nasal packing in place, or potentially life-threatening underlying diseases. Further reasons for inpatient treatment include postoperative nausea, dizziness, pain or bleeding, less-than-normal intake of fluids, an anesthetic hangover, or uncertain domestic circumstances [564]. If this procedure is followed, it is reported that only around 1% of outpatient or day cases have to be readmitted postoperatively because of nasal bleeding [503].

It is up to the national professional bodies to prepare recommendations for outpatient surgery on the basis of the current legal situation in the respective countries. The legislation in Germany, with a far-reaching definition of the medical responsibilities following outpatient procedures, makes no concessions to the surgeon. For this reason, a reluctance to perform ethmoid surgery on an outpatient or day-case basis must in principle be considered appropriate [960]. In addition to the exclusion criteria mentioned, all patients undergoing pansinus surgery or concomitant procedures, for example to the turbinates, should be given inpatient care postoperatively.

8 Postoperative Care following Endoscopic Procedures

Surgery in the paranasal sinus area leaves relatively extensive areas of raw bone, which are left to heal spontaneously. The location and extent of wound areas vary individually and depend on the preoperative anatomy and on the nature and extent of the operation. Only the systematic use of endoscopy in postoperative aftercare revealed the importance of undisturbed wound healing for the success of surgery. At the same time, however, it became clear how limited our knowledge still is of what constitutes normal and disturbed wound healing and how comparatively little knowledge is available on the ways of influencing regeneration therapeutically.

Wound Healing after Paranasal Sinus Surgery

After rather more extensive ethmoid surgery, the regular tissue reactions in the wound bed lead to an initially rapid sequence of changes in the endoscopic appearance of the operative field (Table 8.**1**). The main feature initially is crust formation, followed by the edematous swelling of remaining areas of mucosa and the development of granulation tissue. Wound healing is an individual process and can be delayed or accelerated by local or systemic factors. Local infections have a particularly deleterious effect. A striking feature is the involvement of neighboring intact areas of mucosa in the changes taking place in the wound area [347, 965, 971].

The respiratory wound closes uniformly from all sides without regard to the direction of blood and lymph flow or mucociliary clearance [345]. New bone growth at the area of the base of the wound is observed after one week. This can lead to stenoses, for example, in the frontal sinus recess. In normal cases, new bone growth ceases after around two months [227].

After completion of wound healing, following extensive ethmoid surgery, detailed examination of the mucociliary flow shows a very varied pattern with normal zones and disruptions due to delay or stasis, recirculation, or reverse flow. Healing observed endoscopically does not necessarily equate with complete recovery of local mucociliary flow. Persistent or new foci of inflammation, however, are generally also locations of disrupted mucociliary clearance [945]. In the maxillary sinuses, even after removal of large areas of tissue, the geometry of the transport pathways is basically restored [37, 343]. General recovery of the mucociliary apparatus after healing of chronic rhinosinusitis can be determined by performing a saccharin test [628].

It is known from radical surgery that regenerated respiratory mucosa consists of connective tissue originating from the endosteum that is initially covered by mostly immature and functionally poor quality epithelium. New gland formation is incomplete and late [79, 285, 592, 593]. Where tissue removal is more limited, the functional deficits of the regenerated tissue are less pronounced [326, 345, 598]. However, after optimization of ventilation and drainage, the remaining, intact mucosa of the paranasal sinuses still shows specific histological changes even months after macroscopic healing. The density of the glands is increased, a fact that is probably responsible for persistent disorders of nasal secretion [213]. The inflammatory infiltration of the mucosa often decreases only slightly postoperatively and indicates a continuously activated state [228].

The course of wound healing is generally less satisfactory in patients with a respiratory allergy or aspirin intolerance, and in smokers [37, 742]. Particular problem areas for healing include the anterior vertical lamella of the middle turbinate close to the agger nasi [927]. Scar formation occurring in the anterior superior ethmoid shaft may restrict access to the frontal

Table 8.**1** Endoscopic appearance of wound healing stages after paranasal sinus surgery (Hosemann [347])

Wound healing stage	Characteristics (Endoscopy)	Time after ooperation
1. Blood crust formation	Crust	up to 10 days
2. Obstructive lymphedema	Edema (pale yellow)	up to 30 days
3. Mesenchymal transformation	Granulations (reddish)	up to 3 months
4. Scar formation	Regenerated mucosa with scars	> 3 months

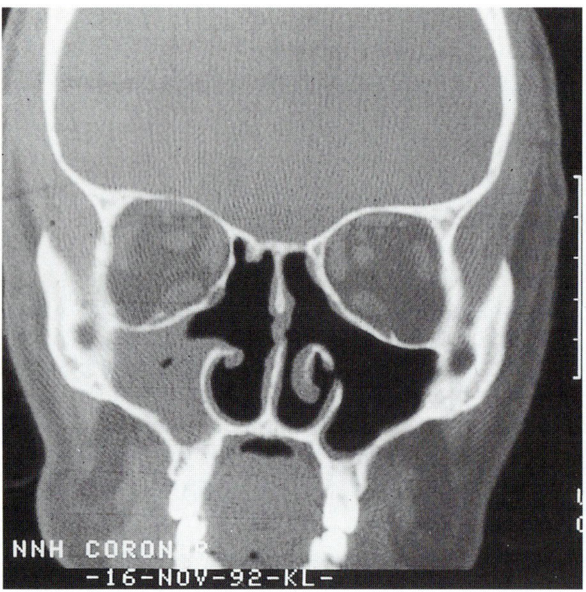

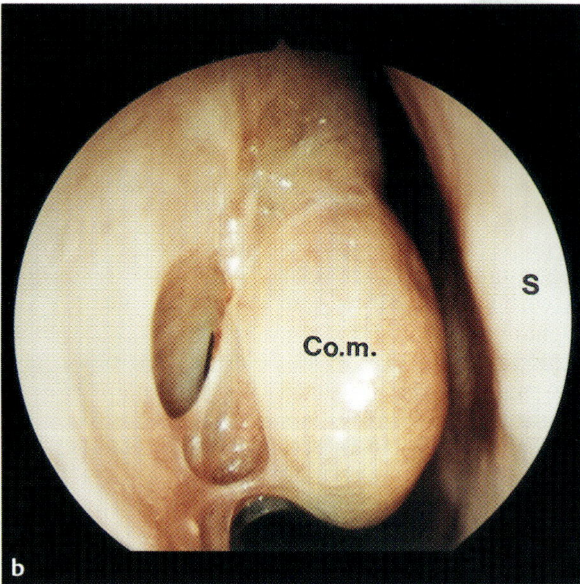

Fig. 8.**1a,b** **Problems of wound healing after paranasal sinus surgery**
(**a**) Coronal CT after a pansinus operation: in spite of maximum ventilation of the right maxillary sinus, persistent swelling of the right-side maxillary sinus mucosa persists.
(**b**) Pronounced adhesions obstruct the view into the middle meatus after limited intervention. Co.m., middle turbinate (concha media)

sinus. These scars in the area of the frontonasal recess [478] are more often the cause of a drainage problem from the frontal sinus than scar formation in the neoostium of the frontal sinus itself [347, 358]. In the maxillary sinus, persistent mucosal edema may be seen for the first time postoperatively [347] (Fig. 8.**1a**). There is increasing evidence that this is caused by secondary lymphedema, since the natural lymph drainage from the maxillary sinus is via the maxillary ostium and fontanelles [293] and can be permanently disturbed after extensive antrostomy. Animal experiments have shown that lymphatic vessels of the paranasal mucosa regenerate very slowly, if at all [349]. Hosemann et al. have investigated the lymphatic drainage pathways in the middle nasal meatus histochemically [359]. Both the nasal and the maxillary sinus mucosa showed a distinct superficial and deep longitudinal lymphatic capillary network with an orientation toward the natural maxillary sinus ostium. The density of the network increased from cranial to caudal, from dorsal to ventral, and reached maximum density at the natural ostium. Lymphatic vessels are relatively scarce in the posterior and superior sections of the middle meatus. Because of this, the natural ostium of the maxillary sinus should be enlarged into the posterior nasal fontanelle to minimize secondary lymphedema.

Schedule for Follow-up Investigations and Aftercare

There is no uniform agreement in the world literature as to which method of postoperative care is best to produce optimal results of endonasal sinus surgery [971, 975]. The period during which intensive, endoscopically assisted topical aftercare is required is generally three months. The frequency of treatment varies from one individual to another, decreasing from daily care in the first 10 days to twice weekly and then to one follow-up examination per week. Visits are then determined by the specialist as required. A final follow-up investigation by the surgeon should be performed nine months after the operation. Further check-ups are to be carried out by the specialist approximately annually or as required.

Kennedy prefers personal aftercare on the first, third, and fourth postoperative days, followed by weekly visits until healing is complete [433]. Other authors use a similar schedule [291, 779]. Kuhn and Citardi [475] described a detailed concept combining topical drug therapy, systemic medication, and mechanical cleaning at the first and fourth days, and after one week, three weeks and seven weeks. Because patients do not like cleaning of the nasal cavity very well, Ryan et al. [768] performed a minimal follow-up with the first cleaning two weeks after surgery and a second and final visit at about three months. With a mean number of follow-up visits of 2.8, a success rate of 78% (n = 120 patients) was reported.

It is certainly inappropriate to prescribe a rigid regimen of aftercare. The schedule will depend on the disease, the nature and scope of the operation, and the length of stay in hospital. During the hospitalization period, daily wound care is the rule for some surgeons.

In the early phases of wound healing, topical wound care under endoscopic guidance is the main feature. Secondary infections are treated specifically. The local treatment is supplemented by topical or systemic administration of drugs.

The patient should avoid physical exertion for 14 days and swimming and diving for around six weeks. After limited procedures, a sick note for about eight days should be issued. In individual cases, however, it may even be possible for the patient to resume work after two days [865]. More extensive operations require 14 days for recovery. An extension of seven days is normal in the event of the relevant symptoms or findings. The further procedure depends on the individual case.

Aftercare in Children

Children generally do not tolerate the usual aftercare. Examination may be possible under sedation in individual cases. For other children, depending on the operation performed, 1–3 visits must be arranged for aftercare under general anesthesia, so-called "second-look nasal endoscopy SLE" [291, 543]. The first of these visits should preferably be 10–14 days after the operation [289, 492]. Walner et al [950] pointed out that no prospective studies performed have been to ascertain the necessity and/or benefit of SLE. They examined the need for revision sinus surgery in two groups of children, 94 who underwent SLE 2–3 weeks after FESS and 53 who did not. There was no significant difference in terms of clinical outcome between the two groups. The authors concluded that SLE is not necessary in all children and the usefulness and application of SLE need to be considered carefully.

Intraoperative packing is avoided in children where possible. Children over six years of age are prescribed a corticosteroid spray (e.g., beclomethasone, flunisolide, fluocortin butyl). In general, they are given decongestant nasal drops and a saline spray, supplemented with oral antibiotics [289]. Antibiotic treatment is often continued for four weeks [536].

The use of Gelfilm is very common internationally. This is a gelatin film that is rolled into a spiral and used to keep the middle meatus open; it is changed at the follow-up visits and later removed [136, 536, 543]. It should be noted that gelatin sponge may lead to pronounced granulations and subsequent scar formation [320], which may interfere with the intended free drainage and ventilation of the sinuses.

Packing and Stents

The use of packing after sinus surgery remains controversial. A large range of materials and durations (a few hours up to seven days) are utilized and some authors use stents for the maxillary or frontal sinus or the ethmoid cavity that are left in situ for weeks to months.

The materials most commonly used for nasal packing are gauze strips impregnated with chlortetracycline or petrolatum [993], rubber finger stalls [175], and special sponges (Merocel; Americal Corp., Mystic, CT, USA) [433]. Ointment-impregnated gauze strips are easy to mold and inexpensive, but their removal is unpleasant. The problem of petrolatum granulomas was mentioned on p. 94 as affecting the adjacent soft tissues of the face and petrolatum packing should be avoided. Sponges can be placed easily and accurately in the middle meatus but their removal is also unpleasant where wound areas are large and may cause troublesome bleeding. Two (to four) rubber finger stalls per side can be positioned quickly and almost painlessly and can be removed without provoking bleeding. However, inadvertent aspiration of this form of packing is life-threatening. For this reason, they must have sutures attached that are then knotted loosely in front of the columella. The ends of the sutures are secured on the bridge of the nose with plaster and trimmed. Rubber finger stalls work as occlusive dressings that promote wound healing in general [6].

Many operators attempt to manage without postoperative packing [437]. This is reportedly possible in half to three-quarters of patients, presumably after limited procedures under local anesthesia [433, 883]. If this is one of the treatment objectives, septal correction is preferably not carried out [437]. About 5% of the patients of Friedman et al. [238] required secondary treatment for bleeding from the operative area.

In addition to ointment-impregnated gauze strips, Wigand also used special tubes to assist breathing, which can remove the patient's fear of complete obstruction of the nasal passages [993]. These are useful in patients with sleep apnea. Daily cleaning is necessary [372].

Instillation of an ointment containing antibiotics and corticosteroids has been suggested after procedures involving minimal tissue trauma [503] Stammberger and Hawke [866] abandoned routine use of this procedure because of the often unpleasant taste, secondary fungal colonization, and observation of residues of ointment in the operative field. Rather less usual packing materials include gelatin [162] and cotton pledgets with microfibrillary collagen and oxymetazoline that are inserted for a short period [291].

Packing is usually removed on the second postoperative day [9, 763, 993]. However, a number of authors remove the material one day earlier [433,

Table 8.2 Use of stents and drainage systems in paranasal sinus surgery

Author	Stent	Location	Period of use
Amble et al. [8]	Silicone strips	Frontal sinus (Jansen-Ritter operation)	6–8 weeks, sometimes longer
Kaschke and Behrbohm [416]	Nasal splint with oval support area on nasal septum and channel for the lower edge of the middle turbinate	Middle turbinate	1–2 weeks
Brennan [77]	U-shaped polyurethane "glove" (Boomerang Turbinate Glove™)	Middle turbinate	14 days
Bumm [84]	Plastic, collar stud	Maxillary sinus, inferior meatus	6 weeks
Christmas and Krouse [109]	Gelfilm	Ethmoid sinus	2 weeks
Deitmer and Rath [151]	Silicone	Frontal sinus (eyebrow incision)	122 days on average
Hoyt [362]	Plastic tubing	Frontal sinus ostium	Approximately 8 weeks (mean)
Lusk and Muntz [536]	Silastic stent Gelfilm	Ethmoid sinus	7–10 days 2–3 weeks
Messingschlager [603]	Plastic, collar stud	Maxillary sinus, inferior meatus	2 months
Milewski [618]	Balloon catheter Ethmo™	Ethmoid sinus	1–2 weeks
Neel et al. [655, 656]	Silicone strips or tubes	Frontal sinus (Jansen-Ritter op.)	6–8 weeks
Parsons and Chambers [696]	Gelfilm	Ethmoid sinus	2 weeks
Rains [727]	Rains frontal sinus stent	Frontal sinus	> 3 weeks "until the ethmoidectomy sites have healed and tissue edema is decreasing"
Rubin et al. [762]	Polyethylene tube	Frontal sinus (eyebrow incision)	5 months
Schaefer and Close [781]	Silicone catheter	Frontal sinus	6 weeks
Shikani [824]	Silicone	Maxillary sinus, middle meatus	10–14 days
Stammberger [861]	Polyethylene tube	Frontal sinus (eyebrow incision)	3–6 months
Toffel et al. [918, 919]	Silastic stent + Merocel	Ethmoid sinus	1 week
Weber et al. [973]	Silicone stent	Frontal sinus	6 months

829] or one [175], three [919] or five days later [444]. If packing is left in place for more than two days, antibiotic cover is generally recommended.

A number of aids are recommended for packing the middle meatus, i.e., for prevention of lateralization of the middle turbinate and formation of local adhesions (Fig. 8.**1 b**): in addition to gelatin, ointments, sponges, and rubber finger stalls, special silicone disks (e.g. Salman stent, Boston Med. Products) [516, 774], modified septum support films [433], U-shaped gelatin films [589], and special polyethylene oxide gel disks [771] are used. Milewski proposed a special balloon catheter (Ethmo balloon catheter; Spiggle & Theis GmbH, Germany). Brennan developed a septum film with a flap to retain and fix the middle turbinate ("boomerang turbinate glove") and inserts this for 14 days. The same purpose is served by a special stent in the neoostium of the middle turbinate (Shikani stent; Spiggle & Theis GmbH, Germany) [824]. This is also left in place for 14 days. A similar spacer is described by Kaschke and Behrbohm (Primed, Bess, Berlin, Germany) [416].

A summary of the currently available stents and drainage systems is shown in Table 8.**2**.

Toxic Shock Syndrome

Toxic shock syndrome (TSS) represents a very rare but life-threatening complication in rhinology resulting from the postoperative packing. It is caused by microbial colonization, particularly by staphylococci, with the production of specific toxins. The cardinal symptoms are fever above 38.9 °C, a rash or enanthema, desquamation of skin, and circulatory failure with hypotension and transition to multiorgan disease. The diagnosis is confirmed by a nasal smear.

Recommended treatment is immediate removal of the packing, specific antibiotic treatment, and treatment for shock if necessary. Early administration of steroids can shorten the course of the illness [1].

A number of cases of TSS following paranasal sinus surgery have been reported [1]. In general, patients become symptomatic shortly after the operation. In one patient, however, the syndrome developed 25 days after endoscopic sphenoethmoidectomy as a result of infection of the crusts in the operative field [619]. Furthermore Younis and Lazar [1017] reported TSS in five patients five days to five weeks after FESS without application of any nasal packing. Younis et al. [1015] reported toxic shock syndrome after postoperative nasal packing with gelatin (Gelfilm/Gelfoam). Since gelatin (Gelfoam) promotes microbial colonization, it is suggested that it should not be used routinely as packing material. Further preventive measures include coating of the usual nasal packings with appropriate antibiotic ointment. Even though nasal packing materials or spacers may increase the probability of TSS, their exact role is unclear so far. However, neither topical nor systemic, nonspecific antibiotic prophylaxis can entirely prevent development of this condition [379].

Local Care of the Operative Field

Local care of the operative field consists of

- Mechanical cleaning
- Application of topical steroids
- Inhalation and irrigation of the nose
- Application of ointments, gels, or solutions

Most authors recommend *local (mechanical) care of the operative area* under endoscopic guidance with thorough cleansing [750, 996]. Prior local anesthesia e.g., with amethocaine or cocaine, is advisable [433]. Topical wound care may include the following.

- Removal of fibrin clots, devitalized bone fragments, and occlusive crusts or scabs.
- Breaking down of adhesions or synechiae.
- Aspiration of secretions from the nose, sinus ostia, and maxillary and frontal sinuses.
- During this process the middle turbinate is held in position and the neo-ostia are suctioned.
- Edema of remaining areas of mucosa, hyperplastic granulations, or small polyps may be treated with topical corticosteroids or removed under visual guidance (through cutting instruments, powered instruments) or treated with silver nitrate (25%) [128, 291].
- Instillation of ointments containing antibiotics and steroids [601, 763, 996].

Meticulous endoscopic aftercare is time-consuming [475] and requires patience and an accurate knowledge of the procedure that has been undertaken and the current anatomy. Perhaps this is why it has not generally become routine practice amongst the doctors caring for patients after their discharge [521]. In carrying out these measures, the altered anatomy should be respected and the regenerating mucosa spared as far as possible. It is imperative not to start new bleeding [475].

The fear of disrupting wound healing by removing scabs has not been confirmed in histological investigations in earlier studies [291, 630]. However, Kühnel et al. [476] showed that local debridement of crusts avulsed parts of epithelium in 23% of cases during the first postoperative week. There was no histological evidence of avulsed epithelium with crusts removed in the second week. This figure later increased to 16%. In principle, large crusts may disturb ventilation and drainage, causing secondary mucositis. Mechanical cleaning must respect the time-dependent irritability of the healing wound, with little risk of impairing epithelialization during the second week after surgery.

If, after 2–3 weeks, there are areas of pronounced tissue contact between the middle turbinate and the lateral nasal wall obstructing entry to the ethmoid cavity, these should be divided to prevent later scar adhesions. Limited surgical measures may also be necessary to remove persistent edema or granulations. Use of sharp cutting instruments, shaver systems, or a microresector is to be preferred.

Topical Cortisone Treatment

Several investigations have demonstrated the favorable effect of long-term administration on the recurrence rate of nasal polyps [414, 767, 941]. Irritation and obstruction of the nose is also favorably influenced; less so the often troublesome symptom nasal secretion [157].

Observation of wound healing processes after topical application of budesonide shows a favorable effect, with reduction of swelling and faster healing [968–971]. Although corticosteroids are known to have an inhibitory action on almost all stages of wound healing [216, 587, 736] and topical corticosteroids can impair cutaneous wound healing [5, 52, 189], results suggest a different clinical experience regarding healing of the respiratory mucosa. This may be explained by the positive effects of steroids on the underlying pathological process leading to chronic sinus inflammation and polyp formation. As a whole, the very

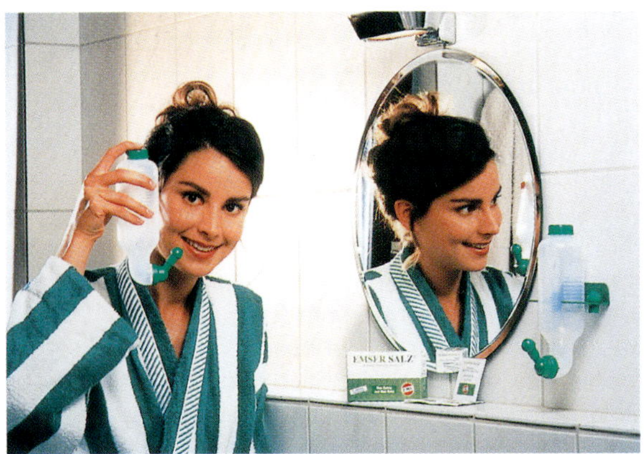

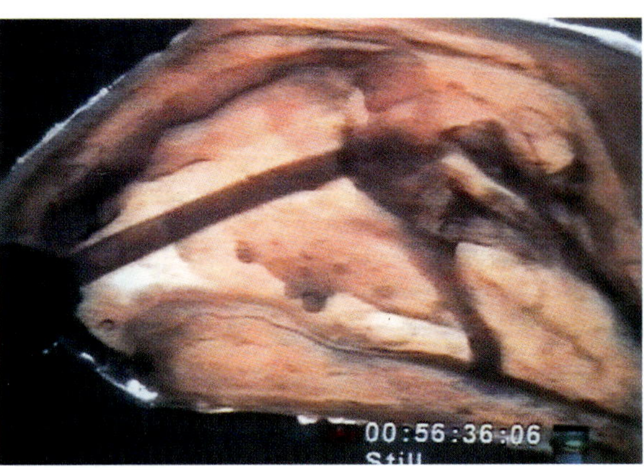

Fig. 8.**2a,b** Nasal irrigation after endonasal sinus surgery with a nasal douche and Ems salt (RhinoCare, Siemens & Co., Bad Ems, Germany) (**a**) View of the appliance. (**b**) Intranasal distribution of fluid demonstrated in a nose model

different courses of wound healing observed in patients treated with corticosteroids may be explained by different disease entities with correspondingly different corticosteroid sensitivities, despite the uniform appearance of polyposis [862]. Furthermore, the clinical effect of topical steroids depends on the intranasal distribution of the administered drug [974]. Hosemann [346] also demonstrated the favorable effect of prednisolone 2 mg/kg intramuscularly on the healing process in the rabbit maxillary sinus. On the whole, it led to quicker and more complete wound closure. A decreased rate was seen only in the first 96 hours. The wound showed less tendency toward hyperplastic granulation and bony apposition.

The administration of newer preparations (budesonide, flunisolide, fluticasone) is unequivocally preferred over beclomethasone, for example, since these have a higher potency and fewer systemic side effects [76, 392].

Treatment should initially be given for one year, there being no risk of damage to the mucosa. The mucociliary apparatus is not affected [945]. Particularly in allergy sufferers, systematic long term treatment is desirable [9, 742].

The application of moisture is particularly important for the nose postoperatively [163]. Intensive *postoperative inhalation treatment* (e. g., inhalation with Ems salts, particle size 10–30 µm, temperature 34–38 °C, three times daily for 10 minutes) has a favorable effect on swelling, crust formation and inflammation in the operative field [614]. Treatment should begin immediately after the operation, depending on the findings and the procedure.

Nasal irrigation with saline solution is recommended by most rhinologists worldwide to remove secretions and crusts and to moisten the mucosa in order to obtain a faster and better healing. From a physiological standpoint saline solutions seems to be superior to sodium chloride solutions if they contain additionally potassium, calcium, and other ions [429]. For this reason, some authors recommend Ems salt (Siemens & Co., Bad Ems, Germany) for nasal irrigation [175, 178, 429]. Ems Brine not only has no toxic effect on mucociliary clearance [27, 158, 1000] but appears to influence regenerative processes favorably [614]. It is important that the solution should be at body temperature. Cool or cold douches produce inflammation-inducing trauma on the nasal mucosa [880].

Keerl et al. [429] found that nasal irrigation after endonasal sinus surgery is judged positively by 95% of their patients and is integrated well into the daily routine (Fig. 8.**2a**). Examinations using a nasal model showed a very good distribution pattern of irrigation fluid using the nasal douche (RhinoCare, Siemens & Co., Bad Ems, Germany, Fig. 8.**2b**). After the middle meatus has been reached, the whole nasal cavity is rinsed in a gentle way and could be cleaned. Seppey et al. [809] use isotonic sea water for nasal irrigation (Rhinomer, Novartis, Munich, Germany).

The use of water jet dental douches was recommended in Britain and the United States [779]. Kuhn and Citardi [475] advise against dental irrigation devices for fear that the device may become colonized with bacteria such as Pseudomonas. Irrigation using the hand should also be avoided because the number of times that Enterobacteriaceae were isolated was significantly higher when irrigation was done using the palm than when the RhinoCare nasal douche was used [391].

After limited procedures, irrigation can start immediately [503]. Where the wound is large, the start of treatment is postponed until about three days, when it is no longer likely to provoke oozing of blood [763].

Nasal irrigation is harmless and can be continued for the rest of the patient's life. Its use is particularly important, for example, in smokers or patients with postoperative rhinitis sicca [742].

A number of *ointments and solutions* are specifically designed for postoperative care; these contain, for example, acetylcysteine; bromhexine, glucose, and vitamins A and E. Use of a slightly hyperosmolar ointment provokes a nonviscous mucosal secretion. A "soft space" is created between the mucosa or wound base and the scab so that the scab adheres less firmly [200]. Covering respiratory wounds with ointment promotes reepithelialization [346]. In addition to proprietary products, pharmacy formulated *nasal emulsions* are still popular. A number of other formulations containing a tetracycline, naphazoline, glucose, or Fortecortin (dexamethasone) as the active ingredient are described by Plinkert [715]. Gleich et al. [272] prepare an autologous fibrin glue and spread this over the wound surfaces. Gross and Gross [291] inject triamcinolone suspension into recurrent polyps or cushions of edema.

The application of ointments is problematic on two grounds:

- If applied by patients themselves, the ointment will never reach the middle nasal meatus or the sinuses (Fig. 8.**3**).
- Ointments and some emulsions contain paraffin, which may cause lung damage in case of (silent) aspiration.

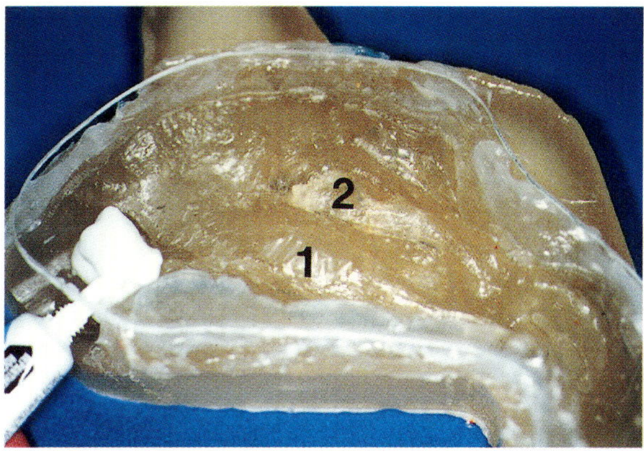

Fig. 8.**3** **Application of a nasal ointment**. Intranasal distribution demonstrated in a nose model. The ointment only reaches the anterior, nonciliated part of the nose. 1, inferior turbinate, 2, middle turbinate

Sinus Irrigation

Moss and King described a combined treatment consisting of endoscopic surgery and serial antimicrobial lavage (ESSAL) to reduce the rate of recurrence of polyposis [642, 643].

For topical antibacterial treatment, the sinuses are irrigated three times daily with antibiotic through an indwelling catheter in the maxillary sinus. Tobramycin 40 mg is added to the irrigating solution three times daily. The catheter is removed 10 days after the operation. During outpatient follow-up, further irrigations are performed every 2–4 weeks using temporary catheters. In acute episodes of infection, topical treatment is again intensified.

Klossek et al. [462] performed postoperative frontal irrigation in cases of diffuse nasal polyposis. The frontal sinus was irrigated three times daily through frontal needles with 250 mL saline solution. Nasal washings and topical corticoid solutions (4 mg prednisolone) were introduced into the sinus twice daily after irrigation. Irrigation was continued for a few weeks. Because a temporary inflammation is encountered routinely after any functional endosopic sinus surgery, the use of postoperative frontal irrigation appears to be helpful [462].

Systemic Medication

Systemic Steroids and Antibiotics

There is some controversy in the literature on the use of systemic steroids and antibiotics. The spectrum ranges from no systemic drugs at all, through administration of steroids or antibiotics in individual cases, to routine prescription of both. Duration, dosage, and drug also vary widely.

There is no evidence that any particular therapeutic regime works best. The following points should be kept in mind:

- Steroids effectively reduce granulation tissue, edema, and scarring. These processes are part of normal wound healing, especially in the first postoperative weeks. However, steroids are often effective in treating the underlying disease, chronic (polypoid) rhinosinusitis.
- After surgery there is a large wound surface that does not drain well. Crust formation (blood clot in the first days, crusts thereafter) with bacterial adhesion cannot be avoided. Bacterial infection is a major cause of delayed wound healing in general.

Therefore, the possibility of using systemic drugs should be kept in mind, especially in extensive disease and surgery.

Corticosteroids

Bumm [85] described a cortisone regime for systemic treatment following ethmoid surgery: Oral treatment begins on the fourth postoperative day with 50 mg prednisolone. The dose is then tapered to 2.5 mg over five weeks (Table 8.**3**). Other authors start cortisone treatment preoperatively (see p. 15). Von Ilberg prescribes 50 mg prednisone daily preoperatively for a week, 50 mg on the day of the operation, and 40 mg on the first postoperative day. This is followed by 30 mg, 20 mg, 10 mg, 5 mg. This final dose is maintained for a maximum of three months [369]. Bearing

Table 8.**3** Cortisone treatment (dosage) following endonasal sinus surgery in nasal polyposis (Bumm [85])

Postoperative day	4	5	6	7	8	9	10	11	12	13–31	For a further 7 days
Prednisolone (mg)	50	40	35	30	25	20	15	12.25	10	7.5–5	2.5

in mind the contraindications, cortisone treatment is indicated in all patients with massive nasal polyposis and following operations for polyp recurrence. Draf and Weber [175, 178] give corticosteroids together with an antihistamine preparation when tissue eosinophilia is detected and have observed a favorable effect on the rate of polyp recurrence [455].

Antibiotics

An intraoperative smear in chronic rhinosinusitis gives positive results in 88% of cases, with mixed flora in 30%. The results of the smears depend on the specific disease, the location and technique of collection, and the treatment that has been given. The majority show coagulase-negative staphylococci, Staphylococcus aureus, Gram-negative bacilli, or streptococci. No anaerobes were found in Hoyt's investigation [361]. The pathogens found are frequently resistant to the usual antibiotics such as erythromycin, tetracycline, or ampicillin.

The majority of authors recommend postoperative antibiotic treatment. The duration of treatment is around 10 days (three days to three weeks) [370, 433, 437, 601, 750, 763]. The preferred preparations are amoxicillin or amoxicillin-clavulanic acid, and where infection persists a smear is taken and the medication is modified [291, 763]. Draf and Weber [175] do not give antibiotics unless purulent inflammation is demonstrated, in which case they give amoxicillin, cefaclor, or cefuroxime. Levine [503] routinely gives no antibiotic.

Moriyama [631, 636] recommends low-dose treatment with erythromycin for 3–6 months after the operation. The dosage is 600 mg daily for 1–2 months, 400 mg for a further 1–2 months, and 200 mg daily for the last 1–2 months. The outcome of the operation is reported to be clearly improved by this regimen [637].

Leukotriene Receptor Antagonists

Leukotrienes are inflammatory mediators and may be divided into two classes: the nonpeptide leukotrienes (LTA_4, LTB_4) and the cysteinyl leukotrienes (LTC_4, LTD_4, LTE_4). The cysteinyl leukotrienes were formerly collectively known as the slow-reacting substance of anaphylaxis [2, 108].

Cysteinyl leukotrienes induce several pathophysiological effects relevant to asthma including:

- Smooth-muscle contraction leading to bronchoconstriction
- An increase in vascular permeability in vivo
- An increase in mucus production in vitro
- Inflammatory cell infiltration into the lung in vivo [2]

Zafirlukast is a selective cysteinyl leukotriene antagonist that is the first of this new drug family to receive Food and Drug Administration (FDA) approval. Results from clinical trials demonstrate that zafirlukast is effective and safe for the prophylactic treatment of asthma [2, 95, 852]. A more recent approved drug is montelukast [148, 497].

Alternatively, leukotriene metabolism can be inhibited by modulation of 5-lipoxygenase activity [472]. Zileuton, also recently cleared by the FDA, is a prototypical 5-lipoxygenase inhibitor. It is effective for chronic asthma, but zafirlukast is likely to be more convenient and less expensive than zileuton since it requires only twice-daily oral administration and does not require multiple measurements of liver enzymes during the first year of therapy [321, 431].

The relevance of these new drugs for therapy of chronic rhinosinusitis, particularly polypoid sinusitis, is unclear as yet. Two studies showed an effect of leukotriene antagonists on mechanisms of allergic rhinitis. Shirasaki et al. [825] found a significant inhibition of antigen-induced and LTD_4-induced microvascular leakage by oral administration of ONO-1078 (pranlukast, 30 mg/kg). Donelly et al. [169] showed that leukotriene receptor antagonist ICI 204219 (zafirlukast) relieved the symptoms of allergic rhinitis, including both sneezing and rhinorrhea.

There are no published data regarding the effect of leukotriene antagonists on nasal polyps. Preliminary results (A. Schapowal, personal communication) show significantly better results than placebo but significantly worse results than corticosteroids (budesonide).

Other Preparations

Draf and Weber [175] recommend the administration of an antihistamine for six weeks postoperatively where tissue eosinophilia has been demonstrated. The preparation is also given where there is a concomitant allergy [636]. The disadvantage of increased viscosity of nasal secretions must be borne in these cases [128].

Kaschke and Behrbohm [415] and Behrbohm et al. [38] give a myrtol preparation (Gelomyrtol Forte) for 2–4 weeks. The essential oils are thought to have a secretolytic action and to encourage ciliary activity.

Details of concomitant antiallergic therapy were given on p. 4.

Adaptive Desensitization

A stepwise treatment plan from conservative treatment to surgical clearance of the sinuses followed by adaptive desensitization is recommended for patients suffering from ASA-triad [75, 468, 885, 886].

Therapy of aspirin-sensitive rhinosinusitis includes avoidance of aspirin and NSAIDs. A general downregulation of the immune response with glucocorticosteroids is effective, e.g., a maintenance dose of 400 g budesonide a day [785, 786]. If steroids do not work well enough, they can be combined with aspirin desensitization at a maintenance dose of 500 mg a day.

In patients with aspirin-sensitive rhinosinusitis with no signs of asthma, meaning no history of asthma attack, normal lung function, negative histamine or metacholine bronchial provocation to exclude bronchial hyperreactivity, desensitization can be performed very quickly [785, 786]. Schapowal et al. [785] prefer a two-day schedule giving 50 mg aspirin at 8 a. m., 100 mg at 14 a. m. on the first day, 250 mg and 500 mg aspirin the second day. They continue with the maintenance dose of 500 mg aspirin per day. Aspirin desensitization in analgesics-asthma-syndrome is more difficult and dangerous and should be performed only in a specialized clinic with an intensive care unit [785, 786].

The combined treatment of topical nasal steroids and aspirin densitization is effective in 65% of the patients with improvement of hypersecretion, irritation, and blockage, and in 73% with improvement of hyposmia, anosmia, and polyps [785, 786].

After surgery, a further anti-inflammatory treatment is necessary, otherwise polyps reoccur in 90% of the cases after weeks or months [785, 786].

Adaptive desensitization is, in principle, a promising addition to the options available for treatment of the ASA triad. However, the treatment is time-consuming and not without side effects. Around one-third of patients have to discontinue desensitization in the medium term, most of them because of gastrointestinal problems [468, 519]. Twenty percent of the patients with a dose of 500 mg aspirin a day will have gastrointestinal side effects and 46% with a dose of 1300 mg a day [785, 786].

Patriarca et al. [699] gave topical intranasal treatment with lysine acetylsalicylate postoperatively. In patients without aspirin intolerance, the salicylate nasal spray led to a reduction in the recurrence of polyposis. No side effects were observed. Schapowal and Schmitz desensitized 12 patients with aspirin sensitive rhinosinusitis using 100 mg lysine-aspirin intranasally. Only two of 12 patients responded well. One year later, only one was still free of symptoms, so that the authors concluded, that 100 mg lysine-aspirin a day helps only occasionally and is no alternative to the oral desensitization with 500 mg aspirin a day [785, 786].

Diet

A diet without artificial colorings, bulking agents, and preservatives, with no other potential triggers of pseudoallergic reactions and without natural salicylates may help to avoid recurrences in patients with aspirin intolerance [180, 723, 884]. A strict diet is, however, impracticable [850]. Kowalski [468] saw no positive effect in patients with the ASA triad.

The effect of taking highly unsaturated fatty acids is speculative. They are reported to have an anti-inflammatory effect through modification of the regulation of the arachidonic acid metabolism and a consequent change in the spectrum of synthesized prostaglandins and leukotrienes [731, 944]. In the light of initial investigations of the lung in patients with the ASA triad [713] and of the nose in allergic individuals [731], the use of this mechanism in chronic rhinosinusitis appears fundamentally questionable.

9 Technical Innovations

Computer-Assisted Surgery (CAS); Video Navigation

Using a series of technical aids to orientation, it is possible for the surgeon to obtain a clear view of the local anatomy of the paranasal sinuses and the base of the skull. The position of an instrument or endoscope is generally displayed on a screen in CT or MRI sections of the various spatial planes. In the attempt to operate safely, systematically, and without damage, these orientation aids provide assistance, particularly during revisions and in surgery to remove tumors and at the anterior base of the skull. A reduction in surgical complications is possible, particularly for the less experienced surgeon. The length of routine procedures is reportedly not increased [638, 639].

Schlöndorff et al. [797] in 1989 first reported 50 operations, some in the paranasal sinuses, using a computer-assisted orientation system (CAS: computer-assisted surgery). The system is said to be accurate to 1–2 mm [13, 639, 797, 1027].

Anon et al. [13] apparently use the comparable viewing wand system in all extensive ethmoid procedures. The basis is a preoperative CT with a section thickness of 3 mm obtained in 3-mm increments. The patient is placed in a Mayfield head restraint and the procedure is therefore carried out under general anesthesia. The easy identification of the base of the skull and sphenoid sinus was of particular benefit in routine operations. Difficulties arose in manipulating the viewing wand in the area of the frontal sinus access. Draf [174] did not encounter this type of problem with his surgical technique. Klimek et al. [456] reported preliminary findings with the use of an MR angiography technique to improve vascular imaging in diseased paranasal sinuses. In all orientation systems with fixed measuring arms, manipulation of the indicator in the operative field requires practice. For any measuring process, concentration on the operating process must be interrupted. Procedures under local anesthesia are impossible in view of the need to immobilize the patient. The processing of measurement data before and during the procedure can be labor-intensive and time-consuming [1027]. Some of the more recent systems overcome these disadvantages.

Nitsche et al. [665, 666] have proposed a new orientation system based on ultrasound location. The deviations, when tested on an anatomic specimen, were less than 2 mm.

Truppe and Stammberger [925] have proposed a system of "3D navigation". This is based on location of the patient and endoscope by means of an electromagnetic locating system. The video image can display small three-dimensional rectangles as "targets." The system is apparently quickly calibrated; fixation of the patient is unnecessary. However, the locating system is susceptible to disruption of the electromagnets by large metallic objects. Accuracy is said to be 1–2.5 mm [295].

A large number of technical questions concerning locating systems are under constant discussion and there is continuous to new development. These new developments relate to the basic apparatus and equipment, the locating method, e.g., with measuring sensors or crosswires, the positioning and fixation of the patient, and the calibration of the systems [23, 296, 610]. With regard to handling and expense, the present systems are of only limited use for routine paranasal sinus surgery.

Stereo Endoscopy

The first stereo optics have been produced in recent years, initially as a system with two eyepieces. A relatively advanced stage is the development of video systems that use 100-Hz monitors and high-speed shutter systems to produce a 3D image. As with all video techniques (see p. 24), the ergonomics are relatively favorable; the surgeon stands upright and can watch the monitor in a relaxed position. The endoscope eyepiece is not contaminated by contact with the surgeon's eye or spectacles, and the operative field remains largely sterile. The time required to complete a procedure, however, is currently still greater by up to 30% using this special technology [36].

Strutz [893] reported a stereo optic system with a diameter of 6 mm in combination with a video system. In these and in our own series of tests, video stereo endoscopy has not yet proved to be competitive for routine procedures in the paranasal sinuses. Here again, relatively rapid new development is to be expected.

Other Innovations

Bone shavers with integrated suction, as used in arthroscopic surgery of the knee, were used as early as 1988 by Reinert and Fritzmeier [738] for maxillary sinus fenestration. Here, however, conventional instruments proved superior.

Hawke et al. [310] presented this instrument again as a "micro-debrider" or "hummer" for polypectomy under endoscopic guidance. With a 500-rpm oscillating movement of the serrated blade, polyps were removed on an outpatient basis, preserving the bony structures. Setliff and Parsons [816] reported 680 operations in 345 patients with the same instruments under local or general anesthesia. The oscillations were set at 1600 rpm. The serrated blade had an aperture of 3.5 mm for adults and 2.5 mm for children. Using controlled pressure, it was possible also to remove bony septa as a matter of routine. Blood loss was surprisingly low. Exposure of orbital fat led to no further complication. Similar experiences have been reported by Davidson et al. [141], Grevers [287], and Mendelsohn [595].

The current bone shavers are very suitable for bloodless removal of recurrent polyps in patients following ethmoid surgery that has created relatively clear anatomic compartments [815]. Irregular bony septa and ridges hamper manipulation, since for technical reasons clean removal of bone is not possible.

Schuman and Pineyro [800] have developed a technique called "functional aqualaser sinuscopy" (FALS). The operative field in the paranasal sinuses is constantly irrigated with isotonic physiological salt solution heated to 39.7 °C. A special suction-irrigation endoscope has been developed for this purpose. The warm irrigating solution leads to vasoconstriction, an "underwater" magnification effect, and constant clearing of blood and secretions. The polyps, moreover, are macerated and can be removed easily. For some stages of the operation a Nd:YAG laser is used. This leads to very localized heating of the irrigating fluid and denatures the polyp tissue. Obturating polyps are then removed mechanically.

A good overview over using lasers in polypectomy is given by Rathfoot [732] as well as Levine [505]. The CO_2 laser is an excellent instrument for soft-tissue vaporization, with the disadvantage of a rigid device applying the beam. As yet no studies have measured temperature at the site of work. This is even more important for the Nd:YAG as well as well as the holmium:YAG laser, whose light can be transmitted via a flexible tube, because they have deep thermopenetration into tissue that could impair adjacent structures.

Rosenberg [758] uses an ultrasound aspirator for polypectomy. Its use is safe, bloodless, and apparently fast, and local anesthesia is sufficient. However, the polyp capsule is sometimes too solid and must first be incised before the instrument can be introduced inside the polyp.

The development of these last techniques has probably not yet been completed and their effectiveness has not yet been fully exploited.

References

1. Abram AC, Bellian KT, Giles WJ, Gross CW (1994) Toxic shock syndrome after functional endonasal sinus surgery: an all or none phenomenon? Laryngoscope 104:927–931
2. Adkins JC, Brogden RN (1998) Zafirlukast. A review of its pharmacology and therapeutic potential in the management of asthma. Drugs 55:121–144
3. Agrifoglio A, Terrier G, Duvoisin B (1990) Etude anatomique et endoscopique de l'ethmoide antérieur. Ann Oto Laryngol (Paris) 107:249–258
4. Albers FWJ (1990) The clinical use of cocaine in rhinosurgery: a case-report and a review. Rhinology 28:55–59
5. Alvarez, OM, Levendorf KD, Smerbeck RV, Mertz PM, Eaglstein WH (1984a) Effect of topically applied steroidal and nonsteroidal anti-inflammatory agents on skin repair and regeneration. Federation Proc. 43:2793–2798
6. Alvarez, OM, Mertz PM, Eaglstein WH (1984b) The effect of occlusive dressings on collagen synthesis and epithelisation in superficial wounds. J Surg Res 35:142–148
7. Amberson JB (1954) A clinical consideration of abscesses and cavities of the lung. Bull Johns Hopkins Hosp 94:227–237
8. Amble FR, Kern EB, Neel III HB, Facer GW, McDonald TJ, Czaja JM (1996) Nasofrontal Duct Reconstruction With Silicone Rubber Sheeting for Inflammatory Frontal Sinus Disease: Analysis of 164 Cases. Laryngoscope 106:809–815
9. Amedee RG, Mann WJ, Gilsbach JM (1989) Microscopic endonasal surgery of the paranasal sinuses and the parasellar region. Arch Otolaryngol Head Neck Surg 115:1103–1106
10. Amedee RG, Mann WJ, Gilsbach JM (1990) Microscopic endonasal surgery. clinical update for treatment of chronic sinusitis with polyps. Am J Rhinol 4:203–205
11. Amedee RG, Mann WJ, Gilsbach JM (1993) Microscopic endonasal surgery for repair of CSF leaks. Am J Rhinol 7:1–4
12. Anand VK (1993) Practical endoscopic sinus surgery. McGraw-Hill, New York
13. Anon JB, Lipman SP, Oppenheim D, Halt RA (1994) Computer-assisted endoscopic sinus surgery. Laryngoscope 104:901–905
14. Antonelli PJ, Duvall AJ, Teitelbaum SL (1992) Maxillary sinus atelectasis. Ann Otol Rhinol Laryngol 101:977–981
15. April MM, Zinreich SJ, Baroody FM, Naclerio RM (1993) Coronal CT scan abnormalities in children with chronic sinusitis. Laryngoscope 103:985–990
16. Arnes E, Anke IM, Mair IWS (1985) A comparison between middle and inferior meatal antrostomy in the treatment of chronic maxillary sinus infection. Rhinology 23:65–69
17. Arnhold-Schneider M, Minnigerode B (1986) Ist die endonasale Operation maligner Siebbeintumoren im hohen Lebensalter eine statthafte Behandlungsmethode? Laryngol Rhinol Otol 65:671–672
18. Aurbach G, Reck R, Mihm B (1991a) Die endonasale, endoskopisch-mikroskopisch kontrollierte Dekompression des N. opticus. HNO 39:302–306
19. Aurbach G, Ullrich D, Mihm B (1991b) Chirurgische Anatomie des Nervus opticus und der Arteria carotis interna in der lateralen Keilbeinhöhlenwand. HNO 39:467–475
20. Aust R, Drettner B (1974) The functional size of the human maxillary ostium in vivo. Acta Otolaryngol 78:432–435
21. Austin MB, Hicks JN (1993) Two-year follow-up after limited anterior functional endoscopic sinus surgery (FESS). Am J Rhinol 7:95–99
22. Babbel R, Harnsberger HR, Nelson B, Sonkens J, Hunt S (1991) Optimization of techniques in screening CT of the sinuses. AJNR 12:849–854
23. Babbel RW, Harnsberger HR, Sonkens J, Hunt S (1992) Recurring patterns of inflammatory sinonasal disease demonstrated on screening sinus CT. AJNR 13:903–912
24. Bachor E, Weber R, Kahle G, Draf W (1994) Temporary unilateral amaurosis with pneumosinus dilatans of the sphenoid sinus. Skull Base Surg 4:169–175
25. Badia L, Parikh A, Brookes GB (1994a) Pyocele of the middle turbinate. J Laryngol Otol 108:783–784
26. Badia L, Lund VJ (1994b) Vile bodies: an endoscopic approach to nasal myasis. J Laryngol Otol 108:1083–1085
27. Badre R, Dirnagl K, Guillerm R, Hee J, Kummer A, Schnelle K (1970) Untersuchungen über die Wirkung von Bad Emser Quellprodukten auf das Flimmerepithel. Z Angew Bäder Klimaheilkd 17:40–58
28. Bagatella F (1981) Technique for removal of the nasosinusal block at autopsy. Rhinology 19:47–50
29. Bagatella F (1986) Vidian nerve surgery revisited. Laryngoscope 96:194–197
30. Bagatella F, Mazzoni A (1980) Transnasal microsurgical ethmoidectomy in nasal polyposis. Rhinology 18:25–29
31. Bagatella F, Guirado CR (1983) The ethmoid labyrinth: an anatomical and radiological study. Acta Otolaryngol Suppl 403:1–19
32. Bagatella F, Mazzoni A (1986) Microsurgery in nasal polyposis, transnasal ethmoidectomy. Acta Otolaryngol Suppl 431:1–19
33. Bansberg SF, Harner SG, Forbes G (1987) Relationship of the optic nerve to the paranasal sinuses as shown by computed tomography. Otolaryngol Head Neck Surg 96:331–335
34. Bardin PG, van Heerden BB, Joubert JR (1990) Absence of pulmonary aspiration of sinus contents in patients with asthma and sinusitis. J Allergy Clin Immunol 86:82–88
35. Beasley NJP, Jones NS, Downes RN (1995) Enophthalmos secondary to maxillary sinus disease: single-stage operative management. J Laryngol Otol 109:868–870

35a. Becker DG, Moore D, Lindsey WH, Gross WE, Gross CW (1995) Modified transnasal endoscopic Lothrop procedure: further considerations. Laryngoscope 105: 1161–1166

36. Becker H, Melzer A, Schurz MO, Buess G (1992) 3-D video technique in endoscopic surgery. Endoscopy 25:40–46
37. Behrbohm H, Sydow K (1991) Nuklearmedizinische Untersuchungen zum Reparationsverhalten der Kieferhöhlenschleimhaut nach FES. HNO 39:173–176
38. Behrbohm H, Kaschke O, Sydow K (1995) Der Einfluß des pflanzlichen Sekretolytikums Gelomyrtol forte auf die mukoziliäre Clearance der Kieferhöhle. Laryngo-Rhino-Otol 74:733–737
39. Belal A (1978a) Surgical microscopy of the nose. New frontiers in nasal diagnosis and treatment. J Laryngol Otol 92:197–207
40. Belal A (1978b) The nasal:paranasal block technique. Preparation and uses. J Laryngol Otol 92:781–790
41. Benda TJ, Corey JP (1994) Malbranchea pulchella fungal sinusitis. Otolaryngol Head Neck Surg 110:501–504
42. Bendet E, Eyal A, Kronenberg J (1995) Pneumocephalus as a complication of intranasal ethmoidectomy and polypectomy. Ann Otol Rhinol Laryngol 104:326–328

43. Benjamin B (1985) Evaluation of choanal atresia. Ann Otol Rhinol Laryngol 94:429–432
44. Benninger MA (1992) Rhinitis, sinusitis, and their relationships to allergies. Am J Rhinol 6:27–43
45. Benninger MS, Sebek BA, Levine HL (1989) Mucosal regeneration of the maxillary sinus after surgery. Otolaryngol Head Neck Surg 101:33–37
46. Benninger MS, Mickelson SA, Yaremchuk K (1990) Functional endoscopic sinus surgery: morbidity and early results. Henry Ford Med J 38:5–8
47. Benninger MS, Lavertu P, Levine H, Tucker HM (1991a) Conservation surgery for inverted papillomas. Head Neck 13:442–445
48. Benninger MS, Schmidt JL, Crissman JD, Gottlieb C (1991b) Mucociliary function following sinus mucosal regeneration. Otolaryngol Head Neck Surg 105:641–648
49. Benninger MS, Kaczor J, Stone C (1993) Natural ostiotomy vs. inferior antrostomy in the management of sinusitis: an animal model. Otolaryngol Head Neck Surg 109:1034–1042
50. Benninger MS, Marks S (1995) The endoscopic management of sphenoid and ethmoid mucoceles with orbital and intranasal extension. Rhinology 33:157–161
51. Bent JP, Cuilty-Siller C, Kuhn FA (1994) The frontal cell as a cause of frontal sinus obstruction. Am J Rhinol 8:185–191
52. Berliner DL, Williams RJ, Taylor GN, Nabors CJ (1967) Decreased scar formation with topical corticosteroid treatment. Surgery 61:619–625
53. Berman SZ, Mathison DA, Stevenson DD, Usselman JA, Shore S, Tan EM (1974) Maxillary sinusitis and bronchial asthma: correlation of roentgenograms, cultures, and thermograms. J Allergy Clin Immunol 53:311–318
54. Berman SZ, Mathison DA, Stevenson DD, Tan EM, Vaughan JH (1975) Transtracheal aspiration studies in asthmatic patients in relapse with ‚infective' asthma and in subjects without respiratory disease. J Allergy Clin Immunol 56:206–214
55. Biedlingmaier JF, Leveque H (1992) Endoscopic identification of the maxillary sinus ostium. Otolaryngol Head Neck Surg 107:606
56. Bingham B, Shankar L, Hawke M (1991) Pitfalls in computed tomography of the paranasal sinuses. J Otolaryngol 20:414–418
57. Blackwell KE, Goldberg R, Calcaterra TC (1993) Atelectasis of the maxillary sinus with enophthalmos and midface depression. Ann Otol Rhinol Laryngol 102:429–432
58. Blackwell KE, Ross DA, Kapur P, Calcaterra TC (1993) Propofol for maintenance of general anesthesia: a technique to limit blood loss during endoscopic sinus surgery. Am J Otolaryngol 14:262–266
59. Blokmanis A (1994) Endoscopic diagnosis, treatment, and follow-up of tumours of the nose and sinuses. J Otolaryngol 23:366–369
60. Blümcke S (1995) Pathologie. W de Gruyter, Berlin
61. Bogdasarian RS, Kwyer TA, Dauser RC, Chandler WF, Kindt GW (1983) Internal carotid artery blowout as a complication of sphenoid sinus and skull-base surgery. Otolaryngol Head Neck Surg 91:308–312
62. Bolger WE, Parsons DS, Matson RE (1990a) Functional endoscopic sinus surgery in aviators with recurrent sinus barotrauma. Aviat Space Environ Med 61:148–156
63. Bolger WE, Woodruff WW, Morehead J, Parsons DS (1990b) Maxillary sinus hypoplasia: classification and description of associated uncinate process hypoplasia. Otolaryngol Head Neck Surg 103:759–765
64. Bolger WE, Butzin CA, Parsons DS (1991) Paranasal sinus bony anatomic variations and mucosal abnormalities: CT analysis for endoscopic sinus surgery. Laryngoscope 101:56–64
65. Bolger WE, Parsons DS, Mair EA, Kuhn FA (1992) Lacrimal drainage system injury in functional endoscopic sinus surgery. Arch Otolaryngol Head Neck Surg 118:1179–1184
66. Bolt RJ, de Vries N, Middelweerd RJ (1995) Endoscopic sinus surgery for nasal polyps in children: results. Rhinology 33:148–151
67. Borgstein JA (1987) Epistaxis and the flexible nasopharyngoscope. Clin Otolaryngol 12:49–51
68. Borman KR, Brown PM, Mezera KK, Jhaveri H (1992) Occult fever in surgical intensive care unit patients is seldom caused by sinusitis. Am J Surg 164:412–416
69. Bosshard C (1982) Endoskopie der Nase als Hilfe für die Tränenwegschirurgie. Klin Mbl Augenheilk 180:303–307
70. Boush GA, Lemke BN, Dortzbach RK (1994) Results of endonasal laser-assisted dacryocystorhinostomy. Ophthalmology 101:955–959
71. Bouton V (1991) Septoplasties sous endoscopie. Les Cahiers d' ORL 26:33–39
72. Bouton V (1992) Sphénoethmoidectomie intranasale de révision dans les affections naso-sinusiennes récidivantes notamment les polyposes. Ann Oto-Laryng (Paris) 109:245–253
73. Bouton V, Sanson J (1991a) Plaie méningée au cours de la chirurgie ethmoidale: traitement endoscopique par colle chirurgicale. Acta Oto-Rhino-Laryngol Belg 45:319–322
74. Bouton V, Sanson J, Leguerinel J (1991b) Sinusites du cornet moyen. Étude descriptive et traitement. Ann Oto-Laryngol (Paris) 108:234–240
75. Brasch J, Doniec M, Mertens J, Wellbrock M (1994) Azetylsalizylsäureintoleranz bei polypöser Rhinosinusitis. Allergologie 17:197–203
76. Brattsand R, Andersson PT, Edsbäcker S, Ryrfeldt (1987) Development of glucocorticosteroids with lung selectivity. In: Godfrey S (Ed.) Glucocorticosteroids in childhood asthma. Excerpta Medica, pp 9–25
77. Brennan LG (1996) Minimizing postoperative care and adhesions following endoscopic sinus surgery. ENT Journal 75:45–47
78. Brown BL, Harner SG, Van Dellen RG (1979) Nasal polypectomy in patients with asthma and sensitivity to aspirin. Arch Otolaryngol 105:413–416
79. Brownell DH (1936) Postoperative regeneration of the mucous membrane of the paranasal sinuses: a summary of the published investigations. Arch Otolaryngol 24:582–588
80. Buchwald C, Franzmann MB, Tos M (1995) Sinonasal papillomas: a report of 82 cases in Copenhagen county, including a longitudinal epidemiological and clinical study. Laryngoscope 105:72–79
81. Budrovich R, Saetti R (1992) Microscopic and endoscopic ligature of the sphenopalatine artery.
82. Buiter CT (1988) Nasal antrostomy. Rhinology 26:5–18
83. Buiter CT, Straatman NJA (1981) Endoscopic antrostomy in the nasal fontanelle. Rhinology 19:17–24
84. Bumm P (1980) Eine Methode, das nasale Kieferhöhlenfenster offenzuhalten. Arch Otorhinolaryngol 227:643–645
85. Bumm P (1992) Hals-Nasen-Ohrenkrankheiten. In: Kaiser H, Kley HK (Eds.) Cortisontherapie, Corticoide in Klinik und Praxis. Thieme, Stuttgart, pp 390–401
86. Burson JG, Gussack GS, Hudgins PS (1995) Endoscopic approach to the pediatric orbit. Laryngoscope 105:771–773
87. Busch RF (1992) Frontal sinus osteoma: complete removal via endoscopic sinus surgery and frontal trephination. Am J Rhinol 4:139–143
88. Bush RK, Asbury D (1995) Aspirin-sensitive asthma. In: Busse WW, Holgate ST (Eds.) Asthma and rhinitis. Blackwell, Oxford, pp 1429–1429
89. Büttner C, Witschel H (1991) Chronische Lipogranulome der Lider nach Nasennebenhöhlenoperationen. Fortschr Ophthalmol 88:566–568
90. Buus DR, Tse DT, Farris BK (1990) Ophthalmic complications of sinus surgery. Ophthalmology 97:612–619
91. Calcaterra TC, Thompson JW, Paglia DE (1980) Inverting papilloma of the nose and paranasal sinuses. Laryngoscope 90:53–60

92. Caldwell GW (1893) A new operation for the radical cure of obstruction of the nasal duct. N Y Med J 58:476
93. Calhoun KH, Rotzler WH, Stiernberg CM (1990) Surgical anatomy of the lateral nasal wall. Otolaryngol Head Neck Surg 102:156–160
94. Calhoun KH, Waggenspack GA, Simpson B, Hokansson JA, Bailey BJ (1991) CT evaluation of the paranasal sinuses in symptomatic and asymptomatic populations. Otolaryngol Head Neck Surg 104:480–483
95. Calhoun WJ (1998) Summary of clinical trials with zafirlukast. Am J Respir Crit Care Med 157:S238-S246
96. Caliot P, Midy D, Plessis JL (1990) The surgical anatomy of the middle nasal meatus. Surg Radiol Anat 12:97–101
97. Cannon CR (1989) Video documentation of endoscopic sinus surgery. Otolaryngol Head Neck Surg 101:629–632
98. Cannon CR (1994) Endoscopic management of concha bullosa. Otolaryngol Head Neck Surg 110:449–454
99. Chambers DW, Davis WE, Cook PR, Nishioka GJ, Rudman DT (1997) Long-term outcome analysis of functional endoscopic sinus surgery: correlation of symptoms with endoscopic examination findings and potential prognostic variables. Laryngoscope 107:504–510
100. Chen D, Concus AP, Halbach VV, Cheung SW (1998) Epistaxis originating from traumatic pseudoaneurysm of the internal carotid artery: diagnosis and endovascular therapy. Laryngoscope 108:326–331
101. Cheung DK, Martin GF, Rees J (1992) Surgical approaches to the sphenoid sinus. J Otolaryngol 21:1–8
102. Cheung DK, Attia EL, Kirkpatrick DA, Marcarian B, Wright B (1993) An anatomic and CT scan study of the lateral wall of the sphenoid sinus as related to the transnasal transethmoid endoscopic approach. J Otolaryngol 22:63–68
103. Chilla R (1981) Chirurgie der Nerven im HNO-Bereich. Sensorische Nerven- Nervus opticus. Arch Otorhinolaryngol 231:339–352
104. Chow JM (1994) Rhinologic headaches. Otolaryngol Head Neck Surg 111:211–218
105. Chow JM, Mafee MF (1989) Radiologic assessment preoperative to endoscopic sinus surgery. Otolaryngol Clin North Am 22:691–701
106. Chow JM, Leonetti JP, Mafee MF (1993) Epithelial tumors of the paranasal sinuses and nasal cavity. Radiol Clin North Am 31:61–73
107. Christenbury JD (1992) Translacrimal laser dacryocystorhinostomy. Arch Ophthalmol 110:170–171
108. Christie PE, Smith CM, Lee TH (1991) The potent and selective sulfidopeptide leukotriene antagonist, SK&F 104353, inhibits aspirin-induced asthma. Am Rev Respir Dis 144:957–958
109. Christmas DA, Krouse JH (1996) Powered instrumentation in functional endoscopic sinus surgery I: surgical technique. ENT J 75:33–40
110. Chu CT, Lebowitz RA, Jacobs JB (1997) An analysis of sites of disease in revision endoscopic sinus surgery. Am J Rhinol 11:287–291
111. Clark RA, Henson PM (1988) The Molecular and cellular biology of wound repair. Plenum Press, New York
112. Clark ST, Babin RW, Salazar J (1989) The incidence of concha bullosa and its relationship to chronic sinonasal disease. Am J Rhinol 3:11–13
113. Clary RA, Cunningham MJ, Eavey RD (1992) Orbital complications of acute sinusitis: comparison of computed tomography scan and surgical findings. Ann Otol Rhinol Laryngol 101:598–600
114. Clemens A, van Slycken S, Zeyen T, van den Abeele D, van de Heyning P, Schmelzer A, Tassignon MJ (1992) Blindness following paranasal sinus surgery: a report of two cases. Bull Soc Belge Ophthalmol 245:81–84
115. Clement PAR, van der Veken P, Verstraelen J, Buisseret T, Cox A, Frecourt N, Kaufman L, Derde MPR (1989) Some remarks on nasal polyposis. Acta Oto-Rhino-Laryngol Belg 43:267–278
116. Clevens RA, Bradford CR, Wolf GT (1994) Tension pneumocephalus after endoscopic sinus surgery. Ann Otol Rhinol Laryngol 103:235–237
117. Close LG, Lee NK, Leach JL, Manning SC (1994) Endoscopic resection of the intranasal frontal sinus floor. Ann Otol Rhinol Laryngol 103:952–958
118. Cody DT, Neel HB, Ferreiro JA, Roberts GD (1994) Allergic fungal sinusitis: the Mayo clinic experience. Laryngoscope 104:1074–1079
119. Cohen IK, Diegelmann RF, Lindblad WJ (1992) Wound healing. WB Saunders, Philadelphia
120. Colclasure JB, Barber JL, Morris BK, Graham SS (1993) Endoscopic sinus surgery. A 300 case review. J Ark Med Soc 90:106–109
121. Coleman JR, Duncavage JA (1996) Extended middle meatal antrostomy: the treatment of circular flow. Laryngoscope 1996:1214–1217
122. Connolly AP, White P (1995) How I do it: transantral endoscopic removal of maxillary sinus foreign body. J Otolaryngol 24:73–74
123. Cook MW, Levin LA, Joseph MP, Pinczower EF (1996) Traumatic optic neuropathy: a meta-analysis. Arch Otolaryngol Head Neck Surg 122:389–392
124. Cook PR, Davis WE, McDonald R, McKinsey JP (1993) Antrochoanal polyposis. A review of 33 cases. Ear Nose Throat J 72:401–404
125. Cook PR, Nishioka GJ, Davis WE, McKinsey JP (1994) Functional endoscopic sinus surgery in patients with normal computed tomographic scans. Otolaryngol Head Neck Surg 110:505–509
126. Cook PR, Begegni A, Bryant C, Davis WE (1995) Effect of partial middle turbinectomy on nasal airflow and resistance. Otolaryngol Head Neck Surg 113:413–419
127. Cooke LD, Hadley DM (1991) MRI of the paranasal sinuses: incidental abnormalities and their relationship to symptoms. J Laryngol Otol 105:278–281
128. Corey JP, Bumsted RM (1989) Revision endoscopic ethmoidectomy for chronic rhinosinusitis. Otolaryngol Clin North Am 22:801–808
129. Corey JP, Bumsted R, Panje W, Namon A (1993) Orbital complications in functional endoscopic sinus surgery. Otolaryngol Head Neck Surg 109:814–820
130. Corey JP, Delsupehe KG, Ferguson BJ (1995) Allergic fungal sinusitis: allergic, infectious, or both? Otolaryngol Head Neck Surg 113:110–119
131. Coste A, Gilain L, Roger G, Sebbagh G, Lenoir G, Manach Y, Peynegre R (1995) Endoscopic and CT-scan evaluation of rhinosinusitis in cystic fibrosis. Rhinology 33:152–156
132. Crockett DM, McGill TJ, Friedman EM, Healy GB, Salkeld LJ (1987) Nasal and paranasal sinus surgery in children with cystic fibrosis. Ann Otol Rhinol Laryngol 96:367–372
133. Cumberworth VL, Sudderick RM, Mackay IS (1994) Major complications of functional endoscopic sinus surgery. Clin Otolaryngol 19:248–253
134. Cumberworth VL, Djazaeri B, Mackay IS (1995) Endoscopic fenestration of choanal atresia. J Laryngol Otol 109:31–35
135. Cummings C, Goodman ML (1970) Inverted papillomas of the nose and paranasal sinuses. Arch Otolaryngol Head Neck Surg 92:445–449
136. Cuyler JP (1992) Follow-up of endoscopic sinus surgery on children with cystic fibrosis. Arch Otolaryngol Head Neck Surg 118:505–506
137. Cuyler JP, Monaghan AJ (1989) Cystic fibrosis and sinusitis. J Otolaryngol 18:173–175
138. Danielsen A (1992) Functional endoscopic sinus surgery on a day case out-patient basis. Clin Otolaryngol 17:473–477
139. Davidson TM (1994) Endoscopic sinus surgery (Editorial). Ear Nose Throat J 73:443–444
140. Davidson TM, Stearns G (1994) Extended indications for endoscopic sinus surgery. Ear Nose Throat J 73:467–474

141. Davidson TM, Murphy C, Mitchell M, SmithC, Light M (1995) Management of chronic sinusitis in cystic fibrosis. Laryngoscope 105:354–358
142. Davidsson A, Hellquist HB (1993) The so-called 'allergic' nasal polyp. ORL 55:30–35
143. Davis WE, Barbero GJ, LaMear WR, Templer JW, Konig P (1993) Paranasal sinus mucoceles in cystic fibrosis. Am J Rhinol 7:31–35
144. Davis WE, Templer, JW, LaMear WR (1991a) Patency rate of endoscopic middle meatus antrostomy. Laryngoscope 101:416–420
145. Davis WE, Templer, JW, LaMear WR, Davis WE, Craig SB (1991b) Middle meatus antrostomy: patency rates and risk factors. Otolaryngol Head Neck Surg 104:467–472
146. Davis WE, Bleynat ML (1991c) A suction-irrigation system for endoscopic sinus surgery. Ear Nose Throat J 70:759–760
147. De Gaudemat I, Ebbo D, Leconte F, Barrault S, Koubbi G, Laurier JN, Fombeur JP (1993) Les mycoses du sinus maxillaire. A propos de 40 cas. Ann Oto-Laryngol (Paris) 110:198–202
148. De Lepeleire I, Reiss TF, Rochette F, Botto A, Zhang J, Kundu S, Decramer M (1997) Montelukast causes prolonged, potent leukotriene D_4-receptor antagonism in the airways of patients with asthma. Clin Pharmacol Ther 61:83–92
149. Dehaen F, Clement PAR (1985) Endonasal surgical treatment of bilateral choanal atresia under optic control in the infant. J Otolaryngol 14:95–98
150. Deitmer T (1996) Moderne Funktionsdiagnostik der Nase und der Nasennebenhöhlen. Eur Arch Oto-Rhino-Laryngol Suppl 1996/I: 1–71
151. Deitmer T, Rath B (1988), Befunde, Behandlung und Verlauf frontobasaler Frakturen. Laryngol Rhinol Otol 67:13–16
152. Delank KW, Stoll W (1994) Die Riechfunktion vor und nach endonasaler Operation der chronisch-polypösen Sinusitis. HNO 42:619–623
153. Denecke HJ, Denecke MU, Draf W, Ey W (1992) Die Operationen an den Nasennebenhöhlen und der angrenzenden Schädelbasis. In: Zenker R, Heberer G, Pichlmayr R (Hrsg.) Allgmeie und spezielle Operationslehre. Band V, 3. Auflage, Teil 2. Springer, Berlin.
154. Dessi P, Castro F, Triglia JM, Zanaret M, Cannoni M (1994a) Major complications of sinus surgery: a review of 1192 procedures. J Laryngol Otol 108:212–215
155. Dessi P, Moulin G, Castro F, Chagnaud C, Cannoni M (1994b) Protrusion of the optic nerve into the ethmoid and sphenoid sinus: prospective study of 150 CT studies. Neuroradiology 36:515–516
156. Diament MJ, Senac MO, Gilsanz V, Baker S, Gillespie T, Larsson S (1987) Prevalence of incidental paranasal sinuses opacification in pediatric patients. J Comp Ass Tom 11:426–431
157. Dingsor G, Kramer J, Olsholt R, Soderstrom T (1985) Flunisolide nasal spray 0025 % in the prophylactic treatment of nasal polyposis after polypectomy. Rhinology 23:49–59
157a. Diringer H, Braig HR (1989) Infectivity of unconventional viruses in dura mater. Lancet 1,I: 439–440
158. Dirnagl K, Guillerm R, Hee J, Badre R, Schnelle K (1979) Untersuchungen über den Einfluß von Soleverdünnungen unterschiedlichen pH-Wertes auf die ziliäre Transportfunktion. Z Angew Bäder Klimaheilkd 26:5–14
159. Dixon FW (1945) A study of the clinical results of the intranasal ethmoidectomy. Trans Am Laryngol Rhinol Otol Soc 1945:35–44
160. Dixon FW (1958) The clinical significance of the anatomical arrangement of the paranasal sinuses. Ann Otol Rhinol Laryngol 67:736–741
161. Dixon HS (1976) Microscopic antrostomies in children: a review of the literature in chronic sinusitis and a plan of medical and surgical treatment. Laryngoscope 86:1796–1814
162. Dixon HS (1983) Microscopic sinus surgery, transnasal ethmoidectomy and sphenoidectomy. Laryngoscope 93:440–444
163. Dixon HS (1985) The use of the operating microscope in ethmoid surgery. Otolaryngol Clin North Am 18:75–86
164. Dodson EE, Gross CW, Swerdloff JL, Gustafson LM (1994) Transnasal endoscopic repair of cerebrospinal fluid rhinorrhea and skull base defects: a review of twenty-nine cases. Otolaryngol Head Neck Surg 111:600–605
165. Dolman PJ, Glazer LC, Harris GJ, Beatty RL, Massaro BM (1991) Mechanisms of visual loss in severe proptosis. Ophthalmic Plast Reconstr Surg 7:256–260
166. Dölp R (1987) Anästhesiologische Gesichtspunkte zur endonasalen Nebenhöhlenchirurgie. HNO 35:435–438
167. Donald PJ, Gadre AK (1995a) Neuralgia-like symptoms in a patient with an airgun pellet in the ethmoid sinus: a case report. J Laryngol Otol 109:646–649
168. Donald PJ, Gluckman JL, Rice DH (1995b) The sinuses. Raven Press, New York
169. Donelly AL, Glass M, Minkwitz MC, Casale TB (1995) The leukotriene D4-receptor antagonist, ICI 204219, relieves symptoms of acute seasonal allergic rhinitis. Am J Respir Crit Care Med 151:1734–9
170. Downing E, Braman S, Settipane G (1982) Bronchial hyperreactivity in patients with nasal polyps before and after polypectomy (abstract). J Allergy Clin Immunol 69:102
171. Draf W (1978) Endoskopie der Nasennebenhöhlen. Springer, Berlin
172. Draf W (1982) Die chirurgische Behandlung entzündlicher Erkrankungen der Nasennebenhöhlen. Arch Otorhinolaryngol 235:133–305
172a. Draf W (1983) Endoscopy of paranasal sinuses. Springer, New York
173. Draf W (1991) Endonasal micro-endoscopic frontal sinus surgery: the Fulda concept. Op Tech Otolaryngol Head Neck Surg 2:234–240
174. Draf W (1992) Endonasale mikro-endoskopische Pansinusoperation bei chronischer Sinusitis. III. Endonasale mikro-endoskopische Stirnhöhlenchirurgie. Eine Standortbestimmung. Otolaryngol Nova 2:118–125
175. Draf W, Weber R (1992a) Endonasale Chirurgie der Nasennebenhöhlen: Das Fuldaer mikro-endoskopische Konzept. HNO-Praxis Heute 12:59–80
176. Draf W, Weber R (1992b) Endonasale mikro-endoskopische Pansinusoperation bei chronischer Sinusitis. Otorhinolaryngol Nova 2:1–4
177. Draf W, Berghaus A (1993a) Tumoren und Pseudotumoren ("tumorähnliche Läsionen") der frontalen Schädelbasis, ausgehend von der Nase, den Nasennebenhöhlen und dem Nasenrachenraum (einschließlich der operativen Zugänge). Rhinochirurgisches Referat. Eur Arch Oto-Rhino-Laryngol Suppl 1993/I:105–203
178. Draf W, Weber R (1993b) Endonasal micro-endoscopic pansinusoperation in chronic sinusitis. I. Indications and operation technique. Am J Otolaryngol 14:394–398
179. Draf W, Weber R, Keerl R, Constantinidis J (1995) Aspekte zur Stirnhöhlenchirurgie. Teil 1: Die endonasale Stirnhöhlendrainage bei entzündlichen Erkrankungen der Nasennebenhöhlen. HNO 43:352–357
180. Drake-Lee AB (1991) The value of medical treatment in nasal polyps. Clin Otolaryngol 16:237–239
181. Drake-Lee AB, Lowe D, Swanston A, Grace A (1984) Clinical profile and recurrence of nasal polyps. J Laryngol Otol 98:783–793
182. Drake-Lee AB, Morgan DW (1989) Nasal polyps and sinusitis in children with cystic fibrosis. J Laryngol Otol 103:753–755
183. Duplechain JK, White JA, Miller RH (1991) Pediatric sinusitis. The role of endoscopic sinus surgery in cystic fibrosis and other forms of sinonasal disease. Arch Otolaryngol Head Neck Surg 117:422–426
184. Duquesne U, Dohen P, Hennebert D (1993) Chirurgie endoscopique fonctionnelle des sinus. Méthode d'evalua-

tion et résultats. Acta Oto-Rhino-Laryngol Belg 47:417–422
185. Dutton JJ (1986) Orbital complications of paranasal sinus surgery. Ophthalmic Plast Reconstr Surg 2:119–127
186. Duvoisin B, Schnyder P, Agrifoglio A (1988) Evaluation tomodensitométrique (TDM) de l'ethmoide antérieur par des sectiones parallèles et perpendiculaires à l'axe du canal fronto-nasal. J Radiol 69:787–789
187. Duvoisin B, Agrifoglio A (1989) Prevalence of ethmoid sinus abnormalities on brain CT of asymptomatic patients. AJNR 10:599–601
188. Duvoisin B, Schnyder P (1992) Do abnormalities of the frontonasal duct cause frontal sinusitis? AJNR 159:1295–1298
189. Eaglstein WH, Mertz PM (1981) Effect of topical medicaments on the rate of repair of superficial wounds. In: Dineen P, Hildick-Smith G (Eds.) The surgical wound. Lea & Febinger, Philadelphia, pp 150–170
190. Earwaker J (1993) Anatomic variants in sinonasal CT. RadioGraphics 13:381–415
191. East CA, Annis JAD (1992) Preoperative CT-scanning for endoscopic sinus surgery: a rational approach. Clin Otolaryngol 17:60–66
192. Ecke U, Klimek L, Muller W, Ziegler R, Mann W (1998) Virtual reality: preparation and execution of sinus surgery. Comput Aided Surg 3:45–50
193. Eckert-Möbius A (1929) Gutartige Geschwülste der inneren Nase und ihrer Nebenhöhlen. In: Denker A, Kahler O (Eds.) Handbuch der Hals-Nasen-Ohrenheilkunde, Band 5. Springer, Berlin
194. Eichel BS (1972) The intranasal ethmoidectomy procedure: historical, technical and clinical considerations. Laryngoscope 82:1806–1821
195. Eichel BS (1982) The intranasal ethmoidectomy: a 12-year perspective. Otolaryngol Head Neck Surg 90:540–543
196. Eichel BS (1985) Revision sphenoethmoidectomy. Laryngoscope 95:300–304
197. Eichel BS (1995) Simplified method of staging hyperplastic rhinosinusitis. Arch Otolaryngol Head Neck Surg 121:725–728
198. Eitzen JP, Elsas FJ (1991) Strabismus following endoscopic intranasal sinus surgery. J Pediatr Ophthalmol Strabismus 28:168–170
199. El Naggar M, Kale S, Aldren C, Martin F (1995) Effect of Beconase nasal spray on olfactory function in post-nasal polypectomy patients: a prospective controlled trial. J Laryngol Otol 109: 941–944
200. Elberg M (1977) Erfahrungen mit Nisita-Salbe bei Nasenschleimhauteingriffen. MMW 119:445
201. El-Guindy A (1994) Endoscopic transseptal vidian neurectomy. Arch Otolaryngol Head Neck Surg 120:1347–1351
202. El-Guindy A, El-Scherief S, Hagrass M, Gamea A (1992) Endoscopic endonasal surgery of posterior choanal atresia. J Laryngol Otol 106:528–529
203. El-Guindy A, Mansour MH (1994) The role of transcanine surgery in antrochoanal polyps. J Laryngol Otol 108:1055–1057
204. El-Shazly (1991) Endoscopic surgery of the vidian nerve. Ann Otol Rhinol Laryngol 100:536–539
205. El-Silimy O (1995) The place of endonasal endoscopy in the treatment of orbital cellulitis. Rhinology 33:93–96
206. Ence BK, Gourley DS, Jorgensen NL, Shagets FW, Parsons DS (1990) Allergic fungal sinusitis. Am J Rhinol 4:169–178
207. English GM (1986) Nasal polypectomy and sinus surgery in patients with asthma and aspirin idiosyncrasy. Laryngoscope 96:374–380
208. Enzmann H, Rieben FW (1983): Rhinosinusitis polyposa und Analgetikaintoleranz (Aspirinintoleranz). Laryngol Rhinol Otol 62:119–125
209. Evans K, Shankar L (1993) Imaging of paranasal sinuses. In: Stammberger H, Hawke M (Eds.) Essentials of functional endoscopic sinus surgery. Mosby, St Louis, pp 43–57
210. Everland HH, Melheim I, Anke IM (1992) Acute orbit from ethmoiditis drained by endoscopic sinus surgery. Acta Otolaryngol (Stockh) Suppl 492:147–151
211. Fadal RG (1993) Chronic sinusitis, steroid-dependent asthma, and IgG subclass and selective antibody deficiencies. Otolaryngol Head Neck Surg 109:606–610
212. Fairley JW (1991) Patrick Watson-Williams and the concept of focal sepsis in the sinuses: an historical caveat for functional endoscopic surgery. J Laryngol Otol 105:1–6
213. Fang SY (1994) Transformation of mucosal secretory elements in chronic maxillary sinusitis after endoscopic sinus surgery. Ann Otol Rhinol Laryngol 103:439–443
214. Farrell BP (1993) Endoscopic sinus surgery: sinonasal polyposis and allergy. Ear Nose Throat J 72:544–559
215. Fassoulaki A, Pamouktsoglou P (1989) Prolonged nasotracheal intubation and its association with inflammation of paranasal sinusitis. Anesth Analg 69:50–52
216. Fauci A, Dale D, Balow J (1976) Glucocorticosteroid therapy: mechanisms of action and clinical considerations. Ann Intern Med 84:304–15.
217. Fearon B, Edmonds B, Bird R (1979) Orbital-facial complications of sinusitis in children. Laryngoscope 89:947–953
218. Fehle R (1988) Ergebnisse endonasaler, endoskopischer Siebbein-Operationen. Inaugural-Dissertation, Erlangen
219. Ferguson BJ (1998) What role do systemic corticosteroids, immunotherapy, and antifungal drugs play in the therapy of allergic fungal rhinosinusitis? Arch Otolaryngol Head Neck Surg 124:1174–1178
220. Fernandes CMC (1994) Bilateral transnasal vidian neurectomy in the management of chronic rhinitis. J Laryngol Otol 108:569–573
221. Flecker H (1913) Observations upon cases of absence of lacrimal bones and of existence of perilacrimal ossicles. J Anat Physiol 48:52–72
222. Fletscher Ingals E (1905) New operation and instruments for draining the frontal sinus. Ann Otol Rhinol Laryngol 14:515–519
223. Flinn J, Chapman ME, Wightman AJA, Maran AGD (1994) A prospective analysis of incidental paranasal sinus abnormalities on CT head scans. Clin Otolaryngol 19:287–289
224. Flynn JT, Mitchell KB, Fuller DG, London HB, Cohen HH (1979) Ocular motility complications following intranasal surgery. Arch Ophthalmol 97:453–458
225. Folker, RJ, Marple BF, Mabry RL, Mabry CS (1998) Treatment of allergic fungal sinusitis: a comparison trial of postoperative immunotherapy with specific fungal antigens. Laryngoscope 108:1623–1627
226. Forschner L (1950) Über die Gefahr von Blutungen bei Eingriffen am Keilbein. Arch Ohr Nase Kehlk Heilkd 158:270–275
227. Forsgren K, Stierna P, Kumlien J, Carsöö B (1993) Regeneration of maxillary sinus mucosa following surgical removal: experimental study in rabbits. Ann Otol Rhinol Laryngol 102:459–466
228. Forsgren K, Fukami M, Penttilä M, Kumlien J, Stierna P (1995) Endoscopic and Caldwell-Luc approaches in chronic maxillary sinusitis: a comparative histopathologic study on preoperative and postoperative mucosal morphology. Ann Otol Rhinol Laryngol 104:350–357
229. Fortune DS, Duncavage JA (1998) Incidence of frontal sinusitis following partial middle turbinectomy. Ann Otol Rhinol Laryngol 107:447–53
230. Franzén G, Klausen OG (1994) Post-operative evaluation of functional endoscopic sinus surgery with computed tomography. Clin Otolaryngol 19:332–339
231. Freije JE, Donegan JO (1991) Intracranial complications of transnasal ethmoidectomy. Ear Nose Throat J 70:376–380
232. Frenkiel S, Chagnon F, Small P, Rochon L, Cohen C, Black M (1985) The immunological basis of nasal polyp formation. J Otolaryngol 14:89–91
233. Fried MP, Kleefield J, Gopal H, Reardon E, Ho BT, Kuhn FA (1997) Image-guided endoscopic surgery: results of ac-

curacy and performance in a multicenter clinical study using an electromagnetic tracking system. Laryngoscope 107:594–601
234. Friedman M, Toriumi DM (1989) The effect of a temporary nasoantral window on mucociliary clearance. An experimental study. Otolaryngol Clin North Am 22:819–830
235. Friedman M, Venkatesau TK, Lang D, Caldarelli DD (1996) Bupivacaine for postoperative analgesia following endoscopic sinus surgery. Laryngoscope 106:1382–1385
236. Friedman R, Ackerman M, Wald E, Casselbran JM, Friday G, Fireman P (1984) Asthma and bacterial sinusitis in children. J Allergy Clin Immunol 74:185–189
237. Friedman WH (1975) Surgery for chronic hyperplastic rhinosinusitis. Laryngoscope 85:1999–2011
238. Friedman WH, Katsantonis GP, Slavin RG, Kannel P, Linford P (1982) Sphenoethmoidectomy: its role in the asthmatic patient. Otolaryngol Head Neck Surg 90:171–177
239. Friedman WH, Katsantonis GP (1989) The role of standard technique in modern sinus surgery. Otolaryngol Clin North Am 22:759–774
240. Friedman WH, Katsantonis GP (1990a) Intranasal and transantral ethmoidectomy: a 10-year experience. Laryngoscope 100:343–348
241. Friedman WH, Katsantonis GP (1990b) Transantral revision of recurrent maxillary and ethmoidal disease following functional intranasal surgery. Otolaryngol Head Neck Surg 106:367–371
242. Friedman WH, Katsantonis GP, Sivore M, Kay S (1990c) Computed tomography staging of the paranasal sinuses in chronic hyperplastic rhinosinusitis. Laryngoscope 100:1161–1165
243. Friedman WH, Katsantonis GP, London A (1992) Palatal extension of middle meatal antrostomy. Otolaryngol Head Neck Surg 107:751–754
244. Friedman WH, Katsantonis GP, Bumpous JM (1995) Staging of chronic hyperplastic rhinosinusitis: treatment strategies. Otolaryngol Head Neck Surg 112:210–214
245. Friedrich JP (1984) Traitement par méatotomies endoscopiques des sinusites maxillaires chroniques. Méd et Hyg 42:3410–3416
246. Friedrich JP (1985) Apport de la prothèse de Silastic dans la chirurgie de l'infundibulum frontal. Problèmes actuels d'ORL 9:43–47
247. Friedrich JP (1987) Le traitement de la polypose nasoethmoidale par chirurgie endoscopique. Ther Umsch 44:86–92
248. Friedrich JP, Terrier G (1984) La chirurgie sinusale maxillaire endoscopique par voie endonasale. Problèmes actuels d'ORL 7:185–189
249. Friedrich JP, Terrier G (1987) Indications et résultats de l'evidement ethmoidal sous guidage endoscopique. Problèmes actuels d'ORL 10:240–247
250. Fuji K, Chambers SM, Rhoton AL (1979) Neurovascular relationships of the sphenoid sinus. J Neurosurg 50:31–39
251. Fujitani T (1972) Intranasal optic canal decompression technique for traumatic visual disturbance. Otologia (Fukuoka) 18:300–307 [In Japanese]
252. Fujitani T (1974) A proposal of endonasal-transethmoidal operation for optic canal decompression and its clinical evaluation in 16 patients. Auris Nasus Larynx 1:129–139
253. Fujitani T, Inoue K, Takahashi T, Ikushima K, Asai T (1986) Indirect traumatic optic neuropathy: visual outcome of operative and nonoperative cases. Jpn J Ophthalmol 30:125–134
254. Fukuda K, Matsune S, Ushikai M, Imamura Y, Ohyama M (1989) A study on the relationship between adenoid vegetation and rhinosinusitis. Am J Otolaryngol 10:214–216
255. Furukawa CF (1992) The role of allergy in sinusitis in children. J Allergy Clin Immunol 90:515–517
256. Gamble RC (1933) Acute inflammation of the orbit in children. Arch Ophthalmol 10:483–497
257. Gamea A, Fathi M, El-Guindy A (1994) The use of the rigid endoscope in trans-sphenoidal pituitary surgery. J Laryngol Otol 108:19–22
258. Gammert C (1984) Langzeitergebnisse der endonasalen Ethmoidektomie. Aktuelle Probleme der ORL 7:205–210
259. Garcia CE, Cunningham MJ, Clary RA, Joseph MP (1993) The etiologic role of frontal sinusitis in pediatric orbital abscesses. Am J Otolaryngol 14:449–452
260. Gardiner Q, Oluwole M, Tan L, White P (1996) An animal model for training in endoscopic nasal and sinus surgery. J Laryngol Otol 110:425–428
261. Gaskins RE (1989) Use of a modified microdrill in endoscopic sinus surgery for improved exposure and reduced adhesions. Laryngoscope 99:556–557
262. Gaskins RE (1992) A surgical staging system for chronic sinusitis. Am J Rhinol 6:5–12
263. Geiger K, Witschel H, Büttner C (1993) Chronische Lipogranulome (Paraffingranulome) der Lider und der Orbita nach endonasaler Nebenhöhlenoperation. Laryngo-Rhino-Otol 72:356–360
264. Gellrich NC, Greulich W, Gellrich MM, Eysel UT (1995) Flash visual evoked potentials (VEP) and electroretinograms (ERG) in the evaluation of optic nerve trauma. Dtsch Z Mund Kiefer Gesichts-Chir 19:98–101
265. Georgieff M, Schirmer U (1995) Klinische Anästhesiologie. Springer, Berlin
266. Gerber ME, Myer CM, Berger TS, Prenger EC (1994) Endoscopic transsphenoidal drainage of an epidural abscess. Am J Otolaryngol 15:310–314
267. Gilain L, Planquart X, Coste A, Lelievre G, Peynegre R (1992) Résultats du traitement des asperigilloses du sinus maxillaire par voie de méatotomie moyenne exclusive. Ann Oto-Laryng (Paris) 109:289–293
268. Giles WC, Gross CW, Abram AC, Greene WM, Avner TG (1994) Endoscopic septoplasty. Laryngoscope 104:1507–1509
269. Gittelman PD, Jacobs JB, Skorina J (1993) Comparison of functional endoscopic sinus surgery under local and general anesthesia. Ann Otol Rhinol Laryngol 102:289–293
270. Glasier CM, Ascher DP, Williams, KD (1986) Incidental paranasal sinus abnormalities on CT of children: clinical correlation. AJNR 7:861–864
271. Glatt HJ, Chan AC, Barrett L (1991) Computed tomography of nasolacrimal duct obstruction after endoscopic sinus surgery. Arch Otolaryngol Head Neck Surg 117:1059–1060
272. Gleich LL, Rebeiz EE, Pankratov MM, Shapshay SM (1995a) Autologous fibrin tissue adhesive in endoscopic sinus surgery. Otolaryngol Head Neck Surg 112:238–241
273. Gleich LL, Rebeiz EE, Pankratov MM, Shapshay SM (1995b) The Holmium-YAG laser-assisted otolaryngologic procedures. Arch Otolaryngol Head Neck Surg 121:1162–1166
274. Gliklich RE, Metson R (1994) A comparison of sinus computed tomography (CT) staging systems for outcomes research. Am J Rhinol 8:291–297
275. Gliklich RE, Metson R (1995a) Techniques for outcomes research in chronic sinusitis. Laryngoscope 105:387–390
276. Gliklich RE, Metson R (1995b) The health impact of chronic sinusitis in patients seeking otolaryngologic care. Otolaryngol Head Neck Surg 113:104–109
277. Glück U (1991) Die physiologische Bedeutung der Nasennebenhöhlen beim Menschen: Spekulationen seit 1800 Jahren. Schweiz Med Wschr 121:925–931
278. Godbersen GS, Kleeberg J, Lüttges J, Werner JA (1995) Sphärulozytose (Myosphärulose) der Nasennebenhöhlen. HNO 43:552–555
279. Goldsmith AJ, Zahtz GD, Stegnjajic A, Shikowitz M (1993) Middle turbinate headache syndrome. Am J Rhinol 7:17–23
280. Golnik KC, Miller NR (1991) Late recovery of function after oculomotor nerve palsy. Am J Ophthalmol 111:566–570
281. Gonnering RS, Lyon DB, Fisher JC (1991) Endoscopic laser-assisted lacrimal surgery. Am J Ophthalmol 111:152–157

282. Good RH (1907) A simple and safe operation on the frontal sinus by the intranasal route. JAMA 49:753–754
283. Good RH (1908) An intranasal method for opening the frontal sinus establishing the largest possible drainage. Laryngoscope 18:266–274
284. Goodyear HM (1944) Mucocele in frontal and ethmoidal sinuses. Simplified surgical treatment. Ann Otol Rhinol Laryngol 53:242–245
285. Gorham CB, Bacher JA (1930) Regeneration of the human maxillary antral lining. Arch Otolaryngol 11:763–771
286. Greinwald JH, Holtee MR (1996) Absorption of topical cocaine in rhinologic procedures. Laryngoscope 106:1223–1225
287. Grevers G (1995) Ein neues Operationssystem für die endoskopische Nasennebenhöhlenchirurgie. Laryngo-Rhino-Otol 74:266–268
288. Grevers G, Reiterer A (1990) Traumatisch bedingte Fremdkörper der Nasennebenhöhlen. Laryngo-Rhino-Otol 69:155–157
289. Gross CW, Gurucharri MJ, Lazar RH, Long TE (1989) Functional endonasal sinus surgery (FESS) in the pediatric age group. Laryngoscope 99:272–275
290. Gross GW, McGeady SJ, Kerut T, Ehrlich SM (1991) Limited-slice CT in the evaluation of paranasal sinus disease in children. AJR 156:367–369
291. Gross CW, Gross WE (1994) Post-operative care for functional endoscopic sinus surgery. Ear Nose Throat J 73:476–479
292. Gross WE, Gross CW, Becker D, Moore D, Phillips D (1995) Modified transnasal endoscopic Lothrop procedure as an alternative to frontal sinus obliteration. Otolaryngol Head Neck Surg 113:427–434
293. Grünwald L (1910) Die Lymphgefässe der Nebenhöhlen der Nase. Arch Laryngol Rhinol 23:1–5
294. Guerin JM, Meyer P, Habib Y, Levy C (1988) Purulent rhinosinusitis is also a cause of sepsis in critically ill patients. Chest 93:893
295. Gunkel AR, Freysinger W, Thumfart WF, Truppe MJ (1995) Application of the ARTMA image-guided navigation system to endonasal sinus surgery. In: Lemke HU, Inamura K, Jaffe CC, Vannier MW (Eds.) Computer assisted radiology. Springer, Heidelberg 1995; pp 1147–1151
296. Gunkel AR, Freysinger W, Thumfart WF (1997) Computer-assisted surgery in the frontal and maxillary sinus. Laryngoscope 107:631–633
297. Gutiérrez-Ortega A, Sprekelsen-Gasso C, Valles-San Leandro L, Delmperial JM (1995) Endonasal dacryocystorhinostomy. Orbit 14:25–28
298. Habal MB, Maniscaldo JE, Rhoton AL (1977) Microsurgical anatomy of the optic canal: correlates to optic nerve exposure. J Surg Res 22:527–533
299. Hajek M (1926) Pathologie und Therapie der entzündlichen Erkrankungen der Nebenhöhlen der Nase, 5. Auflage. F. Deuticke, Leipzig
300. Halle M (1906) Externe oder interne Operation der Nebenhöhleneiterungen. Berl Klin Wochenschr 43:1369–1372, 1404–1407
301. Halton JR, Cannon CR (1993) Functional endoscopic sinus surgery in children. J Miss State Med Assoc 34:1–6
302. Hammer B (1995) Orbital fractures – diagnosis, operative treatment, secondary corrections. Hogrefe & Huber, Göttingen
303. Hammer G, Radberg C (1961) The sphenoidal sinus: an anatomical and roentgenologic study with reference to transsphenoid hypophysectomy. Acta Radiol 56:401–425
304. Handler LC, Davey IC, Hill JC, Lauryssen C (1991) The acute orbit: differentiation of orbital cellulitis from subperiosteal abscess by computerized tomography. Neuroradiology 33:15–18
305. Hao SP, Wang HS, Lui TN (1995) Transnasal endoscopic management of basal encephalocele – craniotomy is no longer mandatory. Am J Otolaryngol 16:196–199
306. Har-El G (1995) Telescopic extracranial approach to frontal mucoceles with intracranial extension. J Otolaryngol 24:98–101
307. Har-El G, Lucente FE (1995) Endoscopic intranasal frontal sinusotomy. Laryngoscope 105:440–443
308. Harner SG, Newell RC (1969) Treatment of frontal osteomyelitis. Laryngoscope 79:1281–1294
309. Havas TE, Motbey JA, Gullane PJ (1988) Prevalence of incidental abnormalities on computed tomographic scans of the paranasal sinuses. Arch Otolaryngol Head Neck Surg 114:856–859
310. Hawke WM, McCombe AW (1995) How I do it: nasal polypectomy with an arthroscopic bone shaver: the Stryker 'hummer'. J Otolaryngol 24:57–59
311. Healy GB, McGill T, Jako GJ, Strong MS, Vaughan CM (1978) Management of choanal atresia with carbon dioxide laser. Ann Otol 87:658–662
312. Heermann H (1958) Über endonasale Chirurgie unter Verwendung des binocularen Mikroskopes. Arch Ohr Nase Kehlk Heilk 171:295–297
313. Heermann J (1962) Resektion des Bodens und der unteren Vorderwand der Keilbeinhöhle zur Erweiterung bei Choanalatresie. Z Laryngol Rhinol 41:390–393
314. Heermann J (1974) Endonasale mikrochirurgische Resektion der Mukosa des Sinus maxillaris. Laryngo-Rhino-Otol 53:938–941
315. Heermann J (1980) Temporäre Amaurose bei mikrochirurgischer endonasaler Ethmoid- und Saccus lacrimalis-Operation in Lokalanaesthesie. HNO 28:70
316. Heermann J (1991) Rhinochirurgische Aspekte bei Tränenwegstenosen. Otorhinolaryngol Nova 1:227–232
317. Heermann J, Neues D (1986) Intranasal microsurgery of all paranasal sinuses, the septum, and the lacrimal sac with hypotensive anesthesia. Ann Otol Rhinol Laryngol 95:631–638
318. Helal MZ (1995) Combined micro-endoscopic trans-sphenoid excisions of pituitary macroadenomas. Eur Arch Otorhinolaryngol 252:186–189
319. Heller M (1913) Blindness and death following intranasal sinus operation. Laryngoscope 33:66–67
320. Hellström S, Salen B, Stenfors L-E (1983) Absorbable gelatin sponge (Gelfoam[R]) in otosurgery: one cause of undesirable postoperative results? Acta Otolaryngol 96:269–275
321. Hendeles L, Marshik P (1997) Zafirlukast for chronic asthma: convenient and generally safe, but is it effective? Ann Pharmocother 31:1084–1086
322. Herzon GD, Zealear DL (1994) Intraoperative monitoring of the visual evoked potential during endoscopic sinus surgery. Otolaryngol Head Neck Surg 111:575–579
323. Heymann P, Ritter G (1909) Zur Morphologie und Terminologie des mittleren Nasenganges. Z Laryngol Rhinol 1:1–18
324. Hilding A (1933) Experimental surgery of the nose and sinuses. II. Gross results following the removal of the intersinusous septum and of strips of mucous membrane from the frontal sinus of the dog. Arch Otolaryngol 17:321–327
325. Hilding AC (1941) Experimental sinus surgery: effects of operative windows on normal sinuses. Ann Otol 50:379–392
326. Hilding AC (1965) Regeneration of respiratory epithelium after minimal surface trauma. Ann Otol Rhinol 74:903–914
327. Hilding AC, Banovetz J (1963) Occluding scars in the sinuses: relation to bone growth. Laryngoscope 73:1201–1218
328. Hill JN, Gershon NI, Gargiulo PO (1983) Total spinal blockade during local anaesthesia of the nasal passages. Anesthesiology 59:144–146
329. Hillen B (1993) Paranasal sinuses and anterior skull base. Elsevier's Interactive Anatomy, Disc I of Volume I: The Head and Neck. Elsevier Science, Amsterdam

330. Hintschich CR, Beyer-Machule CK, Stefani FH (1995) Paraffinoma of the periorbit - a challenge for the oculoplastic surgeon. Ophthalmic Plast Reconstr Surg 11:39–43
331. Hirsch O (1952) Successful closure of cerebrospinal fluid rhinorrhea by endonasal surgery. Arch Otolaryngol 56:1–12
332. Hoffer ME, Kennedy DW (1994) The endoscopic management of sinus mucoceles following orbital decompression. Am J Rhinol 8:61–65
333. Hoffman SR, Stinziano GD, Goodman D (1984) Microscopic rhinoscopy in the treatment of inverted papillomas. Laryngoscope 94:662–663
334. Hoffman SR, Dersarkissian RM, Buck SH, Stinziano GD, Buck GM (1989) Sinus disease and surgical treatment: a results oriented quality assurance study. Otolaryngol Head Neck Surg 100:573–577
335. Hoffmann D, May M (1989) Endoscopic sinus surgery - experience with the initial 100 patients. Trans Pa Acad Ophthalmol Otolaryngol 41:847–850
336. Hoffmann DF, May M (1991) Endoscopic frontal sinus surgery: frontal trephine permits a 'two sided approach'. Operative Techn Otolaryngol Head Neck Surg 2:257–261
337. Hofmann U (1966) Zwischenfälle während endonasaler Siebbeinausräumung bei Asthmapatienten. HNO 14:26–28
338. Hollis LJ, McGlashan JA, Walsh RM, Bowdler DA (1994) Massive epistaxis following sphenoid sinus exploration. J Laryngol Otol 108:171–173
339. Holzapfel L, Chevret S, Madinier G, Ohen G, Demingeon G, Coupry A, Chaudet M (1993) Influence of long-term oro- or nasotracheal intubation on nosocomial maxillary sinusitis and pneumonia. Critical Care Med 21:1132–1138
340. Hong SC, Leopold DA, Oliverio PJ, Benson ML Mellits D, Quaskey SA, Zinreich SJ (1998) Otolaryngol Head Neck Surg 118:183–186
341. Hosemann W, Wigand ME, Fehle J, Sebastian J, Diepgen DL (1988) Ergebnisse endonasaler Siebbein-Operationen bei diffuser hyperplastischer Sinusitis paranasalis chronica. HNO: 36:54–59
342. Hosemann W, Röckelein G (1989a) Entnahme eines Siebbeinblocks von der Leiche für die mikroanatomische Präparation. Laryngo-Rhino-Otol 68:130–131
343. Hosemann W, Wigand ME, Nikol J (1989b) Klinische und funktionelle Aspekte der endonasalen Kieferhöhlen-Operation. HNO 37:225–230
344. Hosemann W, Michelson A, Weindler J, Mang H, Wigand ME (1990) Einfluß der endonasalen Nasennebenhöhlenchirurgie auf die Lungenfunktion des Patienten mit Asthma bronchiale. Laryngo-Rhino-Otol 69:521–526
345. Hosemann W, Göde U, Länger F, Röckelein G, Wigand ME (1991a) Experimentelle Untersuchungen zur Wundheilung in den Nasennebenhöhlen. I. Ein Modell respiratorischer Wunden in der Kaninchenkieferhöhle. HNO 39:8–12
346. Hosemann W, Göde U, Länger F, Wigand ME (1991b) Experimentelle Untersuchungen zur Wundheilung in den Nasennebenhöhlen. II. Spontaner Wundschluß und medikamentöse Effekte im standardisierten Wundmodell. HNO 39:48–54
347. Hosemann W, Dunker I, Göde U, Wigand ME (1991c) Experimentelle Untersuchungen zur Wundheilung in den Nasennebenhöhlen. III. Endoskopie und Histologie des Operationsgebietes nach einer endonasalen Siebbeinausräumung. HNO 39:111–115
348. Hosemann W, Nitsche N, Rettinger G, Wigand ME (1991d) Die endonasale, endoskopisch kontrollierte Versorgung von Duradefekten der Rhinobasis. Laryngo-Rhino-Otol 70:115–119
349. Hosemann W, Wigand ME, Goede U (1991e) Normal wound healing of the paranasal sinuses: Clinical and experimental investigations. Eur Arch Otorhinolaryngol 248:390–394
350. Hosemann W, Leuwer A, Wigand ME (1992a) Die endonasale, endoskopisch kontrollierte Stirnhöhlenoperation bei Mukopyozelen und Empyemen. Laryngo-Rhino-Otol 71:181–186
351. Hosemann W, Wigand ME, Wessel B, Schellmann B (1992b) Medico-legale Probleme in der endonasalen Nasennebenhöhlenchirurgie. Eur Arch Otorhinolaryngol Suppl 1992/II:284–296
352. Hosemann W, Wigand ME (1992c) Merit and demerit of endoscopic surgery. Rhinology Suppl 14:141–145
353. Hosemann W, Goertzen W, Wohlleben R, Wolf S, Wigand ME (1993a) Olfaction after endoscopic endonasal ethmoidectomy. Am J Rhinol 7:11–15
354. Hosemann W, Gottsauner A, Leuwer A, Farmand M, Wenning W, Göde U, Stenglein C, v Glaß W (1993b) Untersuchungen zur Frakturheilung im Siebbein - Ein Beitrag zur rhinologischen Versorgung nasoethmoidaler Verletzungen. Laryngo-Rhino-Otol 72:383–390
355. Hosemann W, Göde U, Wagner W (1994a) Current review: Nasal epidemiology, pathophysiology and range of endonasal sinus surgery. Am J Otolaryngol 15:85–98
356. Hosemann W, Kühnel T (1994b) Medicolegale Aspekte bei endonasalen Nasennebenhöhlenoperationen. Teil 1 und Teil 2. HNO aktuell 2:315–319, 355–360
357. Hosemann W, Groß R, Göde U, Kühnel T, Röckelein G (1995) The anterior sphenoid wall: relative anatomy for sphenoidotomy. Am J Rhinol 9:137–144
358. Hosemann W, Kühnel T, Held P, Wagner W, Felderhoff A (1997) Endonasal fenestration of the frontal sinus in surgical management of chronic sinusitis - a critical evaluation. Am J Rhinol 11:1–11
359. Hosemann W, Kühnel T, Burchard AK, Werner JA (1998) Histochemical detection of lymphatic drainage pathways in the middle nasal meatus. Rhinology 36:50–54
360. Howland WC, Mathison DA, Bell DN, Stevenson DD (1986) Effect of sinus surgery (SS) on asthma. J Allergy Clin Immunol 77:161
361. Hoyt WH (1992) Bacterial patterns found in surgery patients with chronic sinusitis. J Am Osteopath Assoc 92:205–212
362. Hoyt WH (1993) Endoscopic stenting of nasofrontal communication in frontal sinus disease. Ear Nose Throat J 72:596–597
363. Hudgins PA (1993) Complications of endoscopic sinus surgery. The role of the radiologist in prevention. Radiol Clin North Am 31:21–32
364. Hudgins PA, Browning DG, Gallups J, Gussack GS, Peterman SB, Davis PC, Silverstein AM, Beckett WW, Hoffmann JC (1992) Endoscopic paranasal sinus surgery: radiographic evaluation of severe complications. AJNR 13:1161–1167
365. Huggil PH, Ballantyne JC (1952) An investigation into the relationship between adenoids and sinusitis in children. J Otolaryngol 1952:84–91
366. Hui Y, Gaffney R, Crysdale WS (1995) Sinusitis in patients with cystic fibrosis. Eur Arch Otolaryngol 252:191–196
367. Hulka GF, Kulwin DR, Weeks SM, Cotton RT (1995) Congenital lacrimal sac mucoceles with intranasal extension. Otolaryngol Head Neck Surg 113:651–655
368. Huxley EJ, Viroslav J, Gray WR, Pierce AK (1978) Pharyngeal aspiration in normal adults and patients with depressed consciousness. Am J Med 64:564–568
369. Ilberg C (1994) Die Mikrochirurgie der Nase und der Nebenhöhlen; Konzept, Technik und Ergebnis. Pneumologie 48:93–98
370. Ilberg C, May A, Weber A (1990) Zur Mikrochirurgie der Nasenhaupt- und Nebenhöhlen. Laryngo-Rhino-Otol 69:52–57
371. Illum P (1986) Congenital choanal atresia treated by laser surgery. Rhinology 24:205–209
372. Illum P, Grymer L, Hilberg O (1992) Nasal packing after septoplasty. Clin Otolaryngol 17:158–162
373. Irvin CG (1992) Sinusitis and asthma: an animal model. J Allergy Clin Immunol 90:521–533

374. Isenberg SF (1995) Endoscopic removal of chondromyxoid fibroma of the ethmoid sinus. Am J Otolaryngol 16:205–208
375. Isenberg SF, Scott JA (1994) Management of massive hemorrhage during endoscopic sinus surgery. Otolaryngol Head Neck Surg 111:134–136
376. Iwens P, Clement PAR (1994) Sinusitis in allergic patients. Rhinology 32:65–67
377. Jacobs JB, Lebowitz RA, Lagmay VM, Damiano A (1998) Conservative approach to inflammatory nasofrontal duct disease. Ann Otol Rhinol Laryngol 107:658–61
378. Jacobs RL, Freda A, Culver WG (1983) Primary nasal polyposis. Ann Allergy 51:500–505
379. Jacobson JA, Stevens MH, Kasworm EM (1988) Evaluation of single-dose cefazolin prophylaxis for toxic shock syndrome. Arch Otolaryngol Head Neck Surg 114:326–327
380. Jafek BW (1985) Intranasal ethmoidectomy. Otolaryngol Clin North Am 18:61–74
381. Jafek BW, Moran DT, Eller PM, Rowley JC, Jafek TB (1987) Steroid-dependent anosmia. Arch Otolaryngol Head Neck Surg 113:547–549
382. Jamal A, Maran AGD (1987) Atopy and nasal polyposis. J Laryngol Otol 101:355–358
383. Jankowski R, Lhuillier C, Simon C, Wayoff M (1990) Quelle voie d'abord choisir pour les papillomes inversés nasosinusiens? Revue Laryngol Otol Rhinol 111:71–74
384. Jankowski R, Goetz R, Moneret Vautrin DA, Daures P, Lallemant JG, Wayoff M (1991) Les insuffisances de l'ethmoidectomie dans la prise en charge thérapeutique de la polypose. Ann Oto-Laryngol (Paris) 108:298–306
385. Jankowski R, Auque J, Simon C, Marchal JC, Hepner H, Wayoff M (1992a) Endoscopic pituitary tumor surgery. Laryngoscope 102:198–202
386. Jankowski R, Moneret-Vautin DA, Goetz R, Wayoff M (1992b) Influence of medico-surgical treatment for nasal polyps on the development of associated asthma. Rhinology 30:249–258
387. Jäntti-Alanko S, Holopainen E, Malmberg H (1989) Recurrence of nasal polyps after surgical treatment. Rhinology Suppl 8:59–64
388. Javate RM, Campomanes BSA, Co ND, Dinglasan JL, Go CG, Tan EN, Tan FE (1995) The endoscope and the radiofrequency unit in DCR surgery. Ophthalmic Plast Reconstr Surg 11:54–58
389. Jebeles JA, Hicks JN (1993) The use of Merocel for temporary medialization of the middle turbinate during functional endoscopic sinus surgery. Ear Nose Throat J 72:145–146
390. Jiannetto DF, Pratt MF (1995) Correlation between preoperative computed tomography and operative findings in functional endoscopic sinus surgery. Laryngoscope 105:924–927
391. Johannsen V, Maune S, Erichsen H, Hedderich H, Werner JA (1996) Der Einfluß der postoperativen endonasalen Schleimhautpflege auf die nasale Bakterienflora: prospektive Untersuchung zweier Spülverfahren mit NaCl-Lösung nach Nasennebenhöhlenchirurgie. Laryngo-Rhino-Otol 75:580–583
392. Johansson S-A, Andersson K-E, Brattsand R, Gruvstad E, Hedneř P (1982) Topical and systemic glucocorticoid potencies of budesonide, beclomethasone dipropionate and prednisolone in man. Eur J Respir Dis 63 Suppl 122:74–82
393. John G, Low JM, Tan PE, van Hasselt CA (1995) Plasma catecholamine levels during functional endoscopic sinus surgery. Clin Otolaryngol 20:213–215
394. Jonathan DA, Violaris NS (1988) Comparison of cocaine and lignocaine as intranasal local anaesthetics. J Laryngol Otol 102:628–629
395. Jones JW, Parsons DS, Cuyler JP (1993) The results of functional endoscopic sinus (FES) surgery on the symptoms of patients with cystic fibrosis. Int J Pediatr Otorhinolaryngol 28:25–32
396. Jorgensen RA (1991) Endoscopic and computed tomographic findings in ostiomeatal sinus disease. Arch Otolaryngol Head Neck Surg 117:279–287
397. Jorissen und Feenstra (1992) Optic nerve decompression for indirect posterior optic nerve trauma. Acta Oto-Rhino-Laryngolo Belg 46:311–324
398. Joseph MP (1998) Indications, technique, and results of optic nerve decompression. Curr Opin Otolaryngol Head Neck Surg 6:51–61
399. Jovanovic S (1961) Supernumerary frontal sinuses on the roof of the orbit, their clinical significance. Acta Anat 45:133–142
400. Juntunen K, Tarkkanen J, Makinon J (1984) Caldwell Luc operation in the treatment of childhood asthma. Laryngoscope 94:249–251
401. Kainz J, Stammberger H (1988) Das Dach des vorderen Siebbeines: Ein Locus minoris resistentiae an der Schädelbasis. Laryngol Rhinol Otol 66:142–149
402. Kainz J, Stammberger H (1991) Gefahrenpunkte der hinteren Rhinobasis. Anatomische, histologische und endoskopische Befunde. Laryngo-Rhino-Otol 70:479–486
403. Kainz J, Braun H, Genser P (1993a) Die Haller'schen Zellen: Morphologische Evaluierung und klinisch-chirurgische Bedeutung. Laryngo-Rhino-Otol 72:599–604
404. Kainz J, Klimek L, Anderhuber W (1993b) Vermeidung vaskulärer Komplikationen bei der endonasalen Nasennebenhöhlenchirurgie. HNO 41:146–152
405. Kaluskar SK, Patil NP, Sharkey AN (1993) The role of CT in functional endoscopic sinus surgery. Rhinology 31:49–52
406. Kamel RH (1989) Endoscopic transnasal surgery in chronic maxillary sinusitis. J Laryngol Otol 103:492–501
407. Kamel R (1990) Endoscopic transnasal surgery in antrochoanal polyp. Arch Otolaryngol Head Neck Surg 116:841–843
408. Kamel RH (1992) Conservative endoscopic surgery in inverted papilloma. Arch Otolaryngol Head Neck Surg 118:649–653
409. Kamel R (1994) Transnasal endoscopic approach in congenital choanal atresia. Laryngoscope 104:642–646
410. Kamel RH (1995) Transnasal endoscopic medial maxillectomy in inverted papilloma. Laryngoscope 105:847–853
411. Kamel R, Zaher S (1991) Endoscopic transnasal vidian neurectomy. Laryngoscope 101:316–319
412. Kane K (1993) Australian experience with functional endoscopic sinus surgery and its complications. Ann Otol Rhinol Laryngol 102:613–615
413. Kane KJ (1997) Recirculation of mucus as a cause of persistent sinusitis. Am J Rhinol 11:361–369
414. Karlsson G, Rundcrantz H (1982) A randomized trial of intranasal beclomethasone dipropionate after polypectomy. Rhinology 20:144–148
415. Kaschke O, Behrbohm H (1994) Endoskopische Operation der chronischen Sinusitis. Hoher Stellenwert der Nachbehandlung. Therapiewoche 44:408–412
416. Kaschke O, Behrbohm H (1997) Primed Nasensplint. Productinformation Primed, Halberstadt, Germany
417. Kasper KA (1936) Nasofrontal connections – a study based on one hundred consecutive dissections. Arch Otolaryngol 23:322–343
418. Kass E, Massaro B, Komorowski A, Toohill RJ (1993) Wound healing of KTP and argon laser lesions in the canine nasal cavity. Otolaryngol Head Neck Surg 108:283–292
419. Kassel K (1915) Die Nasenheilkunde des Altertums. Zeitschr f Laryngol 4:573–640
420. Katsantonis GP, Friedman WH, Sivore MC (1990) The role of computed tomography in revision sinus surgery. Laryngoscope 100:811–816
421. Katsantonis GP, Friedman WH, Bruns M (1994) Intranasal sphenoethmoidectomy: an evolution of technique. Otolaryngol Head Neck Surg 111:781–786
422. Kaufman J, Wright GW (1969) The effect of nasal and nasopharyngeal irritation on airway resistance in man. Am Rev Respir Dis 100:626–630

423. Kaufmann J, Chen JC, Wright GW (1970) The effect of trigeminal resection on reflex bronchoconstriction after nasal and nasopharyngeal irritation in man. Am Rev Respir Dis 101:768–769
424. Kautzky M, Bigenzahn B, Steurer M, Susani M, Schenk P (1992) Holmium: YAG – Laserchirurgie. Anwendungsmöglichkeiten bei entzündlichen Nasennebenhöhlenerkrankungen. HNO 40:468–471
425. Kavanagh KT (1995) Software review: paranasal sinuses & anterior skull base; interactive anatomy, volume 1. Ann Otol Rhinol Laryngol 104:488–489
426. Keerl R (1999) Die Bedeutung multimedialer Lernsoftware in der Ausbildung zum Nasennebenhöhlenoperateur. Laryngorhinootologie (in press)
427. Keerl R, Weber R (1995) Operationsweiterbildung mittels Multimediatechnik am Beispiel der endonasalen mikroendoskopischen Pansinusoperation. Laryngo-Rhino-Otol 74:361–364
428. Keerl R, Weber R, Draf W, Kind M, Saha A (1996) Periorbital Paraffingranuloma following Paranasal Sinus Surgery. Am J Otolaryngol 17:264–268
429. Keerl R, Weber R, Müller C, Schick B (1997) Zur Effizienz und Verträglichkeit der Nasenspülung nach endonasaler Nasennebenhöhlenoperation. Laryngo-Rhino-Otol 76: 137–41
430. Keerl R, Weber R, Draf W, Dshambazov K (1998) Verträglichkeit, subjektive Beschwerden und mukoziliare Clearance bei Rhinitis sicca vor und nach Nasenspülung mit Rhinomer R Force 1. Laryngo-Rhino-Otologie 77:196–200.
431. Kelloway J (1997) Zafirlukast: the first leukotriene-receptor antagonist approved for the treatment of asthma. Ann Pharmocother 31:1012–1021
432. Kennedy DW (1985) Functional endoscopic sinus surgery. Technique. Arch Otolaryngol 111:643–649
433. Kennedy DW (1992) Prognostic factors, outcomes and staging in ethmoid sinus surgery. Laryngoscope 102:1–18
434. Kennedy DW, Kennedy EM (1985a) Ambulatory surgery: endoscopic sinus surgery. AORN J 42:932–936
435. Kennedy DW, Zinreich SJ, Rosenbaum AE, Johns ME (1985b) Functional endoscopic sinus surgery. Theory and diagnostic evaluation. Arch Otolaryngol 111:576–582
436. Kennedy DW, Zinreich SJ, Shaalan H, Kuhn F, Naclerio R, Loch E (1987) Endoscopic middle meatal antrostomy – theory, technique, and patency. Laryngoscope Suppl 43: 1–9
437. Kennedy DW, Zinreich SJ (1988) The functional endoscopic approach to inflammatory sinus disease: current perspectives and technique modifications. Am J Rhinol 2:89–96
438. Kennedy DW, Josephson JS, Zinreich SJ, Mattox DE, Goldsmith MM (1989a) Endoscopic sinus surgery for mucoceles: a viable alternative. Laryngoscope 99:885–895
439. Kennedy DW, Shaalan H (1989b) Reevaluation of maxillary sinus surgery: experimental study in rabbits. Ann Otol Rhinol Laryngol 98:901–906
440. Kennedy DW, Goodstein ML, Miller NR, Zinreich SJ (1990a) Endoscopic transnasal orbital decompression. Arch Otolaryngol Head Neck Surg 116:275–282
441. Kennedy DW, Zinreich SJ, Hassab MH (1990b) The internal carotid artery as it relates to endonasal sphenoethmoidectomy. Am J Rhinol 4:7–12
442. Kennedy DW, Shaman P, Han W, Selman H, Deems DA, Lanza DC (1994) Complications of ethmoidectomy: a survey of fellows of the American Academy of Otolaryngology – Head and Neck Surgery. Otolaryngol Head Neck Surg 111:589–599
443. Kennedy TL (1994) Endoscopic surgery for frontal and ethmoid sinus mucoceles. Am J Rhinol 8:107–112
444. Kern EB, O'Halloran GL (1994) Conventional intranasal ethmoidectomy: does the endoscope have a role? In: Sadé J (Ed.) Infections in childhood – ear, nose and throat aspects. Excerpta Medica, Amsterdam, pp 257–262
445. Keros P (1965) Über die praktische Bedeutung der Niveauunterschiede der Lamina cribrosa des Ethmoids. Laryngol-Rhino-Otol 41:808–813
446. Keyser JS, Diaz-Ordaz E, Samson MJ, Kartush JM (1995) Use of intraoperative neuromonitoring to prevent orbital complications in ethmoid sinus surgery. Otolaryngol Head Neck Surg 113:99–103
447. Khan JA, Wagner DV, Tiojanco JK, Hoover LA (1995) Combined transconjunctival and external approach for endoscopic orbital apex decompression in Graves' disease. Laryngoscope 105:203–206
448. Khanobthamchai K, Shankar L, Hawke M, Bingham B (1991a) The secondary middle turbinate. J Otolaryngol 20:412–413
449. Khanobthamchai K, Shankar L, Hawke M, Bingham B (1991b) Ethmomaxillary sinus and hypoplasia of maxillary sinus. J Otolaryngol 20:425–427
450. Kidder TM, Toohill RJ, Unger JD, Lehman RH (1974) Ethmoid sinus surgery. Laryngoscope 84:1525–1534
451. Killian G (1900) Die Krankheiten der Kieferhöhle. In: Heymann P (Ed.) Handbuch der Laryngologie und Rhinologie, Band III, 2. Hälfte. Hölder, Wien; pp 1004–1096
452. King HC, Mabry RL (1993) A practical guide to the management of nasal and sinus disorders. Thieme, New York
453. King JM, Caldarelli DD, Pigato JB (1994) A review of revision functional endoscopic sinus surgery. Laryngoscope 104:404–408
454. Kingdom TT, Lee KC, Cropp GJ (1995) Chronic sinusitis and a negative sweat test in a patient with cystic fibrosis. Am J Rhinol 9:225–228
455. Klima A, Weber A, May A, Knecht R (1992) Allergie und Polyposis nasi. Allergologie 15:351–354
456. Klimek L, Kainz J, Reul J, Mösges R (1993) Vermeidung vaskulärer Komplikationen bei der endonasalen Nasennebenhöhlenchirurgie. Teil II: Prä- und intraoperative Bildgebung. HNO 41:582–586
457. Klimek L, Hummel T, Moll B, Kobal G, Mann WJ (1998) Lateralized and bilateral olfactory function in patients with chronic sinusitis compared with healthy control subjects. Laryngoscope 108:111–114
458. Kloppers SP (1987) Endoscopic examination of the nose and results of functional endoscopic sinus surgery in 50 patients. S Afr Med J 72:622–624
459. Kloppers SP (1989) Functional endoscopic sinus surgery. A critical long-term evaluation. S Afr Med J 76:262–264
460. Klossek JM, Fontanel JP (1992) Chirurgie endonasale sous guidage endoscopique. Masson, Paris
461. Klossek JM, Ferrie JC, Goujon JM, Azais O, Poitout F, Babin P, Fontanel JP (1993) Les schwannomes naso-sinusiens. A propos de deux cas. Intéret de l'endoscopie nasale pour le diagnostic et le traitement. Ann Oto-Laryngol (Paris) 110:341–345
462. Klossek J-M, Peloquin L, Friedman WH, Ferrier J-C, Fontanel J-P (1997) Diffuse nasal polyposis: postoperative long-term results after endoscopic sinus surgery and frontal irrigation. Otolaryngol Head Neck Surg 117:355–361
463. Koay CB, Whittet HN, Ryan RM, Lewis CE, Path MRC (1995) Giant cell reparative granuloma of the concha bullosa. J Laryngol Otol 109:555–558
464. Korchia D, Thomassin JM, Duchon Doris JM, Badier M (1992) Asthme et polypose efficacité et nocivité de l'éthmoidectomie endonasale. Résultats à propos de 70 patients. Ann Oto-Laryngol (Paris) 109:359–363
465. Korzec KR (1992) A self-irrigating system for endoscopic sinus surgery. Otolaryngol Head Neck Surg 107:131–132
466. Kosko R, Pratt F, Chames M, Letterman I (1998) Anisocoria: a rare consequence of endoscopic sinus surgery. Otolaryngol Head Neck Surg 118:242–244
467. Kösling S, Schulz HG, Klöppel R (1992) Computertomographie der Nasennebenhöhlen in koronarer Schnittführung – eine Voraussetzung für die endonasale Operation. Röntgenpraxis 45:265–269

468. Kowalski ML (1992) Management of aspirin-sensitive rhinosinusitis-asthma syndrome: what role for aspirin desensitization? Allergy Proc 13:175–183
469. Kraus DH, Lanzieri CF, Wanamaker JR, Little JR, Lavertu P (1992) Complementary use of computed tomography and magnetic resonance imaging in assessing skull base lesions. Laryngoscope 102:623–629
470. Kreidler JF, Koch H (1975) Endoscopic findings of maxillary sinus after middle face fractures. J Max Fac Surg 3:10–14
471. Krmpotic-Nemanic J, Vinter I, Hat J, Jalsovec D (1993) Variations of the labyrinth and sphenoid sinus and CT imaging. Eur Arch Otorhinolaryngol 250:209–212
472. Kroegel C, König W, Jäger L (1997) Erweiterte Thrapie des Asthma bronchiale. DÄB 94:A 1802–1810
473. Kuhn FA (1996) Chronic frontal sinusitis: the endoscopic frontal recess approach. Op Tech Otolaryngol Head Neck Surg 7:222–229
474. Kuhn FA, Bolger WE, Tisdahl RG (1991) The agger nasi cell in frontal recess obstruction: an anatomic, radiologic and clinical correlation. Op Tech Otolaryngol Head Neck Surg 2:226–231
475. Kuhn FA, Citardi MJ (1997) Advances in postoperative care following functional endoscopic sinus surgery. Otolaryngol Clin North Am 30:479–490
476. Kühnel T, Hosemann W, Wagner W, Fayad K (1996) Wie traumatisierend ist die mechanische Nasenpflege nach Eingriffen an den Nasennebenhöhlen? Laryngo-Rhino-Otol 75:575–579
477. Lamear WR, Davis WE, Templer JW, McKinsey JP, DelPorto H (1992) Partial endoscopic middle turbinectomy augmenting functional endoscopic sinus surgery. Otolaryngol Head Neck Surg 107:382–389
478. Lang J (1988a) Klinische Anatomie der Nase, Nasenhöhle und Nebenhöhlen. Thieme, Stuttgart
479. Lang J (1988b) Über die Cellulae ethmoidales posteriores und ihre Beziehung zum Canalis opticus. HNO 36:49–53
480. Lang J, Schlehahn F, Schäfer K (1979) Über den Inhalt der Canales ethmoidales. Verh Anat Ges 73:87–94
481. Langnickel R (1978) Temporäre Amaurose nach endonasaler Siebbeinoperation. HNO 26:172–173
482. Larsen K, Tos M (1994) Clinical course of patients with primary nasal polyps. Acta Otolaryngol (Stockh) 114:556–559
483. Larsen PL, Tos M (1991) Origin of nasal polyps. Laryngoscope 101:305–312
484. Larsen PL, Tos M, Baer S (1994) En bloc removal of the ethmoid and ostiomeatal complex in cadavers, with a practical application. Rhinology 32:62–64
485. Lawson W (1991) The intranasal ethmoidectomy: an experience with 1077 procedures. Laryngoscope 101:367–371
486. Lawson W (1994) The intranasal ethmoidectomy: evolution and an assessment of the procedure. Laryngoscope Suppl 64:1–49
487. Lawson W, Biller HF, Jacobson A, Som P (1983) The role of conservative surgery in the management of inverted papilloma. Laryngoscope 93:148–155
488. Lawson W, Le Benger J, Som P, Bernard PJ, Biller HF (1989) Inverted papilloma: an analysis of 87 cases. Laryngoscope 99:1117–1124
489. Lawson W, Ho BT, Chaari CM, Biller HF (1995) Inverted papilloma: a report of 112 cases. Laryngoscope 105:282–288
490. Lazar RH, Younis RT, Long TE, Gross CW (1992a) Revision functional endonasal sinus surgery. Ear Nose Throat J 71:131–133
491. Lazar RH, Younis RT, Parvey LS (1992b) Comparison of plain radiographs, coronal CT, and intraoperative findings in children with chronic sinusitis. Otolaryngol Head Neck Surg 107:29–34
492. Lazar RH, Younis RT, Gross CW (1992c) Pediatric functional endonasal sinus surgery: review of 210 cases. Head Neck 14:92–98
493. Lazar RH, Younis RT, Long TE (1993) Functional endonasal sinus surgery in adults and children. Laryngoscope 103:1–5
494. Lazar RH, Younis RT (1995) Transnasal repair of choanal atresia using telescopes. Arch Otolaryngol Head Neck Surg 121:517–520
495. Lebowitz RA, Jacobs JB, Tavin ME (1995) Safe and effective infundibulotomy technique. Otolaryngol Head Neck Surg 113: 266–270
496. Lee WC, Kapur TR, Ramsden WN (1997) Local and regional anesthesia for functional endoscopic sinus surgery. Ann Otol Rhinol Laryngol 106: 767–769
497. Leff JA, Busse WW, Pearlman D, Bronsky EA, Kemp J, Hendeles L, Dockhorn R, Kundu S, Zhang J, Seidenberg B, Reiss TF (1998) Montelukast, a leukotriene-receptor antagonist, for the treatment of mild asthma and exercise-induced bronchoconstriction. N Engl J Med 339:147–152
498. Lenz H, Eichler J, Schäfer G, Salk J, Bettges G (1977) Production of a nasoantral window with an Ar-Laser. J Max Fac Surg 5:314–317
499. Lenz H, Eichler J (1984) Endonasale chirurgische Technik mit dem Argonlaser. Laryng Rhinol Otol 63:534–540
500. Leopold DA (1995) The importance of nasal and sinus symptoms. Curr Opin Otolaryngol Head Neck Surg 3:1–4
501. Lesserson JA, Kieserman SP, Finn DG (1994) The radiographic incidence of chronic sinus disease in the pediatric population. Laryngoscope 104:159–166
502. Levine HL (1989) Endoscopy and the KTP 532 laser for nasal sinus disease. Ann Otol Rhinol Laryngol 98:46–51
503. Levine HL (1990) Functional endoscopic sinus surgery: evaluation, surgery, and follow-up of 250 patients. Laryngoscope 100:79–84
504. Levine HL (1991) Endoscopic diagnosis and management of cerebrospinal fluid rhinorrhea. Op Tech Otolaryngol Head Neck Surg 2:282–284
505. Levine HL (1997) Lasers in endonasal surgery. Otolaryngol Clin North Am 30:451–455
506. Levine HL, May M (1993) Endoscopic sinus surgery. Thieme, New York
507. Li J, Stankiewicz J (1991) The endoscopic approach to the lateral accessory sphenoid sinus. Otolaryngol Head Neck Surg 105:608–612
508. Linberg JV, Anderson RL, Bumsted RM, Barreras R (1982) Study of intranasal ostium external dacryocystorhinostomy. Arch Ophthalmol 100:1758–1762
509. Linden BE, Aguilar EA, Allen SJ (1988) Sinusitis in the nasotracheally intubated patient. Arch Otolaryngol Head Neck Surg 114:860–861
510. Lister JR, Sypert GW (1979) Traumatic false aneurysm and carotid-cavernous fistula: a complication of sphenoidotomy. Neurosurgery 5:473–475
511. Liu CM, Yeh TH, Hsu MM (1994) Clinical evaluation of maxillary diffuse polypoid sinusitis after functional endoscopic sinus surgery. Am J Rhinol 8:7–11
512. Lloyd GAS (1990) CT of the paranasal sinuses: study of a control series in relation to endoscopic sinus surgery. J Laryngol Otol 104:477–481
513. Lloyd GAS, Lund VJ, Scadding GK (1991) CT of the paranasal sinuses and functional endoscopic surgery: a critical analysis of 100 symptomatic patients. J Laryngol Otol 105:181–185
514. Loewe G, Slapke J, Kunath H (1985) Nasal polyposis, bronchial asthma and analgesic intolerance. Rhinology 23:19–26
515. Lopatin AS, Piskunov GZ (1996) FESS with and without the availibility of CT imaging. Am J Rhinol 10:51–54
516. Loury MC (1993) Endoscopic frontal recess and frontal sinus ostium dissection. Laryngoscope 103:455–458
517. Loury MC, Hinkley DK, Wong W (1993) Endoscopic transnasal antrochoanal polypectomy: an alternative to the transantral approach. South Med J 86:18–22
518. Lucente FE, Schoenfeld PS (1990) Calibrated approach to endoscopic sinus surgery. Ann Otol Rhinol Laryngol 99:1–4

519. Lumry WR, Curd JG, Zeiger RS, Pleskow WW, Stevenson DD (1983) Aspirin-sensitive rhinosinusitis: the clinical syndrome and effects of aspirin administration. J Allergy Clin Immunol 71:580–587
520. Lund VJ (1985) Fundamental considerations of the design and function of intranasal antrostomies. Rhinology 23:231–236
521. Lund VJ (1986a) The design and function of intranasal antrostomies. J Laryngol Otol 100:35–39
522. Lund VJ (1986b) Fundamental considerations of the design and function of intranasal antrostomies. J Royal Soc Med 79:646–649
523. Lund VJ (1988) Inferior meatal antrostomy. Fundamental considerations of design and function. J Laryngol Otol Suppl 15:1–18
524. Lund VJ (1998) Endoscopic management of paranasal sinus mucoceles. J Laryngol Otol 112:36–40
525. Lund VJ. What is the place of endonasal surgery in fungal sinusitis? In: Stamm A, Draf W (Eds.) Microscopic and Endoscopic Surgery of the Nose and Sinuses. [In press]
526. Lund VJ, Holmstrom M, Scadding GK (1991) Functional endoscopic sinus surgery in the management of chronic rhinosinusitis. An objective assessment. J Laryngol Otol 105:832–835
527. Lund VJ, Mackay IS (1993) Staging in rhinosinusitis. Rhinology 31:183–184
528. Lund VJ, Mackay IS (1994a) Outcome assessment of endoscopic sinus surgery. J R Soc Med 87:70–72
529. Lund VJ, Scadding GK (1994b) Objective assessment of endoscopic sinus surgery in the management of chronic rhinosinusitis: an update. J Laryngol Otol 108:749–753
530. Lund VJ, Kennedy DW, Draf W, Friedman WH, Gwaltney JM, Hoffman SR, Huizing EG, Jones JG, Jones JK, Lusk RP, Mackay IS, Moriyama H, Naclerio RM, Stankiewicz JA, van Cauwenberge P, Vining EM (1995a) Quantification for staging sinusitis. Ann Otol Rhinol Laryngol Suppl 167:17–21
531. Lund VJ, Neijens H, Clement P, Lusk R, Stammberger H (1995b) The treatment of chronic sinusitis a controversial issue. Int J Pediatr Otorhinolaryngol 32 (Suppl) 21–35
532. Lund VJ, Larkin G, Fells P, Adams G (1997) Endoscopic orbital decompression. J Laryngol Otol 111:1051–1055
533. Lund VJ, Howard DJ, Wei WI, Cheesman D (1998) Craniofacial resection for tumors of the nasal cavity and paranasal sinuses – a seventeen year experience. Head Neck Surg 20:97–105
534. Lusk RP (1992a) Pediatric sinusitis. Raven Press, New York
535. Lusk RP (1992b) Surgical modalities other than ethmoidectomy. J Allergy Clin Immunol 90:538–542
536. Lusk RP, Muntz HR (1990) Endoscopic sinus surgery in children with chronic sinusitis: a pilot study. Laryngoscope 100:654–658
537. Lusk RP, Polmar SH, Muntz HR (1991) Endoscopic ethmoidectomy and maxillary antrostomy in immunodeficient patients. Arch Otolaryngol Head Neck Surg 117:60–63
538. Luxenberger W, Stammberger H, Jebeles JA, Walch C (1998) Endoscopic optic nerve decompression: the Graz experience. Laryngoscope 108:873–882
539. Mac Arthur CJ, Gliklich R, McGill TJI, Perez-Atayde A (1993) Sinus complications in mucopolysaccharidosis I H/S (Hurler-Scheie syndrome). Int J Pediatr Otorhinolaryngol 26:79–87
540. Mac Kenty JE (1929) Blindness due to hemorrhage into orbital fat caused by injury in the intranasal ethmoid operation and by other injuries. Laryngoscope 39:772
541. Mackay IS, Djazaeheri B. (1994) Reduced pneumatistion in cystic fibrosis. J Royal Soc Med 81:17–19.
542. Mafee MF (1991) Endoscopic sinus surgery: role of the radiologist. AJNR 12:855–860
543. Mair EA (1996) Pediatric functional endoscopic sinus surgery. Otolaryngol Clin North Am 29:207–19
544. Mair MEA, Bolger WE, Breisch EA (1995) Sinus and facial growth after pediatric endoscopic sinus surgery. Arch Otolaryngol Head Neck Surg 121:547–552
545. Maisel RH (1993) Sinusitis and the immunocompromised patient. In: McCaffrey TV (Ed.) Systemic disease and the nasal airway. Thieme, New York, pp 41–64
546. Maniglia AJ (1989a) Fatal and major complications secondary to nasal and sinus surgery. Laryngoscope 99:276–283
547. Maniglia AJ (1989b) Letter to the editor. Laryngoscope 99:871
548. Maniglia AJ (1991) Fatal and other major complications of endoscopic sinus surgery. Laryngoscope 101: 349–354
549. Maniglia AJ, Chandler JR, Goodwin WJ, Flynn J (1981) Rare complications following ethmoidectomies: a report of eleven cases. Laryngoscope 91:1234–1244
550. Maniscalco JE, Habal (1978) Microanatomy of the optic canal. J Neurosurg 48:402–406
551. Mann W, Dao Trong H (1979) Vergleichende endoskopischê und histologische Befunde bei chronischer Sinusitis. HNO 27:345–347
552. Mann W, Rochels R, Bleier R (1991) Mikrochirurgische endonasale Dekompression des N. opticus. Fortschr Ophthalmol 88:176–177
553. Mann WJ, Amedee RG, Iemma M (1992) An assessment of radiologic discrepancies in patients with paranasal sinus disease. Am J Rhinol 6:211–213
554. Mann WJ, Amedee RG, Grehn F, Lieb W (1994a) Epiphora secondary to blockage of the lacrimal system: the role of endonasal dacryocystorhinostomy. Am J Rhinol 8:139–141
555. Mann WJ, Kahaly G, Lieb W, Amedee RG (1994b) Orbital decompression for endocrine ophthalmopathy: the endonasal approach. Am J Rhinol 8:123–127
556. Manning SC (1992) Surgical management of sinus disease in children. Ann Otol Rhinol Larnygol 101:42–45
557. Manning SC (1993) Endoscopic management of medial subperiostal orbital abscess. Arch Otolaryngol Head Neck Surg 119:789–791
558. Manning SC, Wasserman RL, Silver R, Phillips DL (1994) Results of endoscopic sinus surgery in pediatric patients with chronic sinusitis and asthma. Arch Otolaryngol Head Neck Surg 120:1142–1145
559. Mannor GE, Millman AL (1992) The prognostic value of preoperative dacryocystography in endoscopic intranasal dacryocystorhinostomy. Am J Ophthalmol 72:134–137
560. Maran AGD (1994) Endoscopic sinus surgery. Eur Arch Otorhinolaryngol 251:309–318
561. Marcus MJ (1990) Nasal endoscopic control of epistaxis – a preliminary report. Otolaryngol Head Neck Surg 102:273–275
562. Marks SC, Smith DM (1995) Endoscopic treatment of maxillary sinus cholesterol granuloma. Laryngoscope 105:551–552
563. Marmolya G, Wiesen EJ, Yagan R, Haria CD, Shah AC (1991) Paranasal sinuses: low-dose CT. Radiology 181:689–691
564. Martin SC, May M (1991) Endoscopic sinus surgery. Is hospitalization justified? Op Tech Otolaryngol Head Neck Surg 2:241–243
565. Masing H, Steiner W (1984) Zur Behandlung von Choanalatresien. Laryngol Rhinol Otol 63:181–183
566. Mason J, Haynes R, Jones N (1998) Interpretation of the dilated pupil during endoscopic sinus surgery. J Laryngol Otol 112:622–627
567. Massaro BM, Gonnering RS, Harris GJ (1990) Endonasal laser dacryocystorhinostomy. Arch Ophthalmol 108:1172–1176
568. Massegur H, Ademà JM, Lluansi J, Fabra JM, Montserrat JM (1995) Endoscopic sinus surgery in sinusitis. Rhinology 33:89–92
569. Massoud TF, Whittet HB, Anslow P (1993) CT-dacryocystography for nasolacrimal duct obstruction following paranasal sinus surgery. Br J Radiol 66:223–227
570. Matthews BL, Smith LE, Jones R, Miller C, Brookschmidt JK (1991) Endoscopic sinus surgery: outcome in 155 cases. Otolaryngol Head Neck Surg 104:244–246

571. Mathews BL, Burke AJ (1997) Recirculation of mucus via accessory ostia causing chronic maxillary sinus disease. Otolaryngol Head Neck Surg 117:422–423
572. Mattox DE, Kennedy DW (1990) Endoscopic management of cerebrospinal fluid leaks and cephaloceles. Laryngoscope 100:857–862
573. Maus M (1995) Lasers in oculoplastic surgery. Curr Opin Ophthalmol 6:37–42
574. May M (1990) Nasopharyngeal balloon catheter enhances endoscopic sinus surgery in the awake patient. Op Tech Otolaryngol Head Neck Surg 1:142–143
575. May M (1991a) Reporting results of sinus surgery. A classification system. Op Tech Otolaryngol Head Neck Surg 2:244–246
576. May M (1991b) Frontal sinus surgery: endonasal endoscopic ostioplasty rather than external osteoplasty. Op Tech Otolaryngol Head Neck Surg 2:247–256
577. May, M, Ogura JH, Schramm V (1970) Nasofrontal duct in frontal sinus fractures. Arch Otolaryngol 92:532–538
578. May M, Hoffmann DF, Sobol SM (1990a) Video endoscopic sinus surgery: a two-handed technique. Laryngoscope 100:430–432
579. May M, Korzec KR, Mester SJ (1990b) Video telescopic sinus surgery techniques for teaching. Trans Pa Acad Ophthalmol Otolaryngol 42:1037–1039
580. May M, Har-El G (1990c) Endoscopic sinus surgery: green, yellow, red color-coded measurements for safety. Op Tech Otolaryngol Head Neck Surg 1:126–127
581. May M, Hillsamer P, Hoffmann DF (1991) Management of orbital hematoma following functional endoscopic sinus surgery. Am J Rhinol 5:47–49
582. May M, Levine HL, Schaitkin B, Mester SJ (1993) Complications of endoscopic sinus surgery. In: Levine HL, May M (Eds.) Endoscopic sinus surgery. Thieme, New York, pp 193–243
583. May M, Levine H, Mester SJ, Schaitkin B (1994a) Complications of endoscopic sinus surgery: analysis of 2108 patients – incidence and prevention. Laryngoscope 104:1080–1083
584. May M, Schaitkin B, Kay SL (1994b) Revision endoscopic sinus surgery: six friendly surgical landmarks. Laryngoscope 104:766–767
584aMay M, Schaitkin B (1995) Frontal sinus surgery: endonasal drainage instead of an external osteoplastic approach. Op Tech Otolaryngol Head Neck Surg 6: 184–192
585. Mayer O (1934) Ein Fall von tödlicher Meningitis nach intranasaler Siebbeinoperation. Z f Hals- Nasen- u Ohrenheilk 35:377–384
586. McCary WS, Gross CW, Reibel JF, Cantrell RW (1994) Preliminary report: endoscopic versus external surgery in the management of inverting papilloma. Laryngoscope 104:415–419
587. McCoy BJ, Diegelmann RF, Cohen IK (1980) In vitro inhibition of cell growth, collagen synthesis, and prolyl hydroxylase activity by triamcinolone acetonide. Pro Soc Exp Biol Med 163:216–22
588. McDonogh M, Meiring JH (1989) Endoscopic transnasal dacryocystorhinostomy. J Laryngol Otol 103:585–587
589. McDonogh MB (1990) Prevention of adhesions after functional endoscopic sinus surgery. S Afr Med J 77:111
590. McFadden EA, Kany RJ, Fink JN, Toohill FJ (1990) Sugery for sinusitis and aspirin triad. Laryngoscope 100:1043–1046
591. McGarry GW (1991) Nasal endoscope in posterior epistaxis: a preliminary evaluation. J Laryngol Otol 105:428–431
592. McGregor G (1931) Further proof ot the regeneration of mucous membrane in the human antrum. Arch Otolaryng 14:309–326
593. McGregor G (1932) The reformation of mucous membrane in twenty reoperative cases of chronic maxillary sinusitis. Trans Am Acad Ophthalmol Otolaryngol 37:407–414
594. Mehta D (1993) Atlas of endoscopic sinonasal surgery. Lea & Febiger, London
595. Mendelsohn MG, Gross CW (1997) Soft-tissue shavers in pediatric sinus surgery. Otolaryngol Clin North Am 30:443–449
596. Merck W (1974) Über den pathogenetischen Zusammenhang zwischen Adenoiden Vegetationen und kindlicher Sinusitis maxillaris. HNO 22:198–199
597. Merrit RM, Bent JP, Kuhn FA (1996) The intersinus septal cell: anatomic, radiologic, and clinical correlation. Am J Rhinol 10:299–302
598. Messerklinger W (1966) Über die Drainage der menschlichen Nasennebenhöhlen unter normalen und pathologischen Bedingungen. 1. Mitteilung. Mschr Ohrenheilk 100:56–68
599. Messerklinger W (1978) Endoscopy of the nose. Urban & Schwarzenberg, München
600. Messerklinger W (1981) Endoskopie der Nase bei Erkrankungen der Tränenorgane. In: Hanselmeyer H (Hrsg) Neue Erkenntnisse bei Erkrankungen der Tränenwege. Klin Mbl Augenheilk (Beih 84):14–18
601. Messerklinger W (1987) Die Rolle der lateralen Nasenwand in der Pathogenese, Diagnose und Therapie der rezidivierenden und chronischen Rhinosinusitis. Laryngol Rhinol Otol 66:293–299
602. Messerklinger W, Naumann HH (1995) Chirurgie des Nasennebenhöhlen-Systems. In: Naumann HH (Ed.) Kopf- und Hals-Chirurgie Band 1/II. Thieme, Stuttgart, pp 447–554
603. Messingschlager W (1981) Prothesen zum Offenhalten der Kieferhöhlenfenster. Laryngol Rhinol Otol 60:525–526
604. Metson R (1990) The endoscopic approach for revision dacryocystorhinostomy. Laryngoscope 100:1344–1347
605. Metson R (1991) Endoscopic surgery for lacrimal obstruction. Otolaryngol Head Neck Surg 104:473–479
606. Metson R (1992) Endoscopic treatment of frontal sinusitis. Laryngoscope 102:712–716
607. Metson R (1996) Holmium: YAG laser endoscopic sinus surgery – a randomized, controlled study. Laryngoscope 106 (Suppl 77) 1–18
608. Metson R, Dallow RL, Shore JW (1994a) Endoscopic orbital decompression. Laryngoscope 104:950–957
609. Metson R, Woog JJ, Puliafito CA (1994b) Endoscopic laser dacryocystorhinostomy. Laryngoscope 104:269–274
610. Metson R, Gliklich RE, Cosenza M (1998) A comparison of image guidance systems for sinus surgery. Laryngoscope 108:1164–1170
611. Michel O (1993) Isolierte mediale Orbitawandfrakturen: Ergebnisse einer minimal invasiven endoskopisch-kontrollierten endonasalen Operationstechnik. Laryngo-Rhino-Otol 72:450–454
612. Michel O (1994) Endonasal surgery in children. In: Sadé J (Ed.) Infections in childhood – ear, nose and throat aspects. Excerpta Medica, Amsterdam, pp 263–268
613. Michel O, Bresgen K, Rüssmann W, Thumfart WF, Stennert E (1991a) Endoskopisch kontrollierte endonasale Orbitadekompression beim malignen Ophthalmus. Laryngo-Rhino-Otol 70:656–662
614. Michel O, Charon J (1991b) Postoperative Inhalationsbehandlung nach Nasennebenhöhleneingriffen. HNO 39:433–438
615. Milbrath MM, Madiedo G, Toohill RJ (1994) Histopathological analysis of the middle turbinate after ethmoidectomy. Am J Rhinol 8:37–42
616. Milczuk HA, Dalley RW, Wessbacher FW, Richardson MA (1993) Nasal and paranasal sinus anomalies in children with chronic sinusitis. Laryngoscope 103:247–252
617. Miles-Lawrence R, Kaplan M, Chang K (1982) Methacholine sensitivity in nasal polyposis and the effects of polypectomy (abstract). J Allergy Clin Immunol 69:102
618. Milewski C (1996) Endonasale endoskopische Ethmoidektomie bei akuter therapieresistenter Sinusitis. Laryngo-Rhino-Otol 75:286–289

619. Miller W, Stankiewicz JA (1994) Delayed toxic shock syndrome in sinus surgery. Otolaryngol Head Neck Surg 111:121–123
620. Min YG, Lee YM, Lee BJ, Jung HW, Chang SO (1993) The effect of ostial opening on experimental maxillary sinusitis in rabbits. Rhinology 31:101–105
621. Min YG, Kim IT, Park SH (1994) Mucociliary activity and ultrastructural abnormalities of regenerated sinus mucosa in rabbits. Laryngoscope 104:1482–1486
622. Min YG, Shin JS, Lee CH (1995a) Trans-superior meatal approach to the sphenoid sinus. ORL 57:289–292
623. Min YG, Yun YS, Song BH, Cho YS, Lee KS (1995b) Recovery of nasal physiology after functional endoscopic sinus surgery: olfaction and mucociliary transport. ORL 57:264–268
624. Mings R, Friedman WH, Linford PA, Slavin RG (1988) Five-year follow-up of the effects of bilateral intranasal sphenoethmoidectomy in patients with sinusitis and asthma. Am J Rhinol 71:123–132
625. Minnigerode B (1972) Zur Anatomie und klinischen Bedeutung des Canalis ethmoidalis. Laryngo-Rhino-Otol 51:554–559
626. Mladina R (1992) Endoscopic sinus surgery: a metallic foreign body at the sphenoethmoidal junction. J Laryngol Otol 106:998–999
627. Moloney JR (1977) Nasal polyps, nasal polypectomy, asthma, and aspirin sensitivity. J Laryngol Otol 91:837–846
628. Moloney JR, Collins J (1977) Nasal polyps and bronchial asthma. Br J Dis Chest 71:1–6
629. Moore DF, Grogan JB, Lindsey WH, Anand VK, Gross CW (1995) The myospherulotic potential of water-soluble ointments. Am J Rhinol 9:215–218
630. Morgenstein KM (1985) Intranasal sphenoethmoidectomy and antrotomy. Otolaryngol Clin North Am 18:69–74
631. Moriyama H (1992) Postoperative care and long term results. Rhinology Suppl 14:156–161
632. Moriyama H, Ozawa M, Honda Y (1991a) Technique for endoscopic endonasal sinus surgery. Am J Rhinol 5:137–141
633. Moriyama H, Ozawa M, Honda Y (1991b) Endoscopic endonasal sinus surgery. Approaches and post-operative evaluation. Rhinology 29:93–98
634. Moriyama H, Hesaka H, Tachibana T, HondaY (1992a) Mucoceles of ethmoid and sphenoid sinus with visual disturbance. Arch Otolaryngol Head Neck Surg 118:142–146
635. Moriyama H, Nakajima R, Honda Y (1992b) Studies on mucoceles of the ethmoid and sphenoid sinuses: analysis of 47 cases. J Laryngol Otol 106:23–27
636. Moriyama H, Fukami M, Yanagi K, Ohtori N, Kaneta K (1994) Endoscopic endonasal treatment of ostium of the frontal sinus and the results of endoscopic surgery. Am J Rhinol 8:67–70
637. Moriyama H, Yanagi K, Ohtori N, Fukami M (1995) Evaluation of endoscopic sinus surgery for chronic sinusitis: postoperative erythromycin therapy. Rhinology 33:166–170
638. Mösges R (1993) Computergestützte Chirurgie (CAS) der Schädelbasisregion. 'Ergänzung, Revolution oder Science-fiction?' Eur Arch Oto-Rhino-Laryngol Suppl 1993/I:373–383
639. Mösges R, Klimek L (1993) Computer-assisted surgery of the paranasal sinuses. J Otolaryngol 22:69–71
640. Mosher HP (1902) Measurements for operating distances in the nose. Ann Surg 36:554–559
641. Mosher HP (1929) The surgical anatomy of the ethmoidal labyrinth. Ann Otol Rhinol Laryngol 38:869–901
642. Moss RB (1994) Sinusitis and nasal polyposis in cystic fibrosis. In: Druce HM (Ed.) Sinusitis – Pathophysiology and treatment. M Dekker, New York, pp 247–281
643. Moss RB, King VV (1995) Management of sinusitis in cystic fibrosis by endscopic surgery and serial antimicrobial lavage. Arch Otolaryngol Head Neck Surg 121:566–572
644. Moure (1923) Le traitement des tumeurs malignes des fosses nasales. Congrès francais d'Oto-Rhino-Laryngologie, Paris 1922. Z Hals-Nasen-Ohrenheilk 2:441
645. Mullin WV, Ryder CT (1920) Experimental lesions of the lungs produced by the inhalation of fluids from the nose and throat. Am Rev Tuberc 4:683–687
646. Muntz HR (1987) Pitfalls to laser correction of choanal atresia. Ann Otol Rhinol Laryngol 96:43–46
647. Muntz HR, Lusk RP (1990) Nasal antral windows in children: a retrospective study. Laryngoscope 100:643–646
648. Murthy PSN, Sahota JS, Nayak DR, Balakrishnan R, Hazarika P (1994) Foreign body in the ethmoid sinus. Int J Oral Maxillofac Surg 23:74–75
649. Müsebeck K, Rosenberg H (1982) Strömungsphysikalische Gesichtspunkte im Therapieplan der chronischen Sinusitis maxillaris. Laryngol Rhinol Otol 61:231–233
650. Myers EN, Petruzzelli GJ (1993) Letters to the editor: Endoscopic sinus surgery for inverting papillomas. Laryngoscope 103:711
651. Myerson MC (1932) The natural orifice of the maxillary sinus. Arch Otolaryngol 15:80–91
652. Nass RL, Holliday RA, Reede DL (1989) Diagnosis of surgical sinusitis using nasal endoscopy and computerized tomography. Laryngoscope 99:1158–1160
653. Naumann H (1965) Pathologische Anatomie der chronischen Rhinitis und Sinusitis. In: Proceedings VIII International Congress of Oto-Rhino-Laryngology, Amsterdam, Excerpta Medica, Int Cong Ser 113:79–87
654. Naumann HH (1987) Neue Trends in der Nebenhöhlen-Chirurgie? Laryngo-Rhino-Otol 66:57–59
655. Neel HB III, Whicker JH, Lake CF (1976) Thin rubber sheeting in frontal sinus surgery: Animal and clinical studies. Laryngoscope 86:524–536
656. Neel HB III, McDonald TJ, Facer GW (1987) Modified Lynch procedure for chronic frontal sinus disease: rationale, technique and long-term results. Laryngoscope 97:1274–1279
657. Neivert H (1925) Morphologic variation as a factor in the symptomatology of paranasal sinus disease. Arch Otolaryngol 1:367–383
658. Neuhaus RW (1990) Orbital complications secondary to endoscopic sinus surgery. Ophthalmology 97:1512–1518
659. Newman LJ, Platts-Mills TAE, Phillips CD, Hazen KC, Gross CW (1994) Chronic sinusitis – relationship of computed tomographic findings to allergy, asthma, and eosinophilia. JAMA 271:363–367
660. Ng M, Rice DH (1993) Revision sinus surgery. Ear Nose Throat J 73:44–46
661. Nigam A, Johnson AP (1993) Suction polypectomy forceps. J Laryngol Otol 107:35
662. Nishioka GJ, Cook PR, Davis WE, McKinsey JP (1994a) Immunotherapy in patients undergoing functional endoscopic sinus surgery. Otolaryngol Head Neck Surg 110:406–412
663. Nishioka GJ, Cook PR, Davis WE, McKinsey JP (1994b) Functional endoscopic sinus surgery in patients with chronic sinusitis and asthma. Otolaryngol Head Neck Surg 110:494–500
664. Nishioka GJ, Barbero GJ, König P, Parsons DS, Cook PR, Davis WE (1995) Symptom outcome after functional endoscopic sinus surgery in patients with cystic fibrosis: a prospective study. Otolaryngol Head Neck Surg 113:440–445
665. Nitsche N, Hilbert M, Strasser G, Tümmler HP, Arnold W (1993a) Einsatz eines berührungsfreien computergestützten Orientierungssystems bei Nasennebenhöhlenoperationen. I. Technische Grundlagen der Sonarstereometrie. Otorhinolaryngol Nova 3:57–64
666. Nitsche N, Hilbert M, Strasser G, Schulz HJ, Wunderlich A, Arnold W (1993b) Einsatz eines berührungsfreien computergestützten Orientierungssystems bei Nasennebenhöhlenoperationen. II. Anatomische Studien und erste klinische Erfahrungen. Otorhinolaryngol Nova 3:173–179

667. Nolte D, Berger D (1983) On vagal bronchoconstriction in asthmatic patients by nasal irritation. Eur J Respir Dis 64:110–114
668. Noorily AD, Otto RA, Noorily SH (1995) Intranasal anesthetic effects of lidocaine and tetracaine compared. Otolaryngol Head Neck Surg 113:370–374
669. Oelsner RP (1989) Sinabrasio – ein neues Verfahren zur operativen Behandlung der chronisch polypös entzündeten Kieferhöhle. Inaugural-Dissertation, Bonn
670. Ogura JH, Nelson JR, Dammkoehler R, Kawasaki M, Togawa K (1964) Experimental observations of the relationships between upper airway obstruction and pulmonary function. Trans Am Laryngol Assoc 85:40–64
671. Ogura JH, Harvey JE (1971) Nasopulmonary mechanics – experimental evidence of the influence of the upper airway upon the lower. Acta Otolaryngol 71:123–132
672. O'Halloran GL, Kern EB (1991) Classical intranasal ethmoidectomy: does the endoscope have a role? J Otolaryngol 20:391–394
673. Ohmae T, Ashikawa R, Ishikawa T (1986) Severe visual disturbance after exposure of the optic canal during intranasal ethmosphenoidectomy. Rhinology 24:211–217
674. Ohnishi T (1981) Bony defects and dehiscences of the roof of the ethmoid cells. Rhinology 19:195–202
675. Ohnishi T, Ashikawa R, Takiguchi K, Kamide Y, Tachibana T (1987) Ethmoidal nerve and artery block in endonasal sinusectomy. Rhinology 25:207–212
676. Ohnishi T, Esaki S, Iwasaki M, Tachibana T (1990) Endoscopic microsurgery of the ethmoid sinus. Am J Rhinol 4:119–127
677. Ohnishi T, Tachibana T, Kaneko, Y, Esaki S (1993) High-risk areas in endoscopic sinus surgery and prevention of complications. Laryngoscope 103:1181–1185
678. O'Leary-Stickney K, Makielski K, Weymuller EA (1992) Rigid endoscopy for the control of epistaxis. Arch Otolaryngol Head Neck Surg 118:966–967
679. Önerci M, Aras T (1995) The effect of a new ostium and sinus mucosal flaps on mucociliary flow of the maxillary sinus. Rhinology 33:144–147
680. Onodi A (1903) Die Dehiszenzen der Nebenhöhlen der Nase. Arch Laryngol Rhinol 15:62–71
681. Ophir D, Schindel D, Halperin D, Marshak G (1992) Long-term follow-up of the effectiveness and safety of inferior turbinectomy. Plast Reconstr Surg 90:980–984
682. Ophir D, Shapiro M, Ruchvarger E, Levit I (1994) Pneumocephalus following nasal polypectomy. Ann Otol Rhinol Laryngol 103:576–577
683. Orcutt JC, Hillel A, Weymuller EA (1990) Endoscopic repair of railed dacryocystorhinostomy. Ophthalmic Plast Reconstr Surg 6:197–202
684. Otori N, Fukami M, Yanagi K, Asai K, Iida M, Moriyama H (1996) Patency of the ostium of the frontal sinus after endoscopic endonasal surgery for chronic sinusitis. Nippon Jibiinkoka Gakkai Kaiho 99:653–60 [In Japanese]
685. Otten FW, van Aarem A, Grote JJ (1992) Long-term follow-up of chronic therapy resistant purulent rhinitis in children. Clin Otolaryngol 17:32–33
686. Owen RG, Kuhn FA (1995) The maxillary sinus ostium: demystifying middle meatal antrostomy. Am J Rhinol 9:313–320
687. Owen RG, Kuhn FA (1997) Supraorbital ethmoidal cell. Otolaryngol Head Neck Surg 116:254–261
688. Ozawa M, Konno H, Kaneko S (1984) Endonasal repair of the medial orbital wall, a report of two cases. Otolaryngology (Tokyo) 56:433–438 [In Japanese]
689. Panis R, Thumfart W, Wigand ME (1979) Die endonasale Kieferhöhlenoperation mit endoskopischer Kontrolle als Therapie der chronisch rezidivierenden Sinusitis im Kindesalter. HNO 27:256–259
690. Panwar SS, Martin FW (1996) Trans-nasal endoscopic holmium: YAG laser correction of choanal atresia. J Laryngol Otol 110:429–431
691. Papay FA, Benninger MS, Levine HL, Lavertu P (1989a) Transnasal transseptal endoscopic repair of sphenoidal cerebral spinal fluid fistula. Otolaryngol Head Neck Surg 101:595–597
692. Papay FA, Maggiano H, Dominquez S, Hassenbusch SJ, Levine HL, Lavertu P (1989b) Rigid endoscopic repair of paranasal sinus cerebrospinal fluid fistulas. Laryngoscope 99:1195–1201
693. Park IY (1988) Improved endonasal sinus surgery by use of an operating microscope and a self-retaining retractor speculum. Acta Otolaryngol Suppl 458:27–33
694. Parsons DS, Greene BA (1993a) A treatment for primary ciliary dyskinesia: efficacy of functional endoscopic sinus surgery. Laryngoscope 103:1269–1272
695. Parsons DS, Phillips SE (1993b) Functional endoscopic surgery in children: a retrospective analysis of results. Laryngoscope 103:899–903
696. Parsons DS, Chambers DW (1995), The care of children with sinusitis. In: Stankiewicz JA (Ed.) Advanced endoscopic sinus surgery. Mosby, St. Louis, pp 33–40
697. Parsons DS, Stivers FE, Talbot AR (1996) The missed ostium sequence and the surgical approach to revision functional endoscopic sinus surgery. Otolaryngol Clin North Am 29:169–183
698. Patriarca G, Romano A, Schiavino D, Venuti A, DiRienzoV, Fais G, Nucera E (1986) ASA disease: the clinical relationship of nasal polyposis to ASA intolerance. Arch Otolaryngol 243:16–19
699. Patriarca G, Bellioni P, Nucera E, Schiavino D, Papa G, Schinco G, Fais G, Pirrotta LR (1991a) Intranasal treatment with lysine acetylsalicylate in patients with nasal polyposis. Ann Allergy 67:588–592
700. Patriarca G, Schiavino D, Nuchera E, Papa G, Schinco G, Fais G (1991b) Prevention of relapse in nasal polyposis. Lancet 337:1488
701. Paulsen K (1995) Endonasale Mikrochirurgie. Thieme, Stuttgart
702. Pearson BW, MacKenzie RG, Goodman WS (1969) The anatomical basis of transantral ligation of the maxillary artery in severe epistaxis. Laryngoscope 79:969–984
703. Pelausa EO, Smith K, Dempsey I (1995) Orbital complications of functional endoscopic sinus surgery. J Otolaryngol 24:154–159
704. Péloquin L, Arcand P, Abela A (1995) Endonasal dacryocystocele of the newborn. J Otolaryngol 24:84–86
705. Penne RB, Flanagan JC, Stefanyszyn MA, Nowinski T (1993) Ocular motility disorders secondary to sinus surgery. Ophthalmic Plast Reconstr Surg 9:53–61
706. Perko D (1989) Endoscopic surgery of the frontal sinus without external approach. Rhinology 27:117–123
707. Perko D, Karin RR (1992) Nasoantral windows: an experimental study in rabbits. Laryngoscope 102:320–326
708. Petruson B (1980) History of the treatment of nasal polyps. Gothenburg: Glaxo Läkemedel AB [Company document]
709. Peynegre R, Rouvier P (1996) Anatomy and anatomical variations of the paranasal sinuses. In: Gershwin ME, Incando GA (Eds.) Diseases of the Sinuses. Humana Press, Totowa, pp. 3–32
710. Pfister R, Lütolf M, Schapowal A, Glatte B, Schmitz M, Menz G (1994) Screening for sinus diesease in patients with asthma: a computed tomography-controlled comparison of A-mode ultrasonography and standard radiography. J Allergy Clin Immunol 94:804–809
711. Phillips CD, Platts-Mills TAE (1995) Chronic sinusitis: relationship between CT findings and clinical history of asthma, allergy, eosinophilia, and infection. AJR 164:185–187
712. Piaton JM, Limon S, Ounnas N, Keller P (1994) Endodacryocystorhinostomie transcanaliculaire au laser Neodymium: YAG. J Fr Ophthalmol 17:555–567
713. Picado C, Castillo JA, Schinca N, Pujades M, Ordinas A, Coronas A, Agusti-Vidal A (1988) Effects of a fish oil enriched diet on aspirin intolerant asthmatic patiens: a pilot study. Thorax 43:93–97

714. Pirsig W (1986) Surgery of choanal atresia in infants and children: historical notes and updated review. Int J Paediatr Otorhinolaryngol 11:153–170
715. Plinkert PK (1993) Praktische Therapie von Hals-Nasen-Ohren-Krankheiten: Nasennebenhöhlen. In: Zenner H-P (Ed.) Praktische Therapie von Hals-Nasen-Ohren-Krankheiten. Schattauer Stuttgart, p 186
716. Pöckler C, Brambs HJ, Plinkert P (1994) Computertomographie der Nasennebenhöhlen vor endonasaler Operation. Radiologie 34:79–83
717. Polmar SH (1992) The role of the immunologist in sinus disease. J Allergy Clin Immunol 90:511–515
718. Poole MD (1992) Pediatric sinusitis is not a surgical disease. Ear Nose Throat J 71:622–623
719. Poole MD (1994) Pediatric endoscopic sinus surgery: the conservative view. Ear Nose Throat J 73:221–227
720. Portmann M, Guillen G, Chabrol A (1982) Electrocoagulation of the vidian nerve via the nasal passage. Laryngoscope 92:453–455
721. Prades J (1970) Microcirugia endonasal. Acta ORL Iber-Amer 21:184–192
722. Premachandra DJ (1991) Management of posterior epistaxis with the use of the fiberoptic nasolaryngoscope. J Laryngol Otol 105:17–19
723. Probst L, Stoney P, Jeney E, Hawke M (1992) Nasal polyps, bronchial asthma and aspirin sensitivity. J Otolaryngol 21:60–65
724. Quine SM, Gray RF, Rudd M, v Blumenthal H (1994) Microscope and hot wire cautery management of 100 consecutive patients with acute epistaxis – a superior method to traditional packing. J Laryngol Otol 108:845–848
725. Rachelefsky GS, Spector SL (1990) Sinusitis and asthma. J Asthma 27:1–3
726. Ragheb S, Duncavage JA (1992) Maxillary sinusitis: value of endoscopic middle meatus antrostomy versus Caldwell-Luc procedure. Op Tech Otolaryngol Head Neck Surg 3:129–133
727. Rains M (1997) Rains frontal sinus stent. Productinformation. Smith & Nephew, Bartlett, TN
728. Rak KM, Newell JD, Yakes WF, Damiano MA, Luethke JM (1991) Paranasal sinuses on MR images of the brain: significance of mucosa thickening. AJR 156:381–384
729. Ramadan HH (1995) Endoscopic treatment of acute frontal sinusitis: indications and limitations. Otolaryngol Head Neck Surg 113:295–300
730. Ramadan HH, Allen GC (1995) Complications of endoscopic sinus surgery in a residency training program. Laryngoscope 105:376–379
731. Rangi SP, Serwonska MH, Lenahan GA, Pickett WC, Blake VA, Sample S, Goetzl EJ (1990) Suppression by ingested eicosapentaenoic acid on the increases in nasal mucosal blood flow and eosinophilia of ryegrass-allergic reactions. J Allergy Clin Immunol 85:184–189
732. Rathfoot C, Duncavage J, Shapshay S (1996) Laser use in the paranasal sinuses. Otolarynol Clin North Am 29:943–948
733. Rauchfuß A (1990) Komplikationen der endonasalen Chirurgie der Nasennebenhöhlen. HNO 38:309–316
734. Rebeiz EE, Shapshay SM, Bowlds JH, Pankratov MM (1992) Anatomic guidelines for dacryocystorhinostomy. Laryngoscope 102:1181–1184
735. Reck R (1986) Die therapeutischen Grenzen der endonasalen Kieferhöhlenfensterung. Laryngol Rhinol Otol 65:673–675
736. Reed BR, Clark RA (1985) Cutaneous tissue repair: Practical implications of current knowledge. J Am Acad Dermatol 13:919–941
737. Reifler DM (1993) Results of endoscopic KTP laser-assisted dacryocystorhinostomy. Ophthalmic Plast Reconstr Surg 9:231–236
738. Reinert S, Fritzmeier CU (1988) Mikrokameragestützte Kieferhöhlen-Operationstechnik. Dtsch Zahnärztl Z 43:1292–1294
739. Reinhart DJ, Anderson JS (1993) Fatal outcome during endoscopic sinus surgery: anesthetic manifestations. Anesth Analg 77:188–190
740. Rettinger G, Gjuric M (1994) Osteoplastic endonasal approach to the maxillary sinus. Rhinology 32:42–44
741. Reusch A (1912) Zur Behandlung und Prognose der entzündlichen Erkrankungen der Nasennebenhöhlen. Zs f Laryngologie 4:705 - 731
742. Rice DH (1989) Endoscopic sinus surgery: results at 2-year follow up. Otolaryngol Head Neck Surg 101:476–479
743. Rice DH (1990a) Endoscopic intranasal dacryocystorhinostomy, results in four patients. Arch Otolaryngol Head Neck Surg 116:1061
744. Rice DH (1990b) Endoscopic sinus surgery: anterior approach. Op Tech Otolaryngol Head Neck Surg 1:99–103
745. Rice DH (1992) Discussion. Laryngoscope 102:1180
746. Rice DH (1993a) Endoscopic sinus surgery. Otolaryngol Clin North Am 26:613–618
747. Rice DH (1993b) Chronic frontal sinus disease. Otolaryngol Clin North Am 26:619–622
748. Rice DH (1993c) Guest editorial: functional endoscopic sinus surgery. Ear Nose Throat J 72:369
749. Rice DH, Kennedy D, Schaefer SD, Weymuller EA (1993a) Difficult decisions in endoscopic sinus surgery. Otolaryngol Clin North Am 26:695–700
750. Rice DH, Schaefer SD (1993b) Endoscopic paranasal sinus surgery, 2nd Edn. Raven Press, New York [1st Edn. 1988]
751. Riegle EV, Gunter JB, Lusk RP, Muntz HR, Weiss KI (1992) Comparison of vasoconstrictors for functional endoscopic sinus surgery in children. Laryngoscope 102:820–823
752. Ritter FN (1982) The middle turbinate and its relationship to the ethmoidal labyrinth and the orbit. Laryngoscope 92:479–482
753. Rivron RP, Maran AGD (1991) The Edinburgh FESS trainer: a cadaver-based bench-top practice system for endoscopic ethmoidal surgery. Clin Otolaryngol 16:426–429
754. Rochels R, Rudert H (1995) Notfalltherapie bei traumatischem Orbitahämatom mit akuter Visusminderung. Laryngo-Rhino-Otol 74:325–327
755. Rodriguez-Martinez F, Mascia AV, Mellins RB (1975) The effect of environmental temperature on airway resistance in the asthmatic child. Pediatr Res 7:627–631
756. Roese HF (1933) Ueber Verletzungen des Orbitainhaltes bei endonasaler Siebbeinausräumung. Klin Mbl Augenheilk 91:95–100
757. Rontal M, Rontal E (1991) Studying whole-mounted sections of the paranasal sinuses to understand the complications of endoscopic sinus surgery. Laryngoscope 101:361–366
758. Rosenberg SI (1994) Use of the ultrasonic aspirator during endoscopic nasal polypectomy. Otolaryngol Head Neck Surg 111:143–145
759. Rosenfeld RM (1995) Pilot study of outcomes in pediatric rhinosinusitis. Arch Otolaryngol Head Neck Surg 121:729–736
760. Rosenhall L (1982) Evaluation of intolerance to analgesics, preservatives and food colorants with challenge tests. Eur J Respir Dis 63:410–419
761. Roth M (1994) Should oral steroids be the primary treatment for allergic fungal sinusitis? Ear Nose Throat J 73:928–930
762. Rubin JS, Lund VJ, Salmon N (1986) Frontoethmoidectomy in the treatment of mucoceles. Arch Otolaryngol Head Neck Surg 112:434–436
763. Rudert H (1988) Mikroskop- und endoskopgestützte Chirurgie der entzündlichen Nasennebenhöhlenerkrankungen. HNO 36:475–482
764. Rudert H, Harder T, Werner JA, Lippert BM (1993) Riesenmukozele der Nasennebenhöhlen mit Ausdehnung in die kontralaterale hintere Schädelgrube und reversibler retrocochleärer Schwerhörigkeit. Laryngo-Rhino-Otol 72:247–251

765. Rudert H, Maune S (1997a) Endonasal coagulation of the sphenopalatine artery in severe posterior epistaxis. Laryngo-Rhino-Otol 76:77–82
766. Rudert H, Maune S, Mahnke CG (1997b) Komplikationen der endonasalen Chirurgie der Nasennebenhöhlen. Inzidenz und Strategien zu ihrer Vermeidung. Laryngo-Rhino-Otol 76:200–15
767. Ruhno J, Andersson B, Denburg J, Anderson M, Hitch D, Lapp P, Vanzieleghem M, Dolovich J (1990) A double-blind comparison of intranasal budesonide with placebo for nasal polyposis. J Allergy Clin Immunol 86:946–953
768. Ryan RM, Whittet HB, Norval C, Marks NJ (1996) Minimal follow-up after functional endoscopic sinus surgery. Does it affect outcome? Rhinology 34:44–45
769. Sacks SH, Lawson W, Edelstein D, Green RP (1988) Surgical treatment of blindness secondary to intraorbital hemorrhage. Arch Otolaryngol Head Neck Surg 114:801–803
770. Salam MA, Cable HR (1993) Middle meatal antrostomy: long-term patency and results in chronic maxillary sinusitis. A prospective study. Clin Otolaryngol 18:135–138
771. Salassa JR (1992) Polyethylene oxide gel: a new dressing after endoscopic sinus surgery. Rhinology 30:25–32
772. Salatich DG (1990) An easy method for suctioning and irrigation during functional endoscopic sinus surgery. Laryngoscope 100:670
773. Salman SD (1991) Complications of endoscopic sinus surgery. Am J Otolaryngol 12:326–328
774. Salman SD (1993) A new stent for endoscopic sinus surgery. Otolaryngol Head Neck Surg 109:780–781
775. Sataloff RT, Zwillenberg D, Myers DL (1988) Middle turbinectomy complicated by cerebrospinal fluid leak secondary to ethmoid encephalocele: transethmoid repair. Am J Rhinol 2:27–31
776. Sawyer R (1991) Nasal approach to the sphenoid sinus after prior septal surgery. Laryngoscope 101:89–91
777. Scadding GK, Lung VJ, Darby YC, Navas-Romero J, Seymour N, Turner MW (1994) IgG subclass levels in chronic rhinosinusitis. Rhinology 32:15–19
778. Schabdach DG, Goldberg SG, Breton M, Griffith JW, Lang M, Cunningham D (1994) An animal model of visual loss from orbital hemorrhage. Ophthalmic Plast Reconstr Surg 10:200–205
779. Schaefer SD (1989) Endoscopic total sphenoethmoidectomy. Otolaryngol Clin North Am 22:727–732
780. Schaefer SD (1992) Letter to the editor. Arch Otolaryngol Head Neck Surg 118:105
781. Schaefer SD, Close LG (1990) Endoscopic management of frontal sinus disease. Laryngoscope 100:155–160
782. Schaefer SD, Manning S, Close LG (1989) Endoscopic paranasal sinus surgery: indications and contraindications. Laryngoscope 99:1–5
783. Schaeffer M (1890) Zur Diagnose und Therapie der Erkrankungen der Nebenhöhlen der Nase mit Ausnahme des Sinus maxillaris. Dtsch Med Wschr 16:905–907
784. Schaitkin B, May M, Shapiro A, Fucci M, Mester SJ (1993) Endoscopic sinus surgery. 4-year follow-up on the first 100 patients. Laryngoscope 103:1117–1120
785. Schapowal AG, Simon H-U, Schmitz-Schumann M (1995) Phenomenology, pathogenesis, diagnosis and treatment of aspirin-sensitive rhinosinusitis. Acta Oto-Rhino-Laryngol Belg. 49:235–50
786. Schapowal AG, Simon H-U, Schmitz-Schumann M (1996) Phänomenologie, Pathogenese, Diagnose und Behandlung der Rhinosinusitis bei Aspirinunverträglichkeit. In: Mösges R, Schlöndorff G (Eds.) Die Folgen der Allergie: Rhinitis, Asthma, Polyposis nasi. Biermann, Zülpich, p 15–43
787. Schauss F, Weber R, Draf W, Keerl R (1996) Surgery of the lacrimal system. Acta Oto-Rhino-Laryngol Belg. 50:143–146
788. Schelhorn P, Zenk W, Reuter W (1985) Endoskopische Spätbefunde nach Mittelgesichtsfrakturen mit Kieferhöhlenbeteiligung. Stomatol DDR 35:702–704
789. Scher RL, Gross CW (1990) Additional applications for transnasal endoscopic surgery. Op Tech Otolaryngol Head Neck Surg 1:84–88
790. Scherrer M, Zeller C (1978) Nasal polypectomy in asthma. Lung 155:161–163
791. Scherrer M, Zeller C, Berger M (1984) Asthma bronchiale, Polyposis nasi und Schmerzmittel-Unverträglichkeit (ASA-Trias). Schweiz Med Wschr 114:337–342
792. Schick B, Weber R, Keerl R, Draf W (1996) Duraplastiken in der Keilbeinhöhle. Laryngo-Rhino-Otol 75:275–279
793. Schick B, Weber R, Kahle G, Draf W, Lackmann GM (1997a) Late manifestations of traumatic lesions of the anterior skull base. Skull Base Surg 7:77–83
794. Schick B, Weber R, Mosler P, Keerl R, Draf W (1997b) Langzeitergebnisse frontobasaler Duraplastiken. HNO 45:117–22
795. Schlenter WW, Mann WJ (1982) Die allergische Genese der chronischen Sinusitis. Laryngo-Rhino-Otol 61:228–230
796. Schlenter WW, Mann WJ (1983) Operative Therapie der chronischen Sinusitis – Erfolge bei allergischen und nichtallergischen Patienten. Laryngo-Rhino-Otol 62:284–288
797. Schlöndorff G, Mösges R, Meyer-Ebrecht D, Krybus W, Adams L (1989) CAS (computer assisted surgery) – ein neuartiges Verfahren in der Kopf- und Halschirurgie. HNO 37:187–190
798. Schmidt W, Fleck K (1992) Haben operative Maßnahmen im Nasen-Rachen-Raum einen Einfluß auf den Verlauf des Asthma bronchiale? Atemw-Lungenkrkh 18:166–174
799. Schumacher MJ, Lota KA, Taussig LM (1986) Pulmonary response to nasal challenge testing of atopic subjects with stable asthma. J Allergy Clin Immunol 78:30–35
800. Schuman DM, Pineyro R (1994) Functional aqualaser sinuscopy: a safe technique for the treatment of severe nasal polyposis. J Clin Laser Med Surg 12:333–337
801. Schuring AG (1989) Claims and suits against otology. Am J Otol 10:327–328
802. Schuring AG (1990) The operative report. Am J Otol 11:71–73
803. Seiden AM (1995) Isolated sphenoid sinusitis: problems in diagnosis and therapy. Am J Rhinol 9:229–235
804. Seiden AM, El Hefny YI (1995) Endoscopic trephination for the removal of frontal sinus osteoma. Otolaryngol Head Neck Surg 112:607–611
805. Seiden AM, Smith DV (1988) Endoscopic intranasal surgery as an approach to restoring olfactory function. Chem Senses 13:736
806. Seiden AM, Stankiewicz JA (1998) Frontal sinus surgery: the state of the art. Am J Otolaryngol 19:183–193
807. Seiffert (1930) Zwei Fälle von retrobulbärer Eiterung, geheilt durch endonasale Eröffnung der Orbita durch das Siebbein hindurch. Zentralbl HNO 15:106
808. Seiffert A (1929) Unterbindung der Arteria maxillaris interna. Z Hals-Nasen- und Ohrenheilkd 22:323–325
809. Seppey M, Schweri T, Häusler R (1996) Comparative randomised clinical study of tolerability and efficacy of Rhinomer[R] Force 3 versus a reference product in postoperative care of the nasal fossae after endonasal surgery. ORL 58:87–92
810. Serdahl CL, Berris CE, Chole RA (1990) Nasolacrimal duct obstruction after endoscopic sinus surgery. Arch Ophthalmol 108:391–392
811. Serrano E, Pessey JJ, Lacomme Y (1992) Les mucocèles sinusiennes: aspects diagnostiques et chirurgicaux (à propos de 8 cas traités par rhino-chirurgie endoscopique). Acta Oto-Rhino-Laryngol Belg 46:287–292
812. Sethi DS, Pillay PK (1995) Endoscopic management of lesions of the sella turcica. J Laryngol Otol 109:956–962
813. Sethi DS, Stanley RE, Pillay PK (1995a) Endoscopic anatomy of the sphenoid sinus and sella turcica. J Laryngol Otol 109:951–955
814. Sethi DS, Winkelstein JA, Lederman H, Loury MC (1995b) Immunologic defects in patients with chronic recurrent

sinusitis: diagnosis and management. Otolaryngol Head Neck Surg 112:242–247
815. Setliff RC III (1996) The hummer: a remedy for apprehension in functional endoscopic sinus surgery. Otolaryngol Clin North Am 29:5–104
816. Setliff RC, Parsons DS (1994) The 'Hummer': new instrumentation for functional endoscopic sinus surgery. Am J Rhinol 8:275–278
817. Settipane GA, Chafee FH (1977) Nasal polyps in asthma and rhinitis. J Allergy Clin Immunol 59:17–23
818. Settipane GA, Klein DE, Lekas MD (1985) Asthma and nasal polyps. In: Myers E (Ed.) New dimensions in otorhinolaryngology – head and neck surgery, Vol. 2. Elsevier, Amsterdam pp. 499–500
819. Settipane GA, Klein DE, Settipane RJ (1991) Nasal polyps: state of the art. Rhinology Suppl 11:33–36
820. Shankar L, Evans K, Hawke M, Stammberger H (1994) Atlas der Nasennebenhöhlen. Chapman & Hall, London
821. Shapshay SM, Rebeiz EE, Bohigian RK, Hybels RL, Aretz HT, Pankratov MM (1991) Holmium: Yttrium Aluminium Garnet Laser-assisted endoscopic sinus surgery: laboratory experience. Laryngoscope 101:142–149
822. Shapshay SM, Rebeiz EE, Pankratov MM (1992) Holmium:Yttrium Aluminium Garnet Laser-assisted endoscopic sinus surgery: clinical experience. Laryngoscope 102:1177–1180
823. Sharpe HR, Rowe-Jones JM, Biring GS, Mackay IS (1997) Endoscopic ligation or diathermy of the sphenopalatine artery in persistent epistaxis. J Laryngol Otol 111:1047–1050
824. Shikani AH (1994) A new middle meatal antrostomy stent for functional endoscopic sinus surgery. Laryngoscope 104:638–641
825. Shirasaki H, Asakura K, Narita S, Kataura A (1998) The effect of a cysteinyl leukotriene antagonist ONO-1078 (pranlukast) on agonist- and antigen-induced nasal microvascular leakage in guinea pigs. Rhinology 36:62–65
826. Shturman-Ellstein R, Zeballos RJ, Buckley JM, Souhrada JF (1978) The beneficial effect of nasal breathing on exercise-induced bronchoconstriction. Am Rev Respir Dis 118:72–76
827. Silk HJ (1990) Sinusitis and asthma: a review. J Asthma 27:5–9
828. Sillers MJ, Kuhn FA, Vickery CL (1995) Radiation exposure in paranasal sinus imaging. Otolaryngol Head Neck Surg 112:248–251
829. Silverstein H, McDaniel AB (1987) Microsurgical sphenoethmoidectomy. In: Goldman JL (Ed.) The principles and practice of rhinology. J Wiley, New York, pp 435–442
830. Simmen D (1997) Endonasale, mikroskopisch kontrollierte Stirnhöhlenchirurgie. Laryngo-Rhino-Otol 76:131–136
831. Simmen D, Schuknecht B (1997) Computertomographie der Nasenebenhöhlen – eine präoperative Checkliste. Laryngo-Rhino-Otologie 76:8–13
832. Simpson GT, Shapshay SM, Vaughn CW, Strong MS (1982) Rhinologic surgery with the carbon dioxide laser. Laryngoscope 92:412–415
833. Singh J (1992) Letter to the editor. Arch Otolaryngol Head Neck Surg 118:105
834. Slavin RG (1982) Relationship of nasal disease and sinusitis to bronchial asthma. Ann Allergy 49:76–80
835. Slavin RG, Linford P, Friedman WH (1982) Sinusitis and bronchial asthma (abstract). J Allergy Clin Immunol 69:102
836. Slavin RG, Linford P, Friedman WH (1983) Sphenoethmoidectomy (SE) in the treatment of nasal polyps, sinusitis and bronchial asthma (abstract). J Allergy Clin Immunol 71:156
837. Small P, Frenkiel S, Blank M (1982) Multifactorial etiology of nasal polyps. Ann Allergy 46:317–320
838. Smith LF, Brindley PC (1993) Indications, evaluation, complications, and results of functional endoscopic sinus surgery in 200 patients. Otolaryngol Head Neck Surg 108:688–696
839. Sogg A (1989) Long-term results of ethmoid surgery. Ann Otol Rhinol Laryngol 98:699–701
840. Sogg A (1992) Letter to the editor. Rhinology 30:77–78
841. Sogg A, Eichel B (1991) Ethmoid surgery complications and their avoidance. Ann Otol Rhinol Laryngol 100:722–724
842. Sogg AJ, Heights M (1982) Intranasal antrostomy – causes of failure. Laryngoscope 92:1038–1041
843. Som PM, Sachdev VP, Biller HF (1983) Sphenoid sinus pneumocele. Report of a case. Arch Otolaryngol 109:761–764
844. Som PM, Lawson W, Biller HF, Lanzieri CF (1986a) Ethmoid sinus disease: CT evaluation in 400 cases. Part I: nonsurgical patients. Radiology 159:591–597
845. Som PM, Lawson W, Biller HF, Lanzieri CF (1986b) Ethmoid sinus disease: CT evaluation in 400 cases. Part II: Postoperative findings. Radiology 159:599–604
846. Som PM, Sacher M, Lawson W, Biller HF (1987) CT appearance distinguishing benign nasal polyps from malignancies. J Comput Assist Tomogr 11:129–133
847. Som PM, Dillon WP, Fullerton GD, Zimmerman RA, Rajagopalan B, Marom Z (1989) Chronically obstructed sinonasal secretions: observations on T1 and T2 shortening. Radiology 172:515–520
848. Som PM, Lawson W, Lidov MW (1991) Simulated aggressive skull base erosion in response to benign sinonasal disease. Radiology 180:755–759
849. Sonkens JW, Harnsberger HR, Blanch GM, Babbel RW, Hunt S (1991) The impact of screening sinus CT on the planning of functional endoscopic sinus surgery. Otolaryngol Head Neck Surg 105:802–813
850. South MA (1979) The so-called salicylate-free diet: one more time. Cutis 24:488–494
851. Sözeri B, Ataman M, Gürsel B (1993) Blindness after intranasal ethmoidectomy. Rhinology 31:85–87
852. Spector SL (1996) Management of asthma with zafirlukast. Drugs 52 (Suppl 6) 36–46
853. Spiess G (1899) Die endonasale Chirurgie des Sinus frontalis. Arch Laryngol 9:285–291
854. Stammberger H (1981) Zum invertierten Papillom der Nasenschleimhaut. HNO 29:128–133
855. Stammberger H (1985) Endoscopic surgery for mycotic and chronic recurring sinusitis. Ann Otol Rhinol Laryngol Suppl 119:1–11
856. Stammberger H (1986a) Nasal and paranasal sinus endoscopy. A diagnostic and surgical approach to recurrent sinusitis. Endoscopy18:213–218
857. Stammberger H (1986b) Endoscopic endonasal surgery – concepts in treatment of recurring rhinosinusitis. Part 1. Anatomic and pathophysiological considerations. Otolaryngol Head Neck Surg 94:143–147
858. Stammberger H (1986c) Endoscopic endonasal surgery – concepts in treatment of recurring rhinosinusitis. Part II. Surgical technique. Otolaryngol Head Neck Surg 94:147–156
859. Stammberger H (1990) Letter to the editor. Acta Otolaryngol (Stockh) 109:320–321
860. Stammberger H (1991) Functional endoscopic sinus surgery. B.C. Decker, Philadelphia
861. Stammberger H (1993) Komplikationen entzündlicher Nasennebenhöhlenerkrankungen einschließlich iatrogen bedingter Komplikationen. Eur Arch Oto-Rhino-Laryngol Suppl 1993/I:61–102
862. Stammberger H (1995) Nasal polyposis: Attempting classification. American Rhinologic Society, Combined Otolaryngology Spring Meeting, Palm Desert, CA, 30.4.-1.5.95, Abstracts, S 13–15
863. Stammberger H: Endoscopic diagnosis and surgery of the paranasal sinuses and anterior skull base – the Messerklinger technique and advanced applications from the Graz school. Karl Storz GmbH, Tuttlingen, Germany

864. Stammberger H, Zinreich SJ, Kopp W, Kennedy DW, Johns ME, Rosenbaum AE (1987) Zur operativen Behandlung der chronisch-rezidivierenden Sinusitis – Caldwell-Luc versus funktionelle endoskopische Technik. HNO 35:93–105
865. Stammberger H, Posawetz W (1990) Functional endoscopic sinus surgery. Concept, indications and results of the Messerklinger technique. Eur Arch Otorhinolaryngol 247:63–76
866. Stammberger H, Hawke M (1993) Essentials of functional endoscopic sinus surgery. Mosby, St. Louis
867. Stammberger H, Kennedy DW, Bolger WE, Clement PAR, Hosemann W, Kuhn FA, Lanza DC, Leopold DA, Ohnishi T, Passali D, Schaefer SD, Wayoff MR, Zinreich SJ (1995) Paranasal sinuses: Anatomic terminology and nomenclature. Ann Otol Rhinol Laryngol Suppl 167:7–16
868. Stammberger H, Greistorfer K, Wolf G, Luxenberger W (1997) Operativer Verschluß von Liquorfisteln der vorderen Schädelbasis unter intrathekaler Natriumfluoreszeinanwendung. Laryngo-Rhino-Otol 76:595–607
869. Stankiewicz JA (1987a) Complications of endoscopic nasal surgery: occurence and treatment. Am J Rhinol 1:45–49
870. Stankiewicz JA (1987b) Complications of endoscopic intranasal ethmoidectomy. Laryngoscope 97:1270–1273
871. Stankiewicz JA (1989a) Complications in endoscopic intranasal ethmoidectomy – an update. Laryngoscope 99:686–690
872. Stankiewicz JA (1989b) Complications of endoscopic sinus surgery. Otolaryngol Clin North Am 22:749–758
873. Stankiewicz JA (1989c) Blindness in intranasal ethmoidectomy: prevention and management. Otolaryngol Head Neck Surg 101:320–329
874. Stankiewicz JA (1989d) The endoscopic approach to the sphenoid sinus. Laryngoscope 99:218–221
875. Stankiewicz JA (1989e) Sphenoid sinus mucocele. Arch Otolaryngol Head Neck Surg 115:735–740
876. Stankiewicz JA (1990) The endoscopic repair of choanal atresia. Otolaryngol Head Neck Surg 103:931–937
877. Stankiewicz JA (1991) Cerebrospinal fluid fistula and endoscopic sinus surgery. Laryngoscope 101:250–256
878. Stankiewicz JA (1995) Pediatric endoscopic nasal and sinus surgery. Otolaryngol Head Neck Surg 113:204–210
879. Stankiewicz JA, Girgis SJ (1993) Endoscopic surgical treatment of nasal and paranasal sinus inverted papilloma. Otolaryngol Head Neck Surg 109:988–995
880. Stark WB (1928) Irrigations with aqueous solution. Their effect on the membranes of the upper respiratory tract of the rabbit. Arch Otolaryngol 8:47–55
881. Steadman MG (1985) Transnasal dacryocystorhinostomy. Otolaryngol Clin North Am 18:107–111
882. Steiner W (1982) Endoskopische Diagnostik der entzündlichen Erkrankungen der Nasennebenhöhlen. Arch Otorhinolaryngol 235:69–131
883. Sterman BM, DeVore RA, Lavertu P, Levine HL (1990) Endoscopic sinus surgery in a residency training program. Am J Rhinol 4:207–210
884. Stevens HE, Blair NJ (1988) Intranasal sphenoethmoidectomy: 10 years experience and literature review. J Otolaryngol 17:254–259
885. Stevenson DD (1994) Aspirin sensitivity in the respiratory system. In: Feinmann SE (Ed.) Beneficial and toxic effects of aspirin. CRC Press, Boca Raton, pp 39–51
886. Stevenson DD, Pleskow WW, Simon RA, Mathison DA, Lumry WR, Schatz M, Zeiger RS (1984) Aspirin-sensitive rhinosinusitis asthma: a double-blind crossover study of treatment with aspirin. J Allergy Clin Immunol 73:500–507
887. Stoll W (1993) Operative Versorgung frontobasaler Verletzungen (inklusive Orbita) durch den HNO-Chirurgen. Eur Arch Oto-Rhino-Laryngol Suppl 1993/I:287–307
888. Stone BD, Georgitis JW, Matthews B (1990) Inflammatory mediators in sinus lavage fluid (abstract). J Allergy Clin Immunol 85:222
889. Stone DJ, Gal TJ (1994) Airway management. In: Miller RD (Ed.) Anesthesia. Vol. 2, 4th Edn. Churchill Livingstone, New York, pp 1403–1436
890. Stoney P, Probst L, Shankar L, Hawke M (1993) CT scanning for functional endoscopic sinus surgery: analysis of 200 cases with reporting scheme. J Otolaryngol 22:72–78
891. Straatman NJA, Buiter CT (1981) Endoscopic surgery of the nasal fontanel. Arch Otolaryngol 107:290–293
892. Streitmann MJ, Otto RA, Sakai CS (1994) Anatomic considerations in complications of endoscopic and intranasal sinus surgery. Ann Otol Rhinol Laryngol 103:105–109
893. Strutz J (1993) Die 3D-Endoskopie. HNO 41:128–130
894. Swanson PB, Lanza DC, Vining EM, Kennedy DW (1995) The effect of middle turbinate resection upon the frontal sinus. Am J Rhinol 9:191–195
895. Szentivanyi A (1968) The beta adrenergic theory of the atopic abnormality in bronchial asthma. J Allergy 42:203–232
896. Takahashi M, Itoh M, Kaneko M, Ishii J, Yoshida A (1989) Microscopic intranasal decompression of the optic nerve. Arch Otorhinolaryngol 246:113–116
897. Takahashi R (1952) Decompression of the optic canal. Surgery 5:300–302 [in Japanese] (cited by Takahashi et al. [896])
898. Talbot AR (1996) Frontal sinus surgery in children. Otolaryngol Clin North Am 29:143–158
899. Tamagawa Y, Kitamura K, Miyata M (1995) Branchial cyst of the nasopharynx: resection via the endonasal approach. J Laryngol Otol 109:139–141
900. Tandon DA, Thakar A, Mahapatra AK, Ghosh P (1994) Trans-ethmoidal optic nerve decompression. Clin Otolaryngol 19:98–104
901. Tarver CP, Noorily AD, Sakai CS (1993) A comparison of cocaine vs. lidocaine with oxymetazoline for use in nasal procedures. Otolaryngol Head Neck Surg 109: 653–659
902. Tasman AJ, Faller U, Möller P (1994) Sklerosierende Lipogranulomatose der Augenlider nach Siebbeinoperation: eine Komplikation nach Salbentamponade! Laryngo-Rhino-Otol 73: 264–267
903. Tasman AJ, Wallner F, Kollin GH, Stammberger H (1998) Is monocular perception of depth through the rigid endoscope a disadvantage compared to binocular vision through the operating microscope in paranasal sinus surgery? Am J Rhinol 12:87–91
904. Tasman AJ, Feldhusen F, Kolling GH, Krastel H, Hosemann W (1999) Video-endoscope vs. endoscope für paranasal sinus surgery: influence in visual acuity and color discriminiation. Am J Rhinol 13:7–10
905. Taylor JS, Crocker PV, Keebler JS (1982) Intranasal ethmoidectomy and concurrent procedures. Laryngoscope 92:739–743
906. Teatini GP, Stomeo F, Bozzo C (1991) Transnasal sinusectomy with combined microscopic and endoscopic technique. J Laryngol Otol 105:635–637
907. Terrier F, Terrier G, Rüfenacht D, Friedrich JP, Weber W (1987) Die Anatomie der Siebbeinregion: topographische, radiologische und endoskopische Leitstrukturen. Therapeutische Umschau 44:75–85
908. Terrier G (1991) Rhinosinusal endoscopy, Diagnosis and surgery. Zambon Group, Milano
909. Terrier G, Weber W, Ruefenacht D, Porcellini (1985) Anatomy of the ethmoid: CT, endoscopic, and macroscopic. AJR 144:493–500
910. Terris MH, Billman GF, Pransky SM (1993) Nasal hamartoma: case report and review of the literature. Int J Pediatr Otorhinolaryngol 28:83–88
911. Thaler ER, Smullen AM, Kennedy DW (1994) Adult cystic fibrosis presenting with nasal polyposis and chronic sinusitis. Am J Rhinol 8:237–239
912. Thaler ER, Gottschalk A, Samaranayake R, Lanza DC, Kennedy DW (1997) Anesthesia in endoscopic sinus surgery. Am J Rhinol 11:409–413

913. Thomassin JM, Korchia D (1991) Polypose naso-sinusienne. Indications. Résultats. A propos de 222 ethmoidectomies. Ann Oto-Laryngol (Paris) 108:455–464
914. Thompson RF, Gluckman JL, Kulwin D, Savoury L (1990) Orbital hemorrhage during ethmoid sinus surgery. Otolaryngol Head Neck Surg102:45–50
915. Thorsch E (1909) Beziehungen der Tränensackgrube zur Nase und ihren Nebenhöhlen. Klin Monatsbl Augenh 1909:530–533
916. Todd J, Fishaut M, Kapral F, Welch T (1978) Toxic shock syndrome associated with phage group 1 staphylococci. Lancet 2:1116–1118
917. Toffel PH (1994) Simultaneous secure endoscopic sinus surgery and rhinoplasty. Ear Nose Throat J 73:554–565
918. Toffel PH (1995) Secure endoscopic sinus surgery with middle meatal stenting. Op Tech Otolaryngol Head Neck Surg 6:157–162
919. Toffel PH, Aroesty DJ, Weinmann RH (1989) Secure endoscopic sinus surgery as an adjunct to functional nasal surgery. Arch Otolaryngol Head Neck Surg 115:822–825
920. Tolsdorff P (1992) Endonasale Nasennebenhöhlenchirurgie unter Lupenbrillenkontrolle. Laryngo-Rhino-Otol 71:552–555
921. Tos M, Drake-Lee AB, Lund VJ, Stammberger H (1989) Treatment of nasal polyps – medication or surgery and which technique. Rhinology Suppl 8:45–49
922. Toselli RM, dePapp A, Harbaugh RE, Saunders RL (1991) Neurosurgical complications after intranasal ethmoidectomy. J Neurol Neurosurg Psychiatry 54:463–465
923. Triglia JM, Dessi P, Cannoni M, Pech A (1992) Intranasal ethmoidectomy in nasal polyposis in children. Indications and results. Int J Pediatr Otorhinolaryngol 23:125–131
924. Trittel C, Möller J, Euler HH, Werner JA (1995) Das Churg-Strauss-Syndrom. Eine Differentialdiagnose bei chronisch polypöser Sinusitis. Laryngo-Rhino-Otol 74:577–580
925. Truppe M, Stammberger H (1994) 3D-Navigation: Eine neue Orientierungshilfe bei endoskopischen NNH- und Schädelbasisoperationen. Vortrag 65. Jahresversammlung der Deutschen Gesellschaft für HNO-Heilkunde, Kopf- und Halschirurgie, Chemnitz
926. Tsutsumi M (1969) Transnasal optic canal decompression. J Jap Rhinol Soc 8:20 (cited by Fujitani [252])
927. Uchida Y, Sugita T (1981) Endonasal findings using a fiberoptic telescope in postoperative cases of chronic sinusitis. Rhinology 19:161–165
928. Ulrik CS, Backer V, Dirksen A (1992) A 10 year follow up of 180 adults with bronchial asthma: factors important for the decline in lung function. Thorax 47:14–18
929. Ummat S, Riding M, Kirkpatrick D (1992) Development of the ostiomeatal unit in childhood: a radiological study. J Otolaryngol 21:307–314
930. Ünlü HH, Akyar S, Caylan R, Nalca Y (1994a) Concha bullosa. J Otolaryngol 23:23–27
931. Ünlü HH, Caylan R, Nalca Y, Akyar S (1994b) An endoscopic and tomographic evaluation of patients with sinusitis after endoscopic sinus surgery and Caldwell Luc Operation: a comparative study. J Otolaryngol 23:197–203
932. Urken M, Som PM, Edelstein D, Lawson W, Weber AL, Biller HF (1987) Abnormally large frontal sinus. II. Nomenclature, Pathology, and symptoms. Laryngoscope 97:606–611
933. van Alyea OE (1939) Ethmoid labyrinth. Anatomic study, with consideration of the clinical significance of its structural characteristics. Arch Otolaryngol 29:881–902
934. van Alyea OE (1941) Sphenoid sinus: anatomic study, with consideration of the clinical significance of the structural characteristics of the sphenoid sinus. Arch Otolaryngol 34:225–253
935. van Alyea OE (1946) Frontal sinus drainage. Ann Otol Rhinol Laryngol 55:267–277
936. van der Veken PJV, Clement PAR, Buisseret T, Desprechins B, Kaufman L, Derde MP (1990) CT-scan study of the incidence of sinus involvement and nasal anatomic variations in 196 children. Rhinology 28:177–184
937. van Dishoeck HAE (1961) Allergy and infection of the paranasal sinuses. Adv Oto-Rhino-Laryngol 10:1–29
938. Vancil ME (1969) A historical survey of treatments for nasal polyposis. Laryngoscope 79:435–445
939. Varney VA, Cumberworth V, Sudderick R, Durham SR, Mackay IS (1994) Rhinitis, sinusitis and the yellow nail syndrome: a review of symptoms and response to treatment in 17 patients. Clin Otolaryngol 19:237–240
940. Vining EM, Yanagisawa K, Yanagisawa E (1993) The importance of preoperative nasal endoscopy in patients with sinonasal disease. Laryngoscope 103:512–519
941. Virolainen E; Puhakka H (1980) The effect of intranasal beclomethasone dipropionate on the recurrence of nasal polyps after ethmoidectomy. Rhinology 18:9–18
942. Vleming M, Middelweerd RJ, de Vries N (1992) Complications of endoscopic sinus surgery. Arch Otolaryngol Head Neck Surg 118:617–623
943. von Glaß W, Hauenstein T (1988) Wound healing in the nose and paranasal sinuses after irradiation with the argon laser. Arch Otorhinolaryngol 245:36–41
944. von Schacky C (1990) Omega-3-Fettsäuren – schon klinisch einsetzbar? Dtsch Med Wschr 115:224–231
945. Waguespack R (1995) Mucociliary clearance patterns following endoscopic sinus surgery. Laryngoscope Suppl 71:1–40
946. Waitz G, Wigand ME (1992) Results of endoscopic sinus surgery for the treatment of inverted papillomas. Laryngoscope 102:917–922
947. Waitzman AA, Birt BD (1994) Fungal Sinusitis. J Otolaryngol 23:244–249
948. Wald ER (1992) Sinusitis in children. N Engl J Med 326:319–323
949. Wallace R, Salazar JE, Cowles S (1990) The relationship between frontal sinus drainage and osteomeatal complex disease. AJNR 11:183–186
950. Walner DL, Falciglia M, Willging P, Myer CM III (1998) The role of second-look nasal endoscopy after pediatric functional endoscopic sinus surgery. Arch Otolaryngol Head Neck Surg 124:425–428
951. Walther EK, Herberhold C, Lippel R (1994) Digitale Subtraktions-Dakryozystographie (DS-DCG) und Ergebnisbilanz endonasaler Tränenwegschirurgie. Laryngo-Rhino-Otol 73:609–613
952. Watson DJ, Griffith MV (1988) The safety and efficacy of intra-nasal ethmoidectomy. J Laryngol Otol 102:802–804
953. Watson-Williams P (1933) Chronic nasal sinusitis and its relation to general medicine, 2nd. Edn. J. Wright & Sons Ltd., Bristol
954. Wayoff M (1992) Letter to the editor. Rhinology 30:78–79
955. Wayoff M, Jankowski R (1991) Medico-legal aspects in sinus surgery. Rhinology 29:257–261
956. Weber A, May A, v Ilberg C, Klima A (1991a) Möglichkeiten der Nasenmuschelbehandlung im Rahmen der endonasalen Mikrochirurgie. Laryngo-Rhino-Otol 70:487–490
957. Weber A, May A, v Ilberg C, Klima A, Halbsguth A (1991b) Die Computertomographie als Standarduntersuchungsverfahren zur Nasennebenhöhlendiagnostik aus der Sicht des Hals-Nasen-Ohren-Arztes. Laryngo-Rhino-Otol 70:289–295
958. Weber BP, Kempf HG, Mayer R, Braunschweig R (1993) Ektope Zähne im Nasennebenhöhlenbereich. HNO 41:317–320
959. Weber R, Draf W (1992a) Endonasale mikro-endoskopische Pansinusoperation bei chronischer Sinusitis. Otorhinolaryngol Nova 2:63–69
960. Weber R, Draf W (1992b) Komplikationen der endonasalen mikroendoskopischen Siebbeinoperation. HNO 40:170–175
961. Weber R, Draf W, Kolb P (1993) Die endonasale mikrochirurgische Behandlung von Tränenwegsstenosen. HNO 41:11–18

962. Weber R, Draf W (1994) Reconstruction of Lacrimal Drainage After Trauma or Tumor Surgery. Am J Otolaryngol 15:329–335
963. Weber R, Draf W, Constantinidis J, Keerl R (1995a) Aktuelle Aspekte zur Stirnhöhlenchirurgie IV – Zur Therapie des Stirnhöhlenosteoms. HNO 43:482–486
964. Weber R, Keerl R, Draf W, Wienke A, Kind M (1995b) Zur Begutachtung: Periorbitales Paraffingranulom nach Nasennebenhöhlenoperation. Otorhinolaryngol Nova 5:87–90
965. Weber R, Keerl R, Huppmann A, Draf W, Saha A (1995c) Wound healing after paranasal sinus surgery by video time lapse sequences. Op Tech Otolaryngol Head Neck Surg 6:237–240
966. Weber R, Draf W, Keerl R, Behm K, Schick B (1996a) Langzeitergebnisse nach endonasaler Stirnhöhlenchirurgie. HNO 44:503–509
967. Weber R, Keerl R, Draf W, Schick B, Mosler P, Saha A (1996b) Management of dural lesions during endonasal sinus surgery. Arch Otolaryngol 122:732–736
968. Weber R, Keerl R, Huppmann, Schick B, Draf W (1996c) Investigation of wound healing following paranasal sinus surgery with time lapse video – a pilot study. Am J Rhinol 10:235–238
969. Weber R, Keerl R, Jaspersen D, Huppmann A, Schick B, Draf W (1996d) Computer-assisted documentation and analysis of wound healing of the nasal and esophageal mucosa. J Laryngol Otol 110:1017–1021
970. Weber R, Keerl R, Schick B, Huppmann A, Draf W (1996e) Der Einfluß der Nachbehandlung auf die Wundheilung nach endonasaler Nasennebenhöhlenoperation. Laryngol Rhinol Otol 75: 208–214
971. Weber R, Keerl R (1996f) Einsatz moderner Bild-Datenverarbeitung in der klinisch rhinologischen Forschung. Eur Arch Otorhinolaryngol Suppl I:271–296
972. Weber R, Draf W, Keerl R, Schick B, Saha A (1997a) Microendoscopic endonasal pansinusoperation in chronic sinusitis. II. Results and complications. Am J Otolaryngol 18:247–253
973. Weber R, Hosemann W, Draf W, Keerl R, Schick B, Schinzel S (1997b) Endonasale Stirnhöhlenchirurgie mit Langzeiteinlage eines Platzhalters. Laryngo-Rhino-Otol 76:728–734
974. Weber R, Leuwer R, Keerl R, Dshambazov K, Mlynski G (1998) Videoendoskopische Analyse der intranasalen Verteilung topisch applizierten Kortisons unter Verwendung eines Nasenmodells. Otorhinolaryngol Nova 7:198–203
975. Weber R, Keerl R, Hosemann W, Leuwer R, Draf W, Lund V, Toffel P (1999) Endonasal sinus surgery. Postoperative care, physiology and pathophysiology. Giebel Verlag, Eiterfeld
976. Weed DT, Cole RR (1994) Maxillary sinus hypoplasia and vertical dystopia of the orbit. Laryngoscope 104:758–762
977. Weidenbecher M (1989) Dacryocystorhinostomia interna. In: Wigand ME (Ed.) Endoskopische Chirurgie der Nasennebenhöhlen und der vorderen Schädelbasis. Thieme, Stuttgart, pp 118–119
978. Weidenbecher M, Hosemann W, Buhr W (1994) Endoscopic endonasal dacryocystorhinostomy: results in 56 patients. Ann Otol Rhinol Laryngol 103: 363–367
979. Weissler MC, Montgomery WW, Turner PA, Montgomery SK, Joseph MP (1986) Inverted papilloma. Ann Otol Rhinol Laryngol 95:215–221
980. Werth GR (1984) The role of sinusitis in severe asthma. Immunol Allergy Prac 7:45–49
981. West JM (1911) Eine Fensterresektion des Ductus nasolacrimalis in Fällen von Stenose. Arch Laryngol Rhinol 24:62–64
982. White PS, Robinson JM, Stewart IA, Doyle T (1990) Computerized tomography mini-series: an alternative to standard paranasal sinus radiographs. Aust NZ J Surg 60:25–29
983. White PS, Cowan IA, Robertson MS (1991) Limited CT scanning techniques of the paranasal sinuses. J Laryngol Otol 105:20–23
984. White PS, Frizelle FA, Hanna GB, Tan LK, Gareliner Q, Cuschiere A (1997) Comparison of direct monocular endoscopic, two- and three-dimensional display systems on surgical task performance in functional endoscopic sinus surgery. Clin Otolaryngol 22:65–67
985. Whitnall SB (1913) The relations of the lacrymal fossa to the ethmoidal cells. Ophthal Rev 32:321–325
986. Whittet HB, Shun-Shin GA, Awdry P (1993) Functional endoscopic transnasal dacryocystorhinostomy. Eye 7:545–549
987. Wiatrak BJ, Willging P, Myer CM, Cotton RT (1991) Functional endoscopic sinus surgery in the immunocompromised child. Otolaryngol Head Neck Surg 105:818–825
988. Wiatrak BJ, Myer CM, Cotton RT (1993) Cystic fibrosis presenting with sinus disease in children. Am J Dis Child 147:258–260
989. Wielgosz R, Hohenhorst W, Fronz T (1995) Die Heermann-Modifikation der intranasalen Mikrochirurgie bei Tränenwegstenosen. Laryngo-Rhino-Otol 74:112–117
990. Wigand ME (1981a) Ein Saug-Spül-Endoskop für die transnasale Chirurgie der Nasennebenhöhlen und der Schädelbasis. HNO 29:102–103
991. Wigand ME (1981b) Transnasale, endoskopische Chirurgie der Nasennebenhöhlen bei chronischer Sinusitis. I. Ein bio-mechanisches Konzept der Schleimhautchirurgie. HNO 29:215–221
992. Wigand ME (1981c) Transnasale, endoskopische Chirurgie der Nasennebenhöhlen bei chronischer Sinusitis. II. Die endonasale Kieferhöhlenoperation. HNO 29:263–269
993. Wigand ME (1981d) Transnasale, endoskopische Chirurgie der Nasennebenhöhlen bei chronischer Sinusitis. III. Die endonasale Siebbeinausräumung. HNO 29:287–293
994. Wigand (1981e) Transnasal ethmoidectomy under endoscopical control. Rhinology 19:7–15
995. Wigand ME, Buiter CT, Griffiths MV, Perko D (1988) Treatment of antral pathology – which surgical route. Rhinology 26:253–255
996. Wigand ME (1989) Endoskopische Chirurgie der Nasennebenhöhlen und der vorderen Schädelbasis. Thieme, Stuttgart
997. Wigand ME, Hosemann W (1991) Endoscopic surgery for frontal sinusitis and its complications. Am J Rhinol 5:85–89
998. Wight RG, Cochrane T (1990) A comparison of the effects of two commonly used vasoconstrictors on nasal mucosal blood flow and nasal airflow. Acta Otolaryngol (Stockh) 109:137–141
999. Willner A, Kantrovitz AB, Cohen AF (1994) Intrasphenoidal encephalocele: diagnosis and management. Otolaryngol Head Neck Surg 111:834–837
1000. Wolf G, Koidl B, Pelzmann B (1991) Zur Regeneration des Zilienschlages humaner Flimmerzellen. Laryngol Rhinol Otol. 70:552–555
1001. Wolf G, Anderhuber W, Kuhn F (1993) Development of the paranasal sinuses in children: implications for paranasal sinus surgery. Ann Otol Rhinol Laryngol 102:705–711
1002. Wolf G, Greistorfer K, Jebeles JA (1995) The endoscopic endonasal surgical technique in the treatment of chronic recurring sinusitis in children. Rhinology 33:97–103
1002a. Wolf G, Greistorfer K, Stammberger H (1997) Der endoskopische Nachweis von Liquorfisteln mittels der Fluoresceintechnik. Ein Erfahrungsbericht über 925 Fälle. Laryngo-Rhino-Otol 76: 588–594.
1003. Wolf SR, Göde U, Hosemann W (1996) Endonasal endoscopic surgery for rhinogen intraorbital abscess – a report of 6 cases. Laryngoscope 106: 105–110

1004. Wolfensberger M (1984) Zur Pathogenese des Pneumosinus maxillaris dilatans. HNO 32:518–520
1005. Woodham JD, Doyle PW (1991a) Conservative endoscopic sinus surgery performed from TV monitor using integrated Nagashima endoscopic sinonasal system. J Otolaryngol 20:248–251
1006. Woodham JD, Doyle PW (1991b) Surgical landmarks and resections for the safe performance of conservative endoscopic sinus surgery. J Otolaryngol 20:451–454
1007. Woog JJ, Metson R, Puliafito CA (1993) Holmium: YAG endonasal laser dacryocystorhinostomy. Am J Ophthalmol 116:1–10
1008. Wright E, Mizerny B, Desrosiers M (1997) Minimal access surgery of the frontonasal duct through a simultaneous transfrontal and intranasal approach. Otolaryngol Head Neck Surg 117:127–130
1009. Wurman LH, Sack JG, Flannery JV, Paulson TO (1988) Selective endoscopic electrocautery for posterior epistaxis. Laryngoscope 98: 1348–1349
1010. Wurster CF, Smith DE (1994) The endoscopic approach to the pituitary gland (letter). Arch Otolaryngol Head Neck Surg 120:674
1011. Yamagishi M, Hasegawa S, Suzuki S, Nakamura H, Nakano Y (1989) Effect of surgical treatment of olfactory disturbance caused by localized ethmoiditis. Clin Otolaryngol 14:405–409
1012. Yamaguchi N, Arai S, Mitani H, Uchida Y (1991) Endoscopic endonasal technique of the blowout fracture of the medial orbital wall. Op Tech Otolaryngol Head Neck Surg 2:269–274
1013. Yellin SA, Weiss MH, O'Malley B, Weingarten K (1994) Massive concha bullosa masquerading as an intranasal tumor. Ann Otol Rhinol Laryngol 103:658–659
1014. Yeoh KH, Tan KK (1994) The optic nerve in the posterior ethmoid in asians. Acta Otolaryngol (Stockh) 114:329–336
1015. Younis RT, Gross CW, Lazar RH (1991) Toxic shock syndrome following functional endonasal sinus surgery: a case report. Head & Neck 13:247–248
1016. Younis RT, Lazar RH (1993) Cavernous sinus thrombosis. Successful treatment using functional endonasal sinus surgery. Arch Otolaryngol Head Neck Surg 119:1368–1372
1017. Younis RT, Lazar RH (1996) Delayed Toxic Shock Syndrome After Functional Endonasal Sinus Surgery. Arch Otolaryngol Head Neck Surg 122:83–85
1018. Yousem DM (1993) Imaging of sinonasal inflammatory disease. Radiology 188:303–314
1019. Yousem DM, Kennedy DW, Rosenberg S (1991) Ostiomeatal complex risk factors for sinusitis: CT evaluation. J Otolaryngol 20:419–424
1020. Yousem DM, Fellows DW, Kennedy DW, Bolger WE, Kashima H, Zinreich SJ (1992) Inverted papilloma: evaluation with MR imaging. Radiology 185:501–505
1021. Yung CW, Moorthy RS, Lindley D, Ringle M, Nunery WR (1994) Efficacy of lateral canthotomy and cantholysis in orbital hemorrhage. Ophthalmic Plast Reconstr Surg 10:137–141
1022. Zeitouni Ag, Frenkiel S, Mohr G (1994) Endoscopic repair of anterior skull base cerebrospinal fluid fistulas: an emphasis on postoperative nasal function maximization. J Otolaryngol 23:225–227
1023. Zinreich SJ (1994) Imaging of inflammatory sinus disease. Otolaryngol Clin North Am 26:535–547
1024. Zinreich SJ, Kennedy DW, Rosenbaum AE, Gayler BW, Kumar AJ, Stammberger H (1987) Paranasal sinuses: CT imaging requirements for endoscopic surgery. Radiology 163:769–775
1025. Zinreich SJ, Kennedy DM, Malat J, Curtin HD, Epstein JI, Huff LC, Kumar AJ, Johns ME, Rosenbaum AE (1988a) Fungal sinusitis: diagnosis with CT and MR imaging. Radiology 169:439–444
1026. Zinreich SJ, Mattox DE, Kennedy DW, Chisholm HL, Diffley DM, Rosenbaum AE (1988b) Concha bullosa: CT evaluation. J Comp Ass Tomogr 12:778–784
1027. Zinreich SJ, Tebo SA, Long DM, Brem H, Mattox DE, Loury ME, VanderKolk CA, Koch WM, Kennedy DM, Bryan RN (1993) Frameless stereotaxic integration of CT imaging data: accuracy and initial applications. Radiology 188:735–742
1028. Zuckerkandl E (1882, 1892) Normale und pathologische Anatomie der Nasenhöhle und ihrer pneumatischen Anhänge, Band 1 and 2. W Braumüller, Wien

Index

Page references in **bold** refer to illustrations.